T0249588

Multiple Myeloma

Editor

KENNETH C. ANDERSON

HEMATOLOGY/ONCOLOGY CLINICS OF NORTH AMERICA

www.hemonc.theclinics.com

Consulting Editors
GEORGE P. CANELLOS
H. FRANKLIN BUNN

October 2014 • Volume 28 • Number 5

ELSEVIER

1600 John F. Kennedy Boulevard • Suite 1800 • Philadelphia, Pennsylvania, 19103-2899

http://www.theclinics.com

HEMATOLOGY/ONCOLOGY CLINICS OF NORTH AMERICA Volume 28, Number 5
October 2014 ISSN 0889-8588, ISBN 13: 978-0-323-32613-1

Editor: Jessica McCool
Developmental Editor: Donald Mumford

Hematology/Oncology Clinics (ISSN 0889-8588) is published bimonthly by Elsevier Inc., 360 Park Avenue South, New York, NY 10010-1710. Months of issue are February, April, June, August, October, and December. Business and Editorial Offices: 1600 John F. Kennedy Blvd., Ste. 1800, Philadelphia, PA 19103–2899. Customer Service Office: 3251 Riverport Lane, Maryland Heights, MO 63043. Periodicals postage paid at New York, NY and at additional mailing offices. Subscription prices are $385.00 per year (domestic individuals), $633.00 per year (domestic institutions), $190.00 per year (domestic students/residents), $440.00 per year (Canadian individuals), $783.00 per year (Canadian institutions) $520.00 per year (international individuals), $783.00 per year (international institutions), and $255.00 per year (international and Canadian students/residents). International air speed delivery is included in all Clinics subscription prices. All prices are subject to change without notice. **POSTMASTER:** Send address changes to Hematology/Oncology Clinics of North America, Elsevier Health Sciences Division, Subscription Customer Service, 3251 Riverport Lane, Maryland Heights, MO 63043. Customer Service (orders, claims, online, change of address): Elsevier Health Sciences Division, Subscription Customer Service, 3251 Riverport Lane, Maryland Heights, MO 63043. Tel: 1-800-654-2452 (U.S. and Canada); 314-447-8871 (outside U.S. and Canada). Fax: 314-447-8029. E-mail: journalscustomerservice-usa@elsevier.com (for print support); journalsonlinesupport-usa@elsevier.com (for online support).

Reprints. For copies of 100 or more, of articles in this publication, please contact the Commercial Reprints Department, Elsevier Inc., 360 Park Avenue South, New York, New York 10010-1710; Tel.: 212-633-3874, Fax: 212-633-3820, E-mail: reprints@elsevier.com.

Hematology/Oncology Clinics of North America is covered in MEDLINE/PubMed (Index Medicus), EMBASE/ Excerpta Medica, and BIOSIS.

Contributors

CONSULTING EDITORS

GEORGE P. CANELLOS, MD
William Rosenberg Professor of Medicine; Department of Medical Oncology, Dana-Farber Cancer Institute, Boston, Massachusetts

H. FRANKLIN BUNN, MD
Professor of Medicine; Division of Hematology, Brigham and Women's Hospital, Harvard Medical School, Boston, Massachusetts

EDITOR

KENNETH C. ANDERSON, MD
Department of Hematology/Oncology, Jerome Lipper Multiple Myeloma Center, Dana-Farber Cancer Institute, Harvard Medical School, Boston, Massachusetts

AUTHORS

KENNETH C. ANDERSON, MD
Department of Hematology/Oncology, Jerome Lipper Multiple Myeloma Center, Dana-Farber Cancer Institute, Harvard Medical School, Boston, Massachusetts

JOOEUN BAE, PhD
Instructor, Dana-Farber Cancer Institute, Harvard Medical School, Boston, Massachusetts

WILLIAM BENSINGER, MD
Member, Fred Hutchinson Cancer Research Center; Professor, Division of Oncology, University of Washington, Seattle, Washington

JORGE J. CASTILLO, MD
Bing Center for Waldenström's Macroglobulinemia, Dana-Farber Cancer Institute, Harvard Medical School, Boston, Massachusetts

DHARMINDER CHAUHAN, PhD
Department of Hematology/Oncology, Jerome Lipper Multiple Myeloma Center, Dana-Farber Cancer Institute, Harvard Medical School, Boston, Massachusetts

THIERRY FACON, MD
Hematology Department, University Hospital, Lille, France

SILVIA GENTILI, MD
Department of Hematology, Azienda Ospedaliero-Universitaria Ospedali Riuniti di Ancona, Ancona, Italy

SERGIO GIRALT, MD
Attending Physician, Adult BMT Service, Memorial Sloan Kettering Cancer Center;
Professor of Medicine, Weill Cornell Medical College, New York, New York

TERU HIDESHIMA, MD, PhD
Department of Hematology/Oncology, Jerome Lipper Multiple Myeloma Center,
Dana-Farber Cancer Institute, Harvard Medical School, Boston, Massachusetts

CYRILLE HULIN, MD
Hematology Department, University Hospital, Nancy, France

ZACHARY R. HUNTER, PhD
Bing Center for Waldenström's Macroglobulinemia, Dana-Farber Cancer Institute,
Harvard Medical School, Boston, Massachusetts

ROBERT A. KYLE, MD
Professor of Medicine and Laboratory Medicine, Division of Hematology, Mayo Clinic,
Rochester, Minnesota

HEATHER LANDAU, MD
Assistant Attending Physician, Adult BMT Service, Memorial Sloan Kettering Cancer
Center; Associate Professor of Medicine, Weill Cornell Medical College, New York,
New York

JACOB LAUBACH, MD
Department of Hematology/Oncology, Jerome Lipper Multiple Myeloma Center,
Dana-Farber Cancer Institute, Harvard Medical School, Boston, Massachusetts

SAGAR LONIAL, MD
Professor, Department of Hematology and Medical Oncology, Winship Cancer Institute of
Emory University, Atlanta, Georgia

MARIA-VICTORIA MATEOS, MD, PhD
Consultant Physician, Hematology Department, University Hospital of Salamanca,
Salamanca, Spain

PHILIP L. MCCARTHY, MD
Professor of Oncology and Internal Medicine, Department of Medicine, Blood and Marrow
Transplant Program, Roswell Park Cancer Institute, State University of New York at
Buffalo, Buffalo, New York

GIAMPAOLO MERLINI, MD
Department of Molecular Medicine, Amyloidosis Research and Treatment Center,
University Hospital Policlinico San Matteo, Pavia, Italy

PHILIPPE MOREAU, MD
Hematology Department, UMR892, University Hospital, Nantes, France

NIKHIL C. MUNSHI, MD
Professor, Dana-Farber Cancer Institute, Harvard Medical School, Boston,
Massachusetts

ANTONIO PALUMBO, MD
Myeloma Unit, Division of Hematology, Azienda Ospedaliero-Universitaria Città della
Salute e della Scienza di Torino, University of Torino, Torino, Italy

S. VINCENT RAJKUMAR, MD
Professor of Medicine and Chair, Myeloma Amyloidosis Dysproteinemia Group, Division of Hematology, Mayo Clinic, Rochester, Minnesota

PAUL G. RICHARDSON, MD
Department of Hematology/Oncology, Jerome Lipper Multiple Myeloma Center, Dana-Farber Cancer Institute, Harvard Medical School, Boston, Massachusetts

JESUS F. SAN-MIGUEL, MD, PhD
Professor and Director, Clinical and Translational Medicine, Hematology Department, Clinica Universidad de Navarra, Pamplona, Navarra, Spain

PIETER SONNEVELD, MD, PhD
Department of Hematology, Erasmus MC Cancer Institute, Rotterdam, The Netherlands

STEVEN P. TREON, MD, MA, PhD
Bing Center for Waldenström's Macroglobulinemia, Dana-Farber Cancer Institute, Harvard Medical School, Boston, Massachusetts

NIELS W.C.J. VAN DE DONK, MD, PhD
Department of Hematology, University Medical Center Utrecht, Utrecht, The Netherlands

CINDY VARGA, MD
Department of Hematology/Oncology, Jerome Lipper Multiple Myeloma Center, Dana-Farber Cancer Institute, Harvard Medical School, Boston, Massachusetts

Contents

Monoclonal gammopathy of undetermined significance (MGUS) is characterized by an M spike less than 3 g/dL and a bone marrow containing fewer than 10% plasma cells without evidence of CRAB (hypercalcemia, renal insufficiency, anemia, or bone lesions). Light chain MGUS has an abnormal free light chain (FLC) ratio, increased level of the involved FLC, no monoclonal heavy chain, and fewer than 10% monoclonal plasma cells in the bone marrow. Smoldering multiple myeloma has an M protein of at least 3 g/dL and/or at least 10% monoclonal plasma cells in the bone marrow without CRAB features.

Multiple myeloma (MM) is a tumor of monoclonal plasma cells, which produce a monoclonal antibody and expand predominantly in the bone marrow. Patients present with hypercalcemia, renal impairment, anemia, and/or bone disease. Only patients with symptomatic MM require therapy, whereas asymptomatic patients receive regular follow-up. Survival of patients with MM is very heterogeneous. The variety in outcome is explained by host factors as well as tumor-related characteristics reflecting biology of the MM clone and tumor burden. The identification of cytogenetic abnormalities by fluorescence in situ hybridization is currently the most important and widely available prognostic factor in MM.

Induction regimens containing a proteasome inhibitor and/or immuno-modulatory agent with dexamethasone result in rapid disease control before autologous stem cell transplantation (ASCT). ASCT followed by consolidation and/or maintenance further improves depth of response following effective induction. Overall survival of transplant-eligible patients has been extended with modern therapeutic strategies. The optimal timing of ASCT and methods to prevent relapse following ASCT are under active investigation. Different patient populations may benefit differentially from currently available treatments.

Considerable progress has been recently made in the treatment of elderly patients with multiple myeloma (MM). In Europe the combination of thalidomide with melphalan and prednisone and of bortezomib with melphalan and prednisone are 2 standards of care for frontline therapy for elderly patients. In United States the combination of lenalidomide and dexamethasone is the preferred option in this setting. This article focuses on more recent therapeutic approaches in older MM patients, not eligible for high-dose therapy and autologous stem cell transplantation.

Multiple myeloma (MM) is a neoplasm typical of the elderly, with median age at diagnosis of 70 years, and approximately 65% of patients older than 65 years. Many advances have been made thanks to the use of autologous hematopoietic stem cell transplantation (AHSCT) and the introduction of the immunomodulatory drugs and the proteasome inhibitors. Incorporation of novel agents into induction has resulted in improved overall survival. Optimal MM maintenance therapy should maintain or increase response after induction and, when possible, AHSCT. Optimal maintenance therapy must be effective with minimal toxicity and should be easily administered.

New treatment options for patients with myeloma have helped to change the natural history of this disease, even in the context of relapsed disease. For standard-risk patients, doublet-based therapy may offer benefit, whereas for patients with aggressive or genetically high-risk disease combinations of agents are needed for adequate disease control. Second-generation agents offer significant activity for patients with refractory myeloma, and new categories of agents provide new targets for future study and clinical use. Combinations of these agents in selected patient populations represent the next stage in the quest to cure myeloma.

Prospective trials comparing tandem autologous stem cell transplantation (ASCT) with ASCT followed by allogeneic stem cell transplantation (AlloSCT) have shown mixed results with regard to progression-free and overall survival rates. Thus, AlloSCT, although a potentially curative treatment, is not regarded as a standard treatment for multiple myeloma by most experts in the field. Strategies to improve the therapeutic index of the conditioning regimens have the potential to improve outcomes. Other approaches to modulate graft-versus-host disease while preserving or improving a graft-versus-myeloma effect could elevate AlloSCT to mainstream treatment. These approaches include vaccines, monoclonal antibodies, and adoptive immunotherapies.

New, next-generation targeted treatment strategies are required to improve outcomes in patients with multiple myeloma (MM). Monoclonal antibodies, cell signaling inhibitors, and selective therapies targeting the bone marrow microenvironment have demonstrated encouraging results with generally manageable toxicity in therapeutic trials of patients with relapsed and refractory disease, each critically informed by preclinical studies. A combination approach of these newer agents with immunomodulators and/or proteasome inhibitors as part of a treatment platform seems to improve the efficacy of anti-MM regimens, even in heavily pretreated patients. Future studies are required to better understand the complex mechanisms of drug resistance in MM.

Multiple myeloma (MM) is a B-cell malignancy characterized by the clonal proliferation of malignant plasma cells in the bone marrow and the development of osteolytic bone lesions. MM has emerged as a paradigm within the cancers for the success of drug discovery and translational medicine. This article discusses immunotherapy as an encouraging option for the goal of inducing effective and long-lasting therapeutic outcome. Divided into two distinct approaches, passive or active, immunotherapy, which targets tumor-associated antigens has shown promising results in multiple preclinical and clinical studies.

Waldenström macroglobulinemia (WM) is an IgM-secreting B-cell lymphoproliferative disorder, with strong familial predisposition. MYD88 L265P and CXCR4 WHIM mutations are common in WM and support the growth and survival of WM cells. Clinical manifestations of disease are related to both tumor cell infiltration and paraprotein production. Current treatment includes monoclonal antibodies, alkylating agents, nucleoside analogs, proteasome inhibitors, immunomodulatory drugs, and signal inhibitors. Short- and long-term toxicities should be weighed in treatment decisions with use of these agents. Elucidation of the signaling pathways involved in WM is helping to advance targeted therapeutics for WM and includes efforts directed at MYD88 and CXCR4 signaling.

Multiple Myeloma

HEMATOLOGY/ONCOLOGY CLINICS OF NORTH AMERICA

ISSUE OF RELATED INTEREST

Clinics in Laboratory Medicine, September 2014 (Vol. 34, Issue 3)
Anticoagulants
Jerrold H. Levy, *Editor*
Available at: http://www.labmed.theclinics.com/

VISIT THE CLINICS ONLINE!
Access your subscription at:
www.theclinics.com

NOW AVAILABLE FOR YOUR iPhone and iPad

Preface

Multiple Myeloma

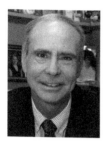

Kenneth C. Anderson, MD
Editor

Remarkable progress has been achieved in our understanding of the biology and pathogenesis of multiple myeloma in its bone marrow microenvironment. Novel agents, including immunomodulatory drugs and proteasome inhibitors, targeting the tumor cell directly, the tumor-host interaction, and the bone marrow milieu can overcome tumor cell resistance to conventional therapy. They have transformed both our therapeutic armamentarium and our patient outcome. The pace of progress is so rapid that up-to-date information on optimal current medical practices, as well as promising developments in diagnosis, prognosis, and treatment, is paramount for both patients and caregivers alike.

This issue of *Hematology/Oncology Clinics of North America* provides cutting-edge information spanning from the bench to the bedside, focusing on current and future clinical advances. Dr Kyle and colleagues, who first described monoclonal gammopathy of undetermined significance and smoldering multiple myeloma, provide new information on mechanisms underlying their evolution to active myeloma as well as treatment protocols to delay or prevent this progression. Dr van de Donk describes current science-based understanding of diagnosis and risk stratification in myeloma, which continues to evolve as our understanding of the genetic complexity of this disease increases. Dr Landau updates management of the newly diagnosed patient with myeloma who is a transplant candidate, and Dr Moreau describes similar advances in the initial management of nontransplant candidates. Dr McCarthy then provides a synthesis of current data on the duration and benefits versus risks of maintenance therapies in transplant recipients as well as elderly nontransplant patients. Despite this progress, myeloma commonly relapses, and Dr Gentili provides information on currently available therapies for relapsed and refractory myeloma. In this context, Dr Bensinger describes the benefits of graft versus myeloma affect versus risk of attendant graft versus host disease associated with allografting in myeloma. Dr Varga and coworkers then describe promising novel therapies in clinical trials at present, new generation immunomodulatory drugs and proteasome inhibitors as well as new

Hematol Oncol Clin N Am 28 (2014) xi–xii
http://dx.doi.org/10.1016/j.hoc.2014.08.001
0889-8588/14/$ – see front matter © 2014 Published by Elsevier Inc.

hemonc.theclinics.com

targeted therapies, which are highly likely to improve patient outcome even further. Dr Bae then summarizes the advances in immune-based therapies, including monoclonal antibodies, vaccines, and checkpoint inhibitors, which have already translated to clinical evaluation in myeloma. Finally, Dr Treon and colleagues describe their seminal finding of MyD88 mutations in a majority of Waldenström macroglobulinemia as well as its important implications for biomarkers and targeted therapy.

Although the last decade has seen amazing progress with a doubling to tripling of patient survival in myeloma, novel agents and immune approaches offer the hope and promise of long-term disease-free survival. This progress has required the selfless commitment of basic and clinical researchers, biotechnology and pharmaceuticals, regulators, National Cancer Institute and Foundation funding, and most importantly, the active participation of patients in clinical trials evaluating new paradigms of therapy. Remarkably, myeloma is already a chronic illness in many patients, and curative potential now a realistic goal.

Kenneth C. Anderson, MD
Department of Hematology/Oncology
Jerome Lipper Multiple Myeloma Center
Dana Farber Cancer Institute
Harvard Medical School
450 Brookline Avenue
Boston, MA 02215, USA

E-mail address:
kenneth_anderson@dfci.harvard.edu

Monoclonal Gammopathy of Undetermined Significance and Smoldering Multiple Myeloma

Robert A. Kyle, MD[a],*, Jesus F. San-Miguel, MD, PhD[b],
Maria-Victoria Mateos, MD, PhD[c], S. Vincent Rajkumar, MD[a]

KEYWORDS

- Monoclonal gammopathy of undetermined significance
- Smoldering multiple myeloma
- Light chain monoclonal gammopathy of undetermined significance
- Multiple myeloma

KEY POINTS

- Monoclonal gammopathy of undetermined significance (MGUS) is characterized by an M spike less than 3 g/dL and a bone marrow containing fewer than 10% plasma cells and no evidence of CRAB (hypercalcemia, renal insufficiency, anemia, or bone lesions). It progresses at a rate of 1% per year.
- Light chain MGUS (LC-MGUS) is characterized by an abnormal free light chain (FLC) ratio, increased level of the involved FLC, no monoclonal heavy chain, and fewer than 10% monoclonal plasma cells in the bone marrow.
- Smoldering multiple myeloma (SMM) has an M protein of at least 3 g/dL and/or at least 10% monoclonal plasma cells in the bone marrow but no evidence of CRAB features. The risk of progression is 10% per year for the first 5 years and then decreases to 3% per year for the next 5 years and finally to 1% to 2% per year for the following 10 years.

INTRODUCTION

More than a half century ago, Jan Waldenström described patients with a small serum protein electrophoretic spike without evidence of multiple myeloma (MM), Waldenström macroglobulinemia (WM), or related disorders as having an essential hyperglobulinemia. He noted the constancy of the size of the protein spike and utilized the term

---

Disclosures: None.
[a] Division of Hematology, Mayo Clinic, 200 First Street Southwest, Rochester, MN 55905, USA;
[b] Hematology Department, Clinica Universidad de Navarra, Avda. Pio XII, No. 36, Pamplona, Navarra 31008, Spain; [c] Hematology Department, University Hospital of Salamanca, Paseo San Vicente, 58-132, Salamanca 37007, Spain
* Corresponding author.
E-mail address: kyle.robert@mayo.edu

Hematol Oncol Clin N Am 28 (2014) 775–790
http://dx.doi.org/10.1016/j.hoc.2014.06.005
0889-8588/14/$ – see front matter © 2014 Elsevier Inc. All rights reserved.

benign monoclonal gammopathy. In contrast, he emphasized that patients with MM or WM had an increasing quantity of monoclonal protein that produced symptomatic disease.[1]

The term monoclonal gammopathy of undetermined significance (MGUS) was introduced more than 35 years ago, because patients with apparently benign monoclonal gammopathy were at risk for the development of symptomatic MM, WM, Light-chain (AL) amyloidosis, or a related disorder during long-term follow-up.[2,3] This article will focus on MGUS, and the related disorder, smoldering multiple myeloma (SMM).

RECOGNITION OF MONOCLONAL GAMMOPATHIES

MGUS and SMM are asymptomatic and are incidentally discovered during work-up of a variety of clinical disorders and symptoms. Typically, a patient suspected to have a clonal plasma cell disorder is screened for the presence of a monoclonal (M) protein using serum protein electrophoresis, serum immunofixation, and the free light chain (FLC) assay.[4] Serum protein electrophoresis is performed on agarose gel or capillary zone electrophoresis.[5] The serum FLC is increasingly being used in place of urine studies during screening.[6] However, if a serum M protein is found, electrophoresis and immunofixation of an aliquot from a 24-hour urine collection are also needed. The amount of M protein provides a measure of the patient's tumor mass and is therefore useful in monitoring the course of one's disease.

The presence of an M protein or an abnormal serum FLC ratio indicates the presence of MGUS, SMM, or a more serious process such as MM, WM, AL, or related plasma cell disorder. MGUS and SMM are diagnosed by excluding the presence of these serious symptomatic disorders, and by the absence of end-organ damage attributable to the underlying plasma cell proliferative process.

MONOCLONAL GAMMOPATHY OF UNDETERMINED SIGNIFICANCE
Definition

MGUS is the most common plasma cell disorder and is the precursor of MM, and almost certainly WM and AL also.[7] It is defined as a monoclonal serum immunoglobulin of no more than 3.0 g/dL, absence of hypercalcemia, renal insufficiency, anemia or bone lesions (CRAB), and fewer than 10% monoclonal plasma cells (PCs) in the bone marrow.[8,9] The most common heavy chain type is immunoglobulin G (IgG) (70%), IgM (15%), IgA (12%), and biclonal gammopathy (3%).[10]

Prevalence

Earlier reports revealed that approximately 1.5% of people older than 50 years and 3% of the population older than 70 years in Sweden, the United States, and western France have an M protein without evidence of MM, WM, AL or a related disorder.[11–13] In a population-based study conducted in Olmsted County, MN, 21,463 (77%) of the 28,038 residents 50 years of age and older were evaluated. The type of MGUS was IgG (69%), IgA (11%), IgM (17%), and biclonal (3%). The prevalence of MGUS was 3.2% (694 patients), with a prevalence of 5.3% in people 70 years of age or older, and in 8.9% in men older than 85 years. The age-adjusted rates were greater in men than in women at 4.0% versus 2.7% (P<.01) (**Table 1** and **Fig. 1**).[14] The size of the M protein was at least 2 g/dL in only 4.5% of MGUS cases, while the M protein was less than 1.5 g/dL in 80% of cases. Reduction of uninvolved immunoglobulins was present in 28% of the 447 patients who were tested. This study was performed in a predominantly white population. The annual incidence of MGUS in men is 120

Table 1
Prevalence of MGUS according to age group and sex among residents of Olmsted County, MN

Age	Men	Women	Total
	Number/Total Number (Percent)[a]		
50–59 y	82/4038 (2.0)	59/4335 (1.4)	141/8373 (1.7)
60–69 y	105/2864 (3.7)	73/3155 (2.3)	178/6019 (3.0)
70–79 y	104/1858 (5.6)	101/2650 (3.8)	205/4508 (4.6)
≥80 y	59/709 (8.3)	111/1854 (6.0)	170/2563 (6.6)
Total	350/9469 (3.7)[b]	344/11,994 (2.9)[b]	694/21,463 (3.2)[b,c]

[a] The percentage was calculated as the number of patients with MGUS divided by the number who were tested.
[b] Prevalence was age-adjusted to the 2000 US total population as follows: men, 4.0% (95% CI, 3.5–4.4); women, 2.7% (95% CI, 2.4–3.0); and total, 3.2% (95% CI, 3.0–3.5).
[c] Prevalence was age- and sex-adjusted to the 2000 US total population.
From Kyle RA, Therneau TM, Rajkumar SV, et al. Prevalence of monoclonal gammopathy of undetermined significance. N Engl J Med 2006;354(13):1366. Copyright © (2006) Massachusetts Medical Society; with permission.

cases per 100,000 population at the age of 50 years, increasing to 530 cases per 100,000 population at the age of 90 years.[15]

The prevalence of MGUS is approximately twice as high in blacks when compared with whites.[16,17] In a study using samples from the National Health and Nutritional Examination Survey (NHANES), among 12,482 people age 50 years and older, the adjusted prevalence of MGUS was significantly higher in blacks (3.7%) compared with whites (2.3%) or Hispanics (1.8%), $P = .001$. The increased prevalence of MGUS is also seen in blacks from Africa; in a study of 917 men (50–74 years) from Ghana, the age-adjusted prevalence of MGUS was 5.84% (95% confidence interval [CI], 4.27–7.40). Compared with white men, the age-adjusted prevalence of MGUS was 1.97-fold (95% CI, 1.94–2.00) higher in Ghanaian men. These studies suggested a genetic predisposition, but a contributing effect of similar socioeconomic status could not be ruled out. In a subsequent study of 1000 black and 996 white women (age 40–79 years) of similar socioeconomic status for MGUS, the racial disparity

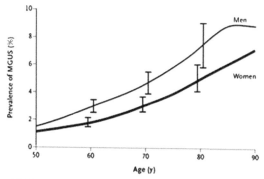

Fig. 1. Prevalence of MGUS According to Age. The I bars represent 95% confidence intervals. Years of age greater than 90 have been collapsed to 90 years of age. (*From* Kyle RA, Therneau TM, Rajkumar SV, et al. Prevalence of monoclonal gammopathy of undetermined significance. N Engl J Med 2006;354(13):1367. Copyright © (2006) Massachusetts Medical Society; with permission.)

persisted; the prevalence of MGUS was 3.9% in blacks versus 2.1% in whites. The presence of racial disparity after adjusting for socioeconomic status strongly suggests a genetic predisposition. In contrast to the increased prevalence seen in blacks, the prevalence of MGUS appears lower in Japan. In 1 study, 2.4% of 52,802 people 50 years of age or older in Nagasaki City, Japan, had MGUS.[18]

First-degree relatives of people with MGUS have an increased risk of developing MGUS and related disorders.[19] In a report of 911 relatives of 232 MM and 97 MGUS patients, there was a 2.0 relative risk (RR) among relatives of MM probands and an RR of 3.3 in MGUS probands.[20]

Light Chain MGUS

Light chain MGUS is defined as the presence of an abnormal FLC ratio (normal 0.26–1.65), no monoclonal immunoglobulin heavy chain, an increased concentration of the involved light chain, absence of end-organ damage, and fewer than 10% monoclonal bone marrow PCs. In a study of 18,353 residents of southeastern Minnesota, light chain MGUS was present in 0.8% residents.[21]

Etiology

The cause of MM is unknown, but both genetic and environmental factors are likely involved.[17,19,22–24] In the study of Nagasaki atomic bomb survivors, people living within 1.5 km of the explosion had a 1.4-fold increase in MGUS compared with those living beyond 3.0 km.[18,25] There was no difference in the prevalence of MGUS in older patients, but those no more than 20 years of age at the time of exposure had an increased prevalence of MGUS.[25] In a report of 555 men from a well-documented prospective cohort of patients applying restricted-use pesticides, 6.8% had MGUS compared with 3.7% of men from Olmsted County, MN. The age-adjusted prevalence of MGUS was 1.9-fold greater among male pesticide workers.[24]

Long-Term Outcome of MGUS

Two hundred and forty-one patients seen at the Mayo Clinic between 1956 and 1970 were followed for 3579 person years (median: 13.7 years, range 0–39 years).[2,3] Fourteen (6%) were alive and had no substantial increase in M protein during a follow-up of 33 years. Twenty-seven percent developed MM, WM, AL, or a lymphoproliferative disorder. Patients in this group were followed for a median of 10.4 years (range 1–32 years) before diagnosis of the malignant lymphoplasmacytic proliferative disorder (**Table 2**). The actuarial risk of progression was 17% at 10 years, 34% at 20 years, and 39% at 25 years (a rate of approximately 1.5% per year) (**Fig. 2**). Sixty-nine percent of

Table 2
Development of multiple myeloma or related disorder in 64 patients with MGUS

	Number (%) of Patients	Interval to Disease (y)	
		Median	Range
Multiple myeloma	44 (69)	10.6	1–32
Macroglobulinemia	7 (11)	10.3	4–16
Amyloidosis	8 (12)	9.0	6–19
Lymphoproliferative disease	5 (8)	8.0	4–19
Total	64 (100)	10.4	1–32

From Kyle RA, Therneau TM, Rajkumar SV, et al. Long-term follow-up of 241 patients with monoclonal gammopathy of undetermined significance: the original Mayo Clinic series 25 years later. Mayo Clin Proc 2004;79(7):862; with permission.

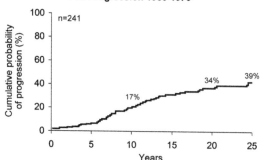

Fig. 2. Rate of development of multiple myeloma or related disorder in 241 patients with monoclonal gammopathy of undetermined significance. (*From* Kyle RA, Therneau TM, Rajkumar SV, et al. Long-term follow-up of 241 patients with monoclonal gammopathy of undetermined significance: the original Mayo Clinic series 25 years later. Mayo Clin Proc 2004;79(7):862; with permission.)

the 64 patients who progressed had MM. AL was found in 8 patients; WM occurred in 7 patients, and a lymphoproliferative disorder occurred in 5 patients.

To eliminate a bias that occurs with referral populations, a separate population-based study of 1384 patients with MGUS from southeastern Minnesota was conducted.[10] The median age at diagnosis was 72 years, in contrast to 64 years for the 241 referred patients. These patients were followed for a median of 15.4 years (range 0–35 years). MM, AL amyloidosis, lymphoma with IgM serum protein, WM, plasmacytoma, or chronic lymphocytic leukemia developed in 115 patients (8%) during follow-up (**Table 3**). The risk of progression was 1% per year (**Fig. 3**). It is important to emphasize that patients with MGUS continue to be at risk for progression as long as they live.

Risk Factors for Progression

Size and type of serum M protein
The size of the M protein is the single most important predictor of progression.[10] At 20 years after recognition of MGUS, 14% with an initial M protein value of no more than 0.5 g/dL and 49% of those presenting with an M protein of 2.5 g/dL progressed. A serum M protein value of 1.5 g/dL had almost twice the risk of progression compared with a value of 0.5 g/dL. At 2.5 g/dL, the risk of progression was 4.6 times that of a value of 0.5 g/dL. A progressive increase in the size of M protein during the first year of follow-up is an important risk factor for progression.[26]

Patients with an IgM or an IgA monoclonal protein have an increased risk of progression compared with patients with an IgG M protein.[10] Varettoni and colleagues[27] found that MGUS patients recognized more recently had a smaller M protein as well as a lower number of bone marrow PCs.

Bone marrow plasma cells
The presence of greater than 5% bone marrow PCs is an independent risk factor for progression.[28] In another study, patients with bone marrow plasmacytosis of 10% to 30% had a malignant transformation rate of 37% compared with 6.8% in patients who had less than 10% PCs.[29]

Table 3
Risk of progression among 1384 residents of southeastern Minnesota in whom MGUS was diagnosed from 1960 through 1994

Type of Progression	Observed Number of Patients	Expected Number of Patients[a]	Relative Risk (95% CI)
Multiple myeloma	75	3.0	25.0 (20–32)
Lymphoma	19[b]	7.8	2.4 (2–4)
Primary amyloidosis	10	1.2	8.4 (4–16)
Macroglobulinemia	7	0.2	46.0 (19–95)
Chronic lymphocytic leukemia	3[c]	3.5	0.9 (0.2–3)
Plasmacytoma	1	0.1	8.5 (0.2–47)
Total	115	15.8	7.3 (6–9)

[a] Expected numbers of cases were derived from the age- and sex-matched white population of the Surveillance, Epidemiology, and End Results program in Iowa, except for primary amyloidosis, for which data are from Kyle, et al.
[b] All 19 patients had serum IgM monoclonal protein. If the 30 patients with IgM, IgA, or IgG monoclonal protein and lymphoma were included, the relative risk would be 3.9 (95% CI, 2.6–5.5).
[c] All 3 patients had serum IgM monoclonal protein. If all 6 patients with IgM, IgA, or IgG monoclonal protein, and chronic lymphocytic leukemia were included, the relative risk would be 17 (95% CI, 0.6–3.7).
From Kyle RA, Therneau TM, Rajkumar SV, et al. A long-term study of prognosis in monoclonal gammopathy of undetermined significance. N Engl J Med 2002;346(8):566. Copyright © (2002) Massachusetts Medical Society; with permission.

Serum FLC ratio

In a study of 1148 people with MGUS from southeastern Minnesota, an abnormal FLC ratio was detected in 33%.[30] The risk of progression in patients with an abnormal FLC ratio was significantly higher (7.6%) compared with those with a normal ratio (hazard ratio 3.5; P<.001). This was independent of the size and type of the serum M protein.[30]

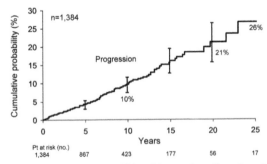

MGUS SE Minnesota
1960-1994

Fig. 3. Probability of progression among 1384 residents of southeastern Minnesota in whom MGUS was diagnosed from 1960 through 1994. The curve shows the probability of progression of MGUS to multiple myeloma, IgM lymphoma, primary amyloidosis, macroglobulinemia, chronic lymphocytic leukemia, or plasmacytoma (115 patients). The bar shows 95% confidence intervals. (*From* Kyle RA, Therneau TM, Rajkumar SV, et al. A long-term study of prognosis in monoclonal gammopathy of undetermined significance. N Engl J Med 2002;346(8):567. Copyright © (2002) Massachusetts Medical Society; with permission.)

Aberrant plasma cells

Perez-Persona[31] reported that the presence of at least 95% aberrant PCs and DNA aneuploidy was associated with a significantly higher risk of progression to MM in a cohort of 407 MGUS and 93 SMM patients. Clonal PCs are discriminated from normal PCs by aberrant phenotypic expressions, typically consisting of simultaneous down-regulation of CD19 and CD45, with or without overexpression of CD56. If CD45 was positively expressed, lack of CD19 and/or bright CD56 staining allowed identification of clonal PCs.

Risk Stratification

The risk of progression of MGUS can be estimated using a simple model that uses the size and type of M protein and the serum FLC ratio. In a study of 1148 people with MGUS, patients with a serum M protein of at least 1.5 g/dL, non-IgG MGUS, and an abnormal serum FLC ratio had a risk of progression at 20 years of 58% (high-risk MGUS) compared with 37% for those with any 2 risk factors (high–intermediate risk), 21% when 1 risk factor was present (low–intermediate risk), and only 5% when none of the risk factors were found (low risk).[30] If one considered the competing causes of death, the risk of progression was only 2% at 20 years in the low-risk group.

Differential Diagnosis

It is critical to differentiate MGUS from MM, Waldenström macroglobulinemia, and AL amyloidosis based on the presence or absence of end organ damage and extent of marrow involvement. A bone marrow aspirate and biopsy, as well as a radiographic bone survey, are indicated in all patients with an M protein value of at least 1.5 g/dL and in all patients with an unexplained abnormality in their hemoglobin, creatinine, or calcium levels. The authors have found the reduction of uninvolved immunoglobulins in serum or the presence of a monoclonal light chain in the urine (Bence Jones proteinuria) is of little help in distinguishing between MGUS and MM.

MM is often associated with circulating monoclonal PCs.[32] The presence of cytogenetic abnormalities with fluorescence in situ hybridization (FISH) may be found in both MGUS and MM.

Secondary MGUS

Secondary MGUS is defined as the emergence of a new M protein different from the original clone during the course of MM. In 1 study, secondary MGUS was found in 6.6% of 1942 patients with MM at a median of 12 months after the diagnosis of MM.[33] It most often occurs in patients who have had a stem cell transplant, and its presence is associated with better survival. More than 1 isotype occurred in approximately one-third of patients. Secondary MGUS is usually transient, with a median duration of 6 months; persistence beyond 1 year is associated with an adverse impact on survival.

Monoclonal gammopathy of renal significance

Monoclonal gammopathy of renal significance (MGRS) is a generic term used to denote patients with MGUS who have renal impairment that is felt to be related to the underlying monoclonal protein.[34] The specific renal pathology may include membranoproliferative glomerulonephritis, C3 glomerulonephritis, and a variety of other renal disorders.[35,36]

Idiopathic Bence Jones proteinuria

Bence Jones proteinuria is frequently present in patients with MM, Waldenström macroglobulinemia, and AL amyloidosis. Patients with Bence Jones protein in the urine without other evidence of lymphoplasmacytic disease are felt to have idiopathic Bence Jones proteinuria. These patients have FLCs that are secreted in quantities large enough to allow detection on urine protein electrophoresis.[37] In this situation, idiopathic Bence Jones proteinuria may be an intermediate stage of disease between LC-MGUS and light chain MM and thus similar to SMM as an intermediate state between MGUS and MM. Some patients with idiopathic Bence Jones proteinuria may remain stable for many years without therapy.

MANAGEMENT OF MGUS

Patients with MGUS must be followed with a history and physical examination, with an emphasis on symptoms and findings that might suggest symptomatic MM, WM, or AL amyloidosis. Serum protein electrophoresis and a complete blood count (CBC) should be repeated 3 to 6 months after recognition of MGUS to exclude the possibility of an evolving MM or WM.

Low-Risk MGUS

If the patient has low-risk MGUS characterized by a serum M spike less than 1.5 g/dL, IgG isotype, and a normal FLC ratio, the risk of progression at 20 years is 5% compared with almost 60% for the high-risk group. Patients with low-risk MGUS do not require a bone marrow examination or skeletal radiography if the clinical evaluation, CBC, and serum creatinine and calcium values are consistent with MGUS.[38] However, a bone marrow examination is needed if there are any CRAB features such as unexplained hypercalcemia, renal insufficiency, or anemia. These patients can probably be followed without laboratory testing until symptoms suggestive of a plasma cell malignancy develop.[39]

Intermediate and High-Risk MGUS

These patients should be followed with a history and physical examination; CBC, calcium, and creatinine values; and measurement of the serum M protein in 6 months. The urinary M protein should also be repeated if abnormal at diagnosis. These studies should be repeated at annual intervals or sooner if the patient develops any symptoms.[39] Treatment is not indicated unless it is part of a clinical trial.[40]

Second Malignancies

Patients with MGUS have been reported to have a higher risk of second cancers, but this is hard to ascertain unless studies are done in the general population.[41] In a population-based study, the risk of acute myelogenous leukemia (AML), acute lymphocytic leukemia (ALL), and myelodysplastic syndrome (MDS) was evaluated in 17,315 people 50 years of age or older who were screened for MGUS and followed for an average of 25 years.[42] People with MGUS had a relative risk of developing MDS of 2.40 and a trend toward increased risk of developing AML, with a relative risk of 1.36, which was not statistically significant. There was no increase in the risk of developing ALL.

SMOLDERING (ASYMPTOMATIC) MULTIPLE MYELOMA
Definition

SMM is an asymptomatic plasma cell disorder defined by the presence of a serum M-protein of at least 3 g/dL and/or at least 10% bone marrow PCs with no evidence of end organ damage.[8,9] The median age of the patients at diagnosis ranges from 65 to 70 years, and the incidence varies from the series, although it usually is between 10%

and 15% of all patients with MM.[43] The annual risk of progression to symptomatic disease is 10% per year for the first 5 years, and it significantly decreases thereafter, 5% per year during the following 5 years and only 1% per year since the 10th year (**Fig. 4**).[44]

Risk Factors Predicting Disease Progression

SMM is not a uniform entity but has a spectrum that ranges from an indolent clinical course similar to MGUS (low risk) to a course characterized by rapid progression to MM.[45] Risk factors for predicting risk of progression are therefore critical in determining optimal management of patients.

Size of M protein and extent of marrow involvement

A systematic study focusing on prognostic factors in SMM was based on retrospective data from 276 patients seen at the Mayo Clinic.[44] In this study, 3 different subgroups of SMM were defined: group 1 with M protein of at least 3 g/dL and at least 10% bone marrow PCs, group 2 with less than 3 g/dL M protein and at least 10% PCs, and group 3 with M protein of at least 3 g/dL but PCs less than 10%. The median time to progression (TTP) to symptomatic MM was significantly different, 2, 8 years, and 19 years, respectively.

In a subsequent study, it was found that only a small fraction of SMM patients have at least 60% bone marrow PCs (21 out of 655 patients, 3.2%), and 95% of them progressed to MM or related malignancy within 2 years of diagnosis.[46]

An increase in the M protein during the disease course allows identification of 2 types of SMM: the so-called evolving and the nonevolving subtypes, with a shorter median TTP (1.3 years) for patients with evolving SMM.[47]

Serum FLC ratio

An abnormal kappa/lambda FLC ratio less than 0.125 or greater than 8 is associated with a significantly higher risk of progression (25% per year in the first 2 years).[48] The risk of progression increases dramatically when the involved/uninvolved FLC ratio rises to at least 100, with a median TTP of 15 months, and a 2-year risk of progression approaching 80%.[49]

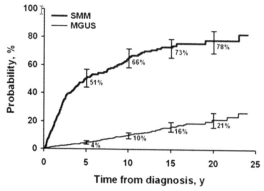

Fig. 4. Probability of progression to active multiple myeloma or primary amyloidosis in patients with SMM or MGUS. I bars denote 95% confidence levels. (*From* Kyle RA, Remstein ED, Therneau TM, et al. Clinical course and prognosis of smoldering (asymptomatic) multiple myeloma. N Engl J Med 2007;356(25):2586. Copyright © (2007) Massachusetts Medical Society; with permission.)

Circulating plasma cells

The presence of increased circulating PCs is a risk factor for progression of SMM. In 1 study increased circulating PCs ($>5 \times 10^6$/L and/or >5% PCs per 100 cytoplasmic immunoglobulin-positive mononuclear cells) was associated with a short median TTP (71% at 2 years).[50]

Immunophenotype and immunoparesis

The Spanish Myeloma Group determined that if clonal PCs represent almost the total population of the bone marrow PC ($\geq$95% phenotypically abnormal PCs), there is a high risk of progression to active MM.[51] In the same study, they showed that the presence of immunoparesis (ie, decrease in 1 or 2 of the uninvolved immunoglobulins) is also a significant prognostic parameter in SMM. Based on these 2 parameters (aberrant PCs and immunoparesis), a scoring system for patients with SMM was proposed, resulting in a prognostic stratification of SMM into 3 risk groups with a median TTP of 23 months when the 2 risk factors were present, compared with 73 months when only 1 risk factor was present; median TTP was not reached when none of the risk factors was present.[51]

Imaging

Novel imaging techniques have also been used to identify patients with SMM at high risk of progression to active MM. Initial studies based on spinal magnetic resonance imaging (MRI) showed that patients with a focal pattern had shorter TTP compared with the diffuse or variegated pattern (median 6 vs 16 vs 22 months).[52] A more recent study conducted in 157 SMM patients with whole MRI showed that the moderate-diffuse pattern was an independent prognostic factor in the prediction of progression to symptomatic MM, and the presence of more than 1 focal lesion was associated with a median TTP to symptomatic disease of 13 months.[53]

Cytogenetic abnormalities

The Mayo Clinic group recently analyzed the prognostic influence of cytogenetic abnormalities in a series of 351 patients with SMM.[54] They identified a high-risk subgroup of patients with t(4;14) and/or del(17p) with a significantly shorter median TTP (24 months) compared with intermediate (trisomies), standard (other cytogenetic abnormalities), and low-risk (no cytogenetic abnormalities) subgroups of patients. Neben and colleagues[55] reported similar results in a study of 249 SMM patients; the presence of t(4;14), gain of 1q21, and hypodiploidy were independent prognostic factors predicting a shorter TTP. Gene expression profiling (GEP) signatures can also identify a subgroup at higher risk of malignant transformation; the combination of GEP70 risk score greater than −0,26 plus elevated involved FLC greater than 25 mg/dL and M protein of at least 3 g/dL were able to identify 3 distinct risk groups.[56] Patients with 2 or 3 risk factors had a 70% progression risk at 2 years, while in patients with 0 or 1 risk factors, the risk of progression at 2 years was 3% and 29%, respectively.

Risk-Stratification of SMM

The risk of progression in SMM varies considerably based on several laboratory parameters (**Table 4**), which directly impact approach to therapy. Ultra-high risk SMM (approximately 80% risk of progression in 2 years) includes patients with greater than 1 focal lesion on MRI studies, at least 60% of clonal bone marrow PCs, or involved/uninvolved serum FLC ratio of at least 100.[45,57–59] High-risk SMM (approximately 50% risk of progression in 2 years) includes patients with M protein of at least 3 g/dL and at least 10% marrow PCs (Mayo Clinic criteria), aberrant phenotype in greater than 95% of clonal PCs plus immunoparesis (Spanish Myeloma Group

Table 4
Risk factors for progression in SMM and management options

Risk Group	Probability of Progression to Myeloma or Related Disorder in First 2 y from Initial Diagnosis of SMM (%)	Recommendation for Therapy
Bone marrow clonal plasma cells ≥60%	90	Treat as myeloma
Serum involved/uninvolved free light chain ratio ≥100	80	Treat as myeloma
Abnormalities on MRI (>1 focal lesion)	70	Treat as myeloma
Abnormal plasma cell immunophenotype ≥95%	50	Consider preventive therapy or trials[a]
Evolving type of SMM[b]	65	Consider preventive therapy or trials[a]
t(4;14) or del 17p	50	Consider preventive therapy or trials
M protein ≥30 g/L and bone marrow clonal plasma cells ≥10%	50	Consider preventive therapy or trials
Serum involved/uninvolved FLC ratio ≥8 and <100	40	Consider clinical trials
No high-risk factors	10–20	Observation or clinical trials

[a] Further efforts to refine cut-offs are ongoing to identify a patient population with 80% or higher risk of progression in first 2 years.
[b] Increase in serum monoclonal protein by ≥10% (increase must be > 0.5 g/dL) on each of 2 successive evaluations within a 6 month period.
Adapted from Rajkumar SV, Kyle RA. Treatment of smoldering multiple myeloma. Nat Rev Clin Oncol 2013;10(10):555; with permission.

criteria), kappa/lambda FLC ratio less than 0.125 or greater than 8, or presence of t(4;14) or del 17p. Additional data are needed to establish specific cut points for circulating PCs and evolving type of SMM.

Management of SMM

The initial work-up investigations in a patient with suspected SMM should include the same tests previously described for MGUS patients with an emphasis to exclude the presence of CRAB. Serum FLC assay and MRI of the spine and pelvis (or ideally whole-body MRI or positron emission tomography) are also recommended.[39,43] The M protein, hemoglobin, calcium, and creatinine should be re-evaluated in 2 to 3 months in order to confirm the stability of these theoretically normal parameters and to plan the follow-up according to the risk of progression to active disease: every 3 to 4 months in high-risk patients, every 6 months in intermediate-risk cases, and every 12 months in low-risk SMM patients.[43]

The standard of care is observation until development of symptomatic MM occurs. Several trials have evaluated the role of early treatment in this group of patients, with conventional and novel agents. Three small studies compared early therapy with melphalan and prednisone (MP) versus observation or deferred MP treatment, showing no significant differences either in TPP or overall survival.[60–62] Two small phase 2 trials evaluated the role of thalidomide as a single agent in SMM patients.[63,64]

The response rate was approximately 35%, and most patients developed peripheral neuropathy. Barlogie and colleagues[65] conducted a phase 2 randomized trial with thalidomide plus pamidronate in 76 patients with SMM that demonstrated a response rate of 42%, with a median TTP to symptomatic disease of 6 years. A randomized trial compared thalidomide plus zoledronic acid versus zoledronic acid in SMM. The response rate was 37% in the thalidomide arm versus 0%, but there were no significant differences in TTP to symptomatic MM (4.3 vs 3.3 years) or overall survival (OS) (74% vs 73% at 5 years).[66] The role of bisphosphonates as single agents has been also analyzed in 3 different trials, including pamidronate as single agent,[67] pamidronate versus observation,[68] and zoledronic acid versus observation.[69] All 3 trials found that bisphosphonates have no antitumor effect, but showed an increase in bone density, decrease in bone resorption markers, and a reduction in the incidence of skeletal-related events. None of the previously mentioned trials supports early treatment in patients with SMM.

The Spanish Myeloma Group (GEM/Pethema) conducted a phase 3 randomized trial in SMM patients at high risk of progression to active disease, comparing treatment with lenalidomide plus dexamethasone versus observation in a series of 120 patients.[70] After a median follow-up of 40 months, median TTP was significantly longer in patients in the treatment group than the observation group (not reached vs 21 months; hazard ratio, 5.59; $P<.001$). Response rate after induction was 82% in the treatment arm, including 26% stringent complete response (sCR) plus CR. Importantly, the 3-year survival rate was significantly higher with lenalidomide-based therapy compared with observation (94% vs 78% at 5 years; hazard ratio, 3.24; $P = .03$). This study shows for the first time the potential to change the treatment paradigm for high-risk SMM patients based on the efficacy of early treatment in terms of TTP to active disease and overall survival as well. Additional trials are ongoing, including a randomized trial of single-agent lenalidomide versus observation in high-risk SMM by the Eastern Cooperative Oncology Group. Recommendations for management of SMM based on risk factors are summarized in **Table 4**. Ultra-high risk patients should be offered therapy, patients with high-risk SMM are candidates for clinical trials, and patients with low-risk SMM should continue to be observed.

SUMMARY

MGUS is present in 3.2% of people 50 years of age and older, and 5.3% of people 70 years or older. The prevalence is twice as high in blacks compared with Caucasians. Light-chain MGUS is a newly defined entity characterized by the presence of an abnormal FLC ratio with no heavy chain expression and increased concentration of the involved light chain. The risk of progression of MGUS is about 1% per year. SMM is an intermediate clinically defined stage with a risk of progression of approximately 10% per year. The clinical course and management of SMM depend on several key biomarkers including M protein level, extent of bone marrow involvement, serum FLC ratio, immunophenotype and immunoparesis. The subset of patients with SMM with ultra-high risk features including more than 1 focal lesion on MRI studies, at least 60% of clonal bone marrow PCs, and involved/uninvolved serum FLC ratio of at least 100 should be considered as having early MM and offered therapy. Clinical trials are indicated in high-risk patients.

REFERENCES

1. Waldenstrom J. Studies on conditions associated with disturbed gamma globulin formation (gammopathies). Harvey Lect 1960–1961;56:211–31.

2. Kyle RA. Monoclonal gammopathy of undetermined significance. Natural history in 241 cases. Am J Med 1978;64:814–26.
3. Kyle RA, Therneau TM, Rajkumar SV, et al. Long-term follow-up of 241 patients with monoclonal gammopathy of undetermined significance: the original Mayo Clinic series 25 years later [see comment]. Mayo Clin Proc 2004;79:859–66.
4. Katzmann JA, Dispenzieri A, Kyle R, et al. Elimination of the need for urine studies in the screening algorithm for monoclonal gammopathies by using serum immunofixation and free light chain assays. Mayo Clin Proc 2006;81:1575–8.
5. Katzmann JA, Kyle RA, Benson J, et al. Screening panels for detection of monoclonal gammopathies. Clin Chem 2009;55:1517–22.
6. Katzmann JA, Clark RJ, Abraham RS, et al. Serum reference intervals and diagnostic ranges for free kappa and free lambda immunoglobulin light chains: relative sensitivity for detection of monoclonal light chains. Clin Chem 2002;48:1437–44.
7. Landgren O, Kyle RA, Pfeiffer RM, et al. Monoclonal gammopathy of undetermined significance (MGUS) consistently precedes multiple myeloma: a prospective study. Blood 2009;113:5412–7.
8. The International Myeloma Working Group. Criteria for the classification of monoclonal gammopathies, multiple myeloma and related disorders: a report of the International Myeloma Working Group. Br J Haematol 2003;121:749–57.
9. Kyle RA, Rajkumar SV. Criteria for diagnosis, staging, risk stratification and response assessment of multiple myeloma. Leukemia 2009;23:3–9.
10. Kyle RA, Therneau TM, Rajkumar SV, et al. A long-term study of prognosis of monoclonal gammopathy of undetermined significance. N Engl J Med 2002;346:564–9.
11. Axelsson U, Bachmann R, Hallen J. Frequency of pathological proteins (M-components) of 6,995 sera from an adult population. Acta Med Scand 1966;179:235–47.
12. Kyle RA, Finkelstein S, Elveback LR, et al. Incidence of monoclonal proteins in a Minnesota community with a cluster of multiple myeloma. Blood 1972;40:719–24.
13. Saleun JP, Vicariot M, Deroff P, et al. Monoclonal gammopathies in the adult population of Finistere, France. J Clin Pathol 1982;35:63–8.
14. Kyle RA, Therneau TM, Rajkumar SV, et al. Prevalence of monoclonal gammopathy of undetermined significance. N Engl J Med 2006;354:1362–9.
15. Therneau TM, Kyle RA, Melton LJ III, et al. Incidence of monoclonal gammopathy of undetermined significance and estimation of duration before first clinical recognition. Mayo Clin Proc 2012;87:1071–9.
16. Cohen HJ, Crawford J, Rao MK, et al. Racial differences in the prevalence of monoclonal gammopathy in a community-based sample of the elderly [Erratum appears in Am J Med 1998;105(4):362]. Am J Med 1998;104:439–44.
17. Landgren O, Graubard BI, Katzmann JA, et al. Racial disparities in the prevalence of monoclonal gammopathies: a population-based study of 12 482 persons from the national health and nutritional examination survey. Leukemia 2014. [Epub ahead of print]. http://dx.doi.org/10.1038/leu.2014.34.
18. Iwanaga M, Tagawa M, Tsukasaki K, et al. Prevalence of monoclonal gammopathy of undetermined significance: study of 52,802 persons in Nagasaki City, Japan. Mayo Clin Proc 2007;82:1474–9.
19. Greenberg AJ, Rajkumar SV, Vachon CM. Familial monoclonal gammopathy of undetermined significance and multiple myeloma: epidemiology, risk factors, and biological characteristics. Blood 2012;119:4771–9.

20. Vachon CM, Kyle RA, Therneau TM, et al. Increased risk of monoclonal gamm-opathy in first-degree relatives of patients with multiple myeloma or monoclonal gammopathy of undetermined significance. Blood 2009;114:785–90.

21. Dispenzieri A, Katzmann JA, Kyle RA, et al. Prevalence and risk of progression of light-chain monoclonal gammopathy of undetermined significance: a retro-spective population-based cohort study. Lancet 2010;375:1721–8.

22. Greenberg AJ, Vachon CM, Rajkumar SV. Disparities in the prevalence, pathogen-esis and progression of monoclonal gammopathy of undetermined significance and multiple myeloma between blacks and whites. Leukemia 2012;26:609–14.

23. Landgren O, Rajkumar SV, Pfeiffer RM, et al. Obesity is associated with an increased risk of monoclonal gammopathy of undetermined significance (MGUS) among African-American and Caucasian women. Blood 2010;116: 1056–9.

24. Landgren O, Kyle RA, Hoppin JA, et al. Pesticide exposure and risk of mono-clonal gammopathy of undetermined significance (MGUS) in the Agricultural Health Study. Blood 2009;25:6386–91.

25. Iwanaga M, Tagawa M, Tsukasaki K, et al. Relationship between monoclonal gammopathy of undetermined significance and radiation exposure in Nagasaki atomic bomb survivors. Blood 2009;113:1639–50.

26. Rosinol L, Cibeira MT, Montoto S, et al. Monoclonal gammopathy of undeter-mined significance: predictors of malignant transformation and recognition of an evolving type characterized by a progressive increase in M protein size. Mayo Clin Proc 2007;82:428–34.

27. Varettoni M, Corso A, Cocito F, et al. Changing pattern of presentation in mono-clonal gammopathy of undetermined significance: a single-center experience with 1400 patients. Medicine (Baltimore) 2010;89:211–6.

28. Cesana C, Klersy C, Barbarano L, et al. Prognostic factors for malignant trans-formation in monoclonal gammopathy of undetermined significance and smol-dering multiple myeloma. J Clin Oncol 2002;20:1625–34.

29. Baldini L, Guffanti A, Cesana BM, et al. Role of different hematologic variables in defining the risk of malignant transformation in monoclonal gammopathy. Blood 1996;87:912–8.

30. Rajkumar SV, Kyle RA, Therneau TM, et al. Serum free light chain ratio is an in-dependent risk factor for progression in monoclonal gammopathy of undeter-mined significance (MGUS). Blood 2005;106:812–7.

31. Pérez-Persona E, Mateo G, García-Sanz R, et al. Risk of progression in smoul-dering myeloma and monoclonal gammopathies of unknown significance: comparative analysis of the evolution of monoclonal component and multipa-rameter flow cytometry of bone marrow plasma cells. Br J Haematol 2009; 148:110–4.

32. Kumar S, Rajkumar SV, Kyle RA, et al. Prognostic value of circulating plasma cells in monoclonal gammopathy of undetermined significance. J Clin Oncol 2005;23:5668–74.

33. Wadhera RK, Kyle RA, Larson DR, et al. Incidence, clinical course, and prog-nosis of secondary monoclonal gammopathy of undetermined significance in patients with multiple myeloma. Blood 2011;118:2985–7.

34. Leung N, Bridoux F, Hutchison CA, et al. Monoclonal gammopathy of renal sig-nificance: when MGUS is no longer undetermined or insignificant. Blood 2012; 120:4292–5.

35. Sethi S, Fervenza FC. Membranoproliferative glomerulonephritis—a new look at an old entity. N Engl J Med 2012;366:1119–31.

36. Sethi S, Rajkumar SV. Monoclonal gammopathy-associated proliferative glomer-ulonephritis. Mayo Clin Proc 2013;88:1284–93.
37. Rajkumar SV, Kyle RA, Buadi FK. Advances in the diagnosis, classification, risk stratification, and management of monoclonal gammopathy of undetermined significance: implications for recategorizing disease entities in the presence of evolving scientific evidence. Mayo Clin Proc 2010;85:945–8.
38. Rajan AM, Rajkumar SV. Diagnostic evaluation of monoclonal gammopathy of undetermined significance. Eur J Haematol 2013;91:561–2.
39. Kyle RA, Durie BG, Rajkumar SV, et al. Monoclonal gammopathy of undeter-mined significance (MGUS) and smoldering (asymptomatic) multiple myeloma: IMWG consensus perspectives risk factors for progression and guidelines for monitoring and management. Leukemia 2010;24:1121–7.
40. Anderson KC, Kyle RA, Rajkumar SV, et al. Clinically relevant end points and new drug approvals for myeloma. Leukemia 2007;22:231–9.
41. Thomas A, Mailankody S, Korde N, et al. Second malignancies after multiple myeloma: from 1960s to 2010s. Blood 2012;119:2731–7.
42. Roeker LE, Larson DR, Kyle RA, et al. Risk of acute leukemia and myelodysplas-tic syndromes in patients with monoclonal gammopathy of undetermined signif-icance (MGUS): a population-based study of 17 315 patients. Leukemia 2013; 27:1391–3.
43. Blade J, Dimopoulos M, Rosinol L, et al. Smoldering (asymptomatic) multiple myeloma: current diagnostic criteria, new predictors of outcome, and follow-up recommendations. J Clin Oncol 2010;28:690–7.
44. Kyle RA, Remstein ED, Therneau TM, et al. Clinical course and prognosis of smoldering (asymptomatic) multiple myeloma. N Engl J Med 2007;356: 2582–90.
45. Rajkumar SV, Merlini G, San Miguel JF. Redefining myeloma. Nat Rev Clin Oncol 2012;9:494–6.
46. Rajkumar SV, Larson D, Kyle RA. Diagnosis of smoldering multiple myeloma. N Engl J Med 2011;365:474–5.
47. Rosinol L, Blade J, Esteve J, et al. Smoldering multiple myeloma: natural history and recognition of an evolving type. Br J Haematol 2003;123:631–6.
48. Dispenzieri A, Kyle RA, Katzmann JA, et al. Immunoglobulin free light chain ratio is an independent risk factor for progression of smoldering (asymptomatic) mul-tiple myeloma. Blood 2008;111:785–9.
49. Larsen JT, Kumar SK, Dispenzieri A, et al. Serum free light chain ratio as a biomarker for high-risk smoldering multiple myeloma. Leukemia 2013;27: 941–6.
50. Bianchi G, Kyle RA, Larson DR, et al. High levels of peripheral blood circulating plasma cells as a specific risk factor for progression of smoldering multiple myeloma. Leukemia 2013;27:680–5.
51. Perez-Persona E, Vidriales MB, Mateo G, et al. New criteria to identify risk of pro-gression in monoclonal gammopathy of uncertain significance and smoldering multiple myeloma based on multiparameter flow cytometry analysis of bone marrow plasma cells. Blood 2007;110:2586–92.
52. Moulopoulos LA, Dimopoulos MA, Smith TL, et al. Prognostic significance of magnetic resonance imaging in patients with asymptomatic multiple myeloma. J Clin Oncol 1995;13:251–6.
53. Hillengass J, Fechtner K, Weber MA, et al. Prognostic significance of focal le-sions in whole-body magnetic resonance imaging in patients with asymptomatic multiple myeloma. J Clin Oncol 2010;28:1606–10.

54. Rajkumar SV, Gupta V, Fonseca R, et al. Impact of primary molecular cytogenetic abnormalities and risk of progression in smoldering multiple myeloma. Leukemia 2013;27:1738–44.

55. Neben K, Jauch A, Hielscher T, et al. Progression in smoldering myeloma is independently determined by the chromosomal abnormalities del(17p), t(4;14), gain 1q, hyperdiploidy, and tumor load. J Clin Oncol 2013;31:4325–32.

56. Dhodapkar MV, Sexton R, Waheed S, et al. Clinical, genomic, and imaging predictors of myeloma progression from asymptomatic monoclonal gammopathies (SWOG S0120). Blood 2014;123:78–85.

57. Rajkumar SV, Kyle RA. Haematological cancer: treatment of smoldering multiple myeloma. Nat Rev Clin Oncol 2013;10:554–5.

58. Dispenzieri A, Stewart AK, Chanan-Khan A, et al. Smoldering multiple myeloma requiring treatment: time for a new definition? Blood 2013;122:4172–81.

59. Mateos MV, San Miguel JF. New approaches to smoldering myeloma. Curr Hematol Malig Rep 2013;8:270–6.

60. Hjorth M, Hellquist L, Holmberg E, et al. Initial versus deferred melphalanprednisone therapy for asymptomatic multiple myeloma stage I–a randomized study. Myeloma Group of Western Sweden. Eur J Haematol 1993;50:95–102.

61. Grignani G, Gobbi PG, Formisano R, et al. A prognostic index for multiple myeloma. Br J Cancer 1996;73:1101–7.

62. Riccardi A, Mora O, Tinelli C, et al. Long-term survival of stage I multiple myeloma given chemotherapy just after diagnosis or at progression of the disease: a multicentre randomized study. Cooperative Group of Study and Treatment of Multiple Myeloma. Br J Cancer 2000;82:1254–60.

63. Rajkumar SV, Gertz MA, Lacy MQ, et al. Thalidomide as initial therapy for early-stage myeloma. Leukemia 2003;17:775–9.

64. Weber D, Rankin K, Gavino M, et al. Thalidomide alone or with dexamethasone for previously untreated multiple myeloma. J Clin Oncol 2003;21:16–9.

65. Barlogie B, van Rhee F, Shaughnessy JD Jr, et al. Seven-year median time to progression with thalidomide for smoldering myeloma: partial response identifies subset requiring earlier salvage therapy for symptomatic disease. Blood 2008;112:3122–5.

66. Witzig TE, Laumann KM, Lacy MQ, et al. A phase III randomized trial of thalidomide plus zoledronic acid versus zoledronic acid alone in patients with asymptomatic multiple myeloma. Leukemia 2013;27:220–5.

67. Martin A, Garcia-Sanz R, Hernandez J, et al. Pamidronate induces bone formation in patients with smouldering or indolent myeloma, with no significant antitumour effect. Br J Haematol 2002;118:239–42.

68. D'Arena G, Gobbi PG, Broglia C, et al. Pamidronate versus observation in asymptomatic myeloma: final results with long-term follow-up of a randomized study. Leuk Lymphoma 2011;52:771–5.

69. Musto P, Petrucci MT, Bringhen S, et al. A multicenter, randomized clinical trial comparing zoledronic acid versus observation in patients with asymptomatic myeloma. Cancer 2008;113:1588–95.

70. Mateos MV, Hernández MT, Giraldo P, et al. Lenalidomide plus dexamethasone for high-risk smoldering multiple myeloma. N Engl J Med 2013;369:438–47.

Diagnosis and Risk Stratification in Multiple Myeloma

Niels W.C.J. van de Donk, MD, PhD[a], Pieter Sonneveld, MD, PhD[b],*

KEYWORDS

- Multiple myeloma • Prognosis • Risk stratification • Diagnostic workup
- Chromosomal abnormalities

KEY POINTS

- Multiple myeloma (MM) is a tumor of monoclonal plasma cells, which produce a monoclonal antibody and expand predominantly in the bone marrow.
- Patients present with hypercalcemia, renal impairment, anemia, and/or bone disease (CRAB criteria). Only patients with symptomatic MM require therapy, whereas asymptomatic patients receive regular follow-up. Survival of patients with MM is very heterogeneous.
- Gene expression profiling is emerging as a prognostic tool to further improve risk stratification.
- Incorporation of imaging techniques, such as positron emission tomography/computed tomography and magnetic resonance imaging, will add valuable information to the standard response assessment.
- New therapeutic strategies for high- and low-risk MM should be explored in the setting of clinical trials.

CLINICAL PRESENTATION

Multiple myeloma (MM) is a tumor of terminally differentiated monoclonal B cells (plasma cells) that produce a monoclonal protein and .expand predominantly in the bone marrow (BM). Hypercalcemia, renal impairment, anemia, and bone disease represent the CRAB criteria for symptomatic MM requiring therapy.

Symptoms of anemia develop as a result of displacement of normal hematopoiesis. Thrombocytopenia occurs rarely with only 5% of patients with newly diagnosed MM presenting with platelets less than 100×10^9/L.[1] Alterations in the BM microenvironment result in reduced bone formation by osteoblasts and increased bone destruction

[a] Department of Hematology, University Medical Center Utrecht, Heidelberglaan 100, Utrecht 3584CX, The Netherlands; [b] Department of Hematology, Erasmus MC Cancer Institute, 's Gravendijkwal 230, Rotterdam 3015CE, The Netherlands
* Corresponding author.
E-mail address: p.sonneveld@erasmusmc.nl

Hematol Oncol Clin N Am 28 (2014) 791–813
http://dx.doi.org/10.1016/j.hoc.2014.06.007
0889-8588/14/$ – see front matter © 2014 Elsevier Inc. All rights reserved.

by osteoclasts, which lead to diffuse osteoporosis, osteolytic lesions, and painful pathologic fractures. There is also a higher incidence of infections because of immune dysfunction, especially during active disease. Approximately 20% of the patients with newly diagnosed MM present with renal impairment (creatinine ≥2 mg/dL); it is most frequently caused by light-chain cast nephropathy, which results in extensive destruction of tubular cells.[1] Several other factors, such as dehydration, hypercalcemia, infections, nephrotoxic drugs, and contrast media, may also contribute to renal impairment.[2] Also amyloidosis and monoclonal immunoglobulin deposition disease are causes of renal impairment in MM, leading to usually nonselective proteinuria.

DIFFERENTIAL DIAGNOSIS

Sixty-three percent of the patients with MM present at more than 65 years of age, and 37% of the patients newly diagnosed with MM are older than 75 years.[3] Therefore, patients may present with renal impairment that is not related to MM but a result of other underlying medical conditions that are prevalent in elderly patients, such as hypertension and diabetes. Similarly, primary hyperparathyroidism should be considered for hypercalcemia; deficiencies of iron, vitamin B_{12}, and folic acid for anemia; and metastatic carcinoma for lytic bone lesions. Other symptomatic plasma cell diseases that have to be excluded include solitary plasmacytoma and primary plasma cell leukemia (pPCL) (**Table 1**). Symptomatic MM is virtually always preceded by monoclonal gammopathy of uncertain significance (MGUS) that progresses to smoldering myeloma (SMM) (see **Table 1**).[4] MGUS and SMM do not require therapy but only clinical observation, except in the setting of clinical trials.

DIAGNOSTIC WORKUP OF MM

At the time of MM diagnosis, the authors obtain a detailed medical history and physical examination and perform laboratory studies, such as full blood count and differential, peripheral blood smear, blood chemistry including tumor lysis parameters, beta-2 microglobulin, serum protein electrophoresis, and free light chains (**Box 1**). Staging procedures should also include the evaluation of urine M protein in 24-hour urine and a skeletal survey. Whole-body radiographs still remain the standard tool for the evaluation of MM bone disease.[5] However, it is well recognized that this imaging technique underevaluates the extent of skeletal lesions. Low-dose whole-body computed tomography (CT), which is faster and has greater sensitivity compared with standard radiography, is a valuable alternative.[5] Magnetic resonance imaging (MRI) is useful for the evaluation of cord compression or a painful area of the skeleton. Furthermore, MRI is recommended in patients with radiographs suggesting a solitary plasmacytoma of the bone.[4]

In addition, the authors perform a BM biopsy and BM aspiration for morphology, immunophenotyping by flow cytometry, and cytogenetic analysis by fluorescence in situ hybridization (FISH), which should include at least t(4;14)(p16;q32), t(14;16)(q32;q23), ampl(1q21), and del(17p13) (see **Box 1**). Lumbar puncture, MRI, or CT is performed when extramedullary (EM) involvement is suspected.

PROGNOSTIC FACTORS

Response to treatment and survival of patients with MM is very heterogeneous, with some patients dying of refractory MM within a few weeks, whereas others live for more than 10 years. This variety in outcome is related to intrinsic tumor cell characteristics, including sensitivity to active MM drugs,[6] tumor burden, and several host factors. Risk stratification of patients with MM is important in order to define which

Table 1
Definitions

	International Myeloma Working Group Consensus Diagnostic Criteria[112] Combined with the Mayo Clinic Criteria[113]
Non-IgM MGUS	• Serum M protein <30 g/L and • Clonal bone marrow plasma cells <10% and • Absence of end-organ damage[a,b]
IgM MGUS	• Serum IgM M protein <30 g/L and • Bone marrow lymphoplasmacytic infiltration <10% and • Absence of end-organ damage[b,c]
Light-chain MGUS	• Abnormal FLC ratio (<0.26 or >1.65) and • Increased level of the involved light-chain and • No immunoglobulin heavy-chain expression on immunofixation and • Clonal bone marrow plasma cells <10% and • Absence of end-organ damage[a,b]
SMM (or asymptomatic MM)	• Serum M protein ≥30 g/L and/or • Clonal bone marrow plasma cells ≥10% and • Absence of end-organ damage[a,b]
Idiopathic Bence Jones proteinuria	• Urinary M protein ≥500 mg/24 h and/or clonal bone marrow plasma cells ≥10% • No immunoglobulin heavy-chain expression on immunofixation • Absence of end-organ damage[a,b]
Symptomatic MM	• Presence of M protein in serum and/or urine (except in patients with nonsecretory multiple myeloma) and • Clonal bone marrow plasma cells ≥10% and • Evidence of end-organ damage[a,b]
Solitary plasmacytoma	• Biopsy-proven solitary lesion of bone or soft tissue with evidence of clonal plasma cells • Normal bone marrow with no evidence of clonal plasma cells • Normal skeletal survey and MRI of spine and pelvis (except for primary solitary lesion) • Absence of end-organ damage[a,b]
pPCL	• >20% circulating plasma cells and/or an absolute level of >2 × 10^9/L • Not arising from preexisting MM

Abbreviations: FLC, free light chain; IgM, immunoglobulin M; MRI, magnetic resonance imaging.
[a] End-organ damage includes hypercalcemia (serum calcium >11.5 mg/dL [>2.65 mM]), renal insufficiency (serum creatinine >2 mg/dL [>177 μM]), anemia (hemoglobin <10 g/dL [<6.2 mM] or >2.0 g/dL [>1.25 mM] less than the lower limit of the normal range), and bone disease (lytic bone lesions, severe osteopenia, or pathologic fractures) (CRAB) that can be attributed to the plasma cell proliferative disorder.
[b] Especially in elderly persons other causes should be considered, such as deficiencies of vitamin B$_{12}$, folic acid, or iron for anemia; primary hyperparathyroidism for hypercalcemia; diabetes and hypertension for renal insufficiency; and metastatic carcinoma for lytic bone lesions.
[c] End-organ damage includes anemia, constitutional symptoms, hyperviscosity, lymphadenopathy, or hepatosplenomegaly that can be attributed to the underlying lymphoproliferative disorder.
Adapted from Kyle RA, Durie BG, Rajkumar SV, et al. Monoclonal gammopathy of undetermined significance (MGUS) and smoldering (asymptomatic) multiple myeloma: IMWG consensus perspectives risk factors for progression and guidelines for monitoring and management. Leukemia 2010;24(6):1121–7; and Kyle RA, Rajkumar SV. Criteria for diagnosis, staging, risk stratification and response assessment of multiple myeloma. Leukemia 2009;23(1):3–9.

Box 1
Diagnostic evaluation for MM

Medical history and physical examination

With emphasis on the presence of comorbidities, frailty, and disability (Charlson index, ADL, and IADL)

Blood

Complete blood count with differential

BUN, creatinine, liver enzymes, bilirubin, alkaline phosphatase, total protein, CRP

LDH, calcium, phosphate

Beta-2 microglobulin and albumin

Serum protein electrophoresis, immunofixation, serum-free light-chain analysis

Urine

24-hour urine collection for electrophoresis and immunofixation

24-hour urine for total protein

Bone marrow

Biopsy for histology

Aspirate for

Morphology

Immunophenotyping

Cytogenetic analysis by FISH[a] at least focused on del(17p13), t(4;14), ampl(1q21), and t(14;16); an extended panel may focus on del(13q), del(1p21), t(11;14), t(14;20), and ploidy status

Radiographic skeletal survey including skull, pelvis, vertebral column, and long bones[b]

Additional investigations, which may be useful under certain circumstances

Lumbar puncture (cell counts, chemistry, cytology, immunophenotyping): suspicion of leptomeningeal involvement

MRI: evaluation of cord compression or painful area of the skeleton (suspicion of soft tissue plasmacytomas arising from bone) as well as in the evaluation of patients with radiographs suggesting a solitary plasmacytoma of the bone

CT or ^{18}F-FDG-PET/CT: suspicion of extramedullary plasmacytomas

Survey for evaluation of AL amyloidosis

Bleeding time, APTT, PT

Cryoglobulins, cold agglutinins

Serum viscosity, fundoscopy: symptoms of hyperviscosity

HLA typing: in case allo-SCT is considered

Abbreviations: ADL, activities of daily living; allo-SCT, allogeneic stem cell transplantation; APTT, activated partial thromboplastin time; BUN, blood urea nitrogen; CRP, C-reactive protein; CT, computed tomography; ^{18}F-FDG-PET, ^{18}F-fluorodeoxyglucose positron emission tomography; FISH, fluorescence in situ hybridization; IADL, instrumental activities of daily living; LDH, lactate dehydrogenase; MRI, magnetic resonance imaging; PT, prothrombin time.
[a] FISH is preferably performed on purified tumor cells or with simultaneous staining of cytoplasmic immunoglobulins.
[b] As alternative to conventional radiography, low-dose whole-body CT can be considered.

patients will have a long-term survival and which patients have high-risk MM, so that the best therapeutic strategy can be defined.

In the next section, the authors describe prognostic factors that reflect myeloma biology and represent MM tumor burden and discuss patient characteristics that have an impact on survival. Because outcome is also associated with quality of response, the authors also discuss several therapy-related factors.

DISEASE CHARACTERISTICS
Conventional Cytogenetics

Conventional cytogenetics reveal karyotypic abnormalities in only 20% to 30% of the patients,[7] whereas more sensitive techniques that are not based on metaphase availability, such as FISH, array comparative genomic hybridization, and single-nucleotide polymorphism (SNP)–based mapping arrays, reveal that virtually all MM tumors have chromosomal abnormalities. This discrepancy is related to the low proliferation index of the tumor cells observed in most patients with MM. The normal karyotype in patients with a low proliferation index probably corresponds with normal BM myeloid cells.

FISH

FISH can detect specific changes in interphase cells, thereby overcoming the problem of the lack of proliferating cells, which are required for conventional cytogenetic analysis. Because of the frequent low percentage of tumor cells in the BM aspirate, plasma cell purification or sorting is required before FISH.

In MM chromosome translocations involving the immunoglobulin heavy chain (IgH) locus and hyperdiploidy, with multiple trisomies of chromosomes 3, 5, 7, 9, 11, 15, 19, and 21, are primary events, whereas other events, such as del(17p) and amp(1q21), are acquired during disease progression (**Table 2**).

Hyperdiploidy occurs in approximately 50% of patients with newly diagnosed MM and is associated with an improved progression-free survival (PFS) and overall survival (OS).[8–11] However, patients with hyperdiploidy represent a heterogeneous group, which is partly explained by the presence of other cytogenetic abnormalities (see later discussion).

Translocation t(4;14) leads to deregulation of fibroblast growth factor receptor 3 (*FGFR3*) and multiple myeloma *SET* domain (*MMSET*). However, because *FGFR3* is not expressed in about one-third of the patients with t(4;14), the target gene is most likely *MMSET*. The t(4;14) is associated with impaired PFS and OS in several

Table 2	
Incidence of chromosomal abnormalities in newly diagnosed MM	
Genomic Aberration	**Incidence (%)**
del(13q)	~50
14q32 Translocations	~50–60
Hyperdiploidy	~50
t(4;14)	~15
t(11;14)	~15
t(14;16)	~5
t(14;20)	~1
del(17p)	~10
amp(1q21)	~30–43
del(1p21)	~20

studies.[8,9,12–19] Importantly, bortezomib seems to overcome part of the negative prognostic impact of t(4;14).[16,18,20–23]

The translocation t(14;16) results in deregulation of the *c-MAF* proto-oncogene and is predictive of a poor outcome.[8,12,15] However, an intergroupe francophone du myelome (IFM) analysis showed no adverse impact of t(14;16), which may be related to treatment differences, with 60% of patients in this study receiving double auto-stem cell transplantation (SCT).[24] The rare translocation t(14;20) results in deregulation of *MAFB* and confers a poor prognosis.[12]

The translocation t(11;14) results in upregulation of cyclinD1 and was identified as a favorable prognostic factor in some studies,[13,25] whereas it has no impact on outcome in others.[8,9,14] This translocation is also associated with CD20 expression on the cell surface and lymphoplasmacytic morphology of the tumor cells.[25]

Del(13q) predicts for impaired PFS and OS; however, the negative prognostic impact of del(13) is mainly related to its frequent association with del(17p) and t(4;14).[7,8,15,16,19,26,27] In patients with del(13q) detected by FISH without t(4;14) or del(17p), del(13q) is no longer predictive of survival.[8,9,12,16,28] However, deletion of chromosome 13 retains its prognostic value when it is detected by conventional cytogenetics.[10,29]

Del(17p) is an important prognostic factor with a negative impact on PFS and OS.[7–9,12,14–16,18,19] The molecular target of del(17) may be *TP53*, which is important in both clonal immortalization and survival of tumor cells after treatment.[6,28] Several studies show that bortezomib or lenalidomide do not overcome the poor prognosis conferred by del(17p). However, in the randomized Hovon-65/GMMG-HD4 study, long-term bortezomib administration during induction and maintenance overcomes part of the adverse impact of del(17p).[16,23] Also incorporation of bortezomib in the Total Therapy 3 (TT3) protocol abrogated the negative prognostic impact of del(17p) in patients with gene-expression profiling (GEP)–defined low-risk disease.[30] These conflicting results may be explained by differences in the cumulative dose of bortezomib administered in the different protocols.

Gain of 1q21 has also been linked to an adverse prognsosis.[12,16] Patients with greater than 3 copies of 1q21 have a worse outcome when compared with patients with 3 copies of 1q21,[16] possibly reflecting a dosage effect of genes located at this chromosomal region. Also del(1p) confers poor prognosis in MM.[31]

Multiple Adverse Cytogenetic Abnormalities

Boyd and colleagues[12] showed that ampl(1q) is very common in patients with adverse IgH translocations. Seventy-two percent of the patients with an adverse IgH translocation also had amp(1q21), whereas this was 32.4% in the group without adverse IgH translocations. The frequency of del(17p) was similar in patients with or without adverse IgH translocations. Importantly, there is an association between the accumulation of adverse lesions and progressive impairment of survival. The median PFS and OS of patients treated in the Medical Research Council (MRC) Myeloma IX trial without adverse genetic lesions (no adverse IgH translocation, no del[17p], and no amp[1q21]), one adverse lesion, and greater than 1 adverse genetic lesion was 23.5, 17.8, and 11.7 months and 60.6, 41.9, 21.7 months, respectively. The median OS was only 9.1 months for the 16 patients with 3 adverse genetic abnormalities.[12]

Good Combined with Adverse Cytogenetic Abnormalities

Within the group of patients with hyperdiploidy, there is a great heterogeneity in survival. Avet-Loiseau and colleagues[32] showed that gain of 5q31 resulted in a better outcome in hyperdiploid MM compared with hyperdiploid cases without this feature.

Another study demonstrated that among patients with hyperdiploidy trisomy 11 confers a favorable prognosis, whereas gain of 1q and loss of chromosome 13 drive poor outcomes.[33] Also GEP identifies subclasses of hyperdiploid MM with different clinical outcomes.[34]

Another study showed that coexistent hyperdiploidy does not abrogate the poor prognosis associated with adverse cytogenetics in MM.[11] In the Myeloma IX study, 58% of the patients had hyperdiploidy. Of these hyperdiploid patients, 61% had one or more adverse lesions (t[14;14], t[14;16], t[14;20], amp[1q], or del[17p]). The OS and PFS were significantly worse in patients with hyperdiploidy with an adverse lesion when compared with those patients with hyperdiploidy alone (median PFS 23.0 vs 15.4 months; median OS 60.9 vs 35.7 months). Alternatively, the outcome of patients with an adverse lesion was independent of the presence or absence of hyperdiploidy.[11]

However, a recent study showed that patients with high-risk chromosomal abnormalities (t[4;14], t[14;16], t[14;20], or del[17p]) have different outcomes depending on the presence (median OS: not reached) or absence of trisomy (median OS: 3 years).[35]

Gene Expression Profiling

Several studies have evaluated myeloma at the transcriptional level by using GEP, which has led to molecular classification systems for MM based on differential gene expression[36–38] but also to improved risk stratification. So far none of these signatures has been introduced into general clinical practice.

Shaughnessy and colleagues[39] evaluated the gene expression profile of newly diagnosed MM patients and identified a 70-gene subset as an independent predictor of outcome. The presence of a high-risk signature (13.1% of the patients) resulted in inferior event-free survival (EFS) (5-year EFS: 18% vs 60%) and OS (5-year OS: 28% vs 78%) compared with a low-risk signature. In this 70-gene high-risk signature, elevated expression levels of genes mapped to chromosome 1q and reduced expression levels of genes mapped to chromosome 1p, which reflects the importance of amp(1q21) and del(1p) in conferring a poor prognosis.[39] However, epigenetic modifications in chromosome 1 cannot be excluded. The same group performed GEP analysis before and 48 hours after a bortezomib test dose in patients treated in bortezomib-based TT3 protocols. Based on changes in expression following the test dose, the University of Arkansas Medical School (UAMS)-80 signature was constructed, which has strong prognostic impact on both PFS and OS. The selected genes in this model were enriched in genes of the protein ubiquitination pathway.[40]

The Erasmus MC-92 signature is derived from patients treated in the Hovon-65/GMMG-HD4 trial, and predicts for impaired PFS and OS in several independent data sets.[41] The survival of high-risk patients in the bortezomib arm of the Hovon-65/GMMG-HD4 study was 30 months, whereas it was 19 months in the vincristine, adriamycin, dexamethasone (VAD) arm.[41] Other GEP-based risk models that predict survival in patients newly diagnosed with MM include the IFM-15[42] and MRC-IX-6[43] gene expression signatures. These different models have to be validated in the context of other treatment approaches because it is to be expected that prognostic factors change with different treatment schedules.

Plasma Cell Proliferation

Several studies using different techniques have demonstrated that proliferation of tumor cells is an important independent adverse prognostic factor in MM. The plasma cell labeling index (PCLI) is a measure of the fraction of cells in S phase and is evaluated by using fluorescence microscopy. The PCLI predicts for impaired PFS and

OS.[1,14,44] Furthermore, reduction of the PCLI after initial therapy is predictive of improved survival.[44]

Use of the PCLI has not gained widespread acceptance because of its labor-intensive slide-based method.[44] However, the fraction of plasma cells in S phase can also be determined by flow cytometry. With this technique, a subgroup of patients with inferior PFS and OS can be identified.[45] A recent study showed that novel agents may overcome the poor prognosis of patients with a high plasma cell proliferation index as determined by flow cytometry.[45]

In another technique, Ki-67 staining identifies proliferating cells in G1, G2, S, and M phases of the cell cycle (but not G0). In MM, it is associated with impaired survival.[46] Also gene-expression–based proliferation assessment identifies patients with significantly inferior EFS and OS.[47]

Lactate Dehydrogenase

Elevated lactate dehydrogenase (LDH) levels are present in 10% to 15% of newly diagnosed patients. Several studies have shown that high LDH serum levels are associated with advanced disease and shorter survival.[21,27,40,45,48–53] LDH retains its prognostic significance in patients treated with novel agents (JCO Moreau, unpublished, 2014).[40,52]

M Protein Isotype

The isotype of the M protein that is produced by the plasma cell clone may have prognostic value. However, this is frequently related to presence of other poor prognostic factors. For example, patients with IgA MM have an inferior outcome when compared with IgG MM, which is related to its association with t(4;14).[13,17,18,27]

IgD MM accounts for approximately 1% to 2% of all MM cases and is associated with a high frequency of undetectable or small M-protein levels.[54,55] IgD MM is characterized by an increased frequency of EM involvement, anemia, renal failure, osteolytic bone lesions, hypercalcemia, and International Staging System (ISS) stage III disease.[54,55] The clustering of these adverse prognostic factors may explain the poor prognosis of IgD MM when compared with IgG or IgA MM.

Similar to IgD MM, IgE M-protein levels are very low in IgE MM. IgE MM is a very rare subgroup and has a poor prognosis.[54]

EM Myeloma and Primary Plasma Cell Leukemia

EM disease is more common in patients with high-risk cytogenetics or high-risk GEP profiles and carries a poor outcome.[56] EM disease occurs more frequently at the time of relapse than at diagnosis.[57]

EM disease (positron emission tomography [PET]–positive lesions not contiguous to bone and arising in soft tissues) was detected by using PET/CT in 6% of patients with newly diagnosed MM who were treated with double auto-SCT.[58] In this study, EM disease was predictive of shorter PFS (4-year PFS: 22% vs 63% for patients with and without EM disease, respectively) and OS (4-year OS: 64% vs 90%).[58] EM disease defined by PET/CT (present in 6% of cases) also had a prognostic impact in patients enrolled in TT3.[59]

The most aggressive plasma cell dyscrasia is pPCL.[60] Compared with MM, pPCL presents more often with anemia, thrombocytopenia, hypercalcemia, EM involvement, impaired renal function, elevated beta-2 microglobulin, high plasma cell labeling index, increased LDH levels, and GEP-defined high-risk disease. Furthermore, the presence of high-risk cytogenetic abnormalities, such as t(4;14), t(14;16), del(17p), del(1p), and amp(1q), is markedly higher in pPCL compared with newly diagnosed

MM.[60] Conversely, the incidence of hyperdiploidy is rare (0%–8.8%). Altogether, this explains the poor prognosis of patients with pPCL.

Imaging Characteristics

Both MRI and PET/CT findings at the time of diagnosis have prognostic value. The number of focal lesions as detected by MRI is a prognostic marker for PFS and OS.[59,61,62] In addition, diffuse BM involvement is associated with more advanced disease and inferior survival.[63]

An Italian study, with patients enrolled in a trial that included double auto-SCT, showed that several characteristics of PET/CT have prognostic value, including the presence of EM disease, degree of fluorodeoxyglucose (FDG) uptake at the time of diagnosis, and type of BM involvement (>3 focal lesions or diffuse BM uptake).[58] The number of focal lesions and degree of uptake before therapy as defined by PET/CT was also predictive of outcome for patients treated in TT3.[59,64]

Higher numbers of focal lesions on MRI and PET, as well as the degree of uptake on PET, are linked to GEP-defined high-risk disease.[65]

Other Factors

Several studies have shown that several variables that reflect tumor burden, including M-protein level,[66] extent of bone lesions,[66] BM plasma cell infiltration,[14,45,66,66] beta-2 microglobulin,[9,14,21,26,27,32,42,45,66] low platelet count,[1,9,42,53,66] and anemia,[9,21,27,45,53,66,67] have prognostic value in patients with newly diagnosed MM. Other factors that are associated with reduced survival include albumin,[1,9,32,66] serum calcium,[53,66,67] and presence of plasmablastic morphology.[68]

PATIENT CHARACTERISTICS
Geriatric Assessment

Aging is associated with an increased frequency of comorbidities, poor performance status, frailty, and disability, which negatively affect treatment tolerability and survival.[26,27,53,66,67,69] Furthermore, a recent meta-analysis showed that nonhematologic toxicity, especially cardiac adverse events and infections, is associated with drug discontinuation and subsequent lower cumulative delivered dose, which translates into decreased efficacy of anti-MM therapy and reduced survival in elderly patients with MM.[3]

For elderly patients with MM, Bringhen and colleagues[69] a scoring system based on age, comorbidities, as well as cognitive and physical condition that categorizes patients into 3 groups (fit, unfit, or frail), with different survival and risk of severe toxicities. In a group of 869 newly diagnosed patients treated with lenalidomide-, bortezomib-, or carfilzomib-based regimens, the cumulative 6-month rate of grade 3 to 5 nonhematologic adverse events was 19.6%, 20.7%, and 29.9% in fit, unfit, and frail patients, respectively. This finding resulted in significantly higher treatment discontinuation in the frail and unfit groups when compared with the fit groups, which translates in impaired PFS (median PFS: 14, 13, and 11 months for fit, unfit, and frail patients, respectively) and OS (1-year OS: 96%, 93%, and 78%).[69]

Altogether this clearly demonstrates the importance of geriatric assessment (see **Box 1**) in predicting survival and also its importance in guiding dose modifications to avoid unacceptable toxicity and drug discontinuation, which may lead to reduced efficacy of anti-MM therapy in elderly patients.[70]

Sociodemographic Factors

Al-Hamadani and colleagues[71] analyzed 27,987 patients with MM diagnosed between 1998 and 2000 and registered in the US National Cancer Data Base. In this cohort, 8% of the patients had an OS of 10 years or more. Factors associated with long-term survival included race, educational level, annual household income, and type of insurance. Furthermore, patients treated in an academic hospital had a higher likelihood of long-term survival compared with patients treated in community hospitals. The major limitation of this study is that it only includes patients diagnosed with MM until 2000; since then, treatment of MM has changed significantly as well as the various sociodemographic factors.

Renal Function

Several studies have shown that renal impairment is associated with poorer survival,[3,27,32] which may be related to higher tumor load, dose reductions, or interruptions because of adverse events. A recent study also showed a higher frequency of high-risk cytogenetic lesions, such as del(17p) and t(4;14), in this subgroup.[72] Patients with measurable light-chain proteinuria more frequently present with impaired renal function.[53]

The use of novel agents, especially bortezomib, has led to high rates of improvements in renal function, when compared with conventional agents.[73,74] Furthermore, in several studies, bortezomib-based therapy abrogates the negative prognostic impact of renal failure both in elderly patients and in patients receiving high-dose therapy.[3,20,23,72,75,76] For example, in the Hovon-65/GMMG-HD4 study, 3-year OS for patients with a creatinine level of 2 mg/dL or greater was only 34% in the VAD arm, whereas it was 74% in the bortezomib, adriamycin, dexamethasone (PAD) arm, which was comparable with the survival of patients with a creatinine level less than 2 mg/dL (3-year OS in the PAD arm: 79%).[72] Altogether, a bortezomib-based regimen should be selected in case of MM-related renal dysfunction. However, thalidomide (no dose reduction needed) and lenalidomide (dose has to be adjusted according to creatinine clearance) may also be considered in case of renal dysfunction and intolerance or resistance to bortezomib.[2,74,77]

Therapy-Related Characteristics

As described in the previous sections, survival depends on both patient- and tumor-related factors. Furthermore, one of the most important prognostic factors for long-term outcomes is response to therapy. Choice of treatment strategy for each individual patient is based on several host factors (such as age and performance status), characteristics of the tumor (presence of cytogenetic abnormalities), and approval status of diverse anti-MM agents. The response that is achieved after the start of therapy depends on various biological characteristics of the tumor.

Importance of Complete Response

In younger patients treated with high-dose therapy and auto-SCT, as well as elderly patients treated with novel agents, the achievement of immunofixation-negative complete response (CR) is associated with improved PFS and OS.[78–81]

A large meta-analysis of 4990 younger patients showed that obtaining CR before or after high-dose therapy results in improved time to progression (TTP) and OS.[79] In addition, a retrospective analysis of 1175 patients with newly diagnosed MM treated with melphalan, prednisone (MP), MP+bortezomib (MPV), MP+thalidomide (MPT), or MP+bortezomib+thalidomide-bortezomib/thalidomide (VMPT-VT) showed that the 3-year PFS was 67% in patients who achieved CR, 27% for patients who obtained very good partial response (VGPR), and 27% for those in partial response (PR). The 3-year OS was 91%, 70%, and 67% for patients that achieved CR, VGPR, or PR, respectively.[78] The impact of CR was similar in patients older or younger than

75 years.[78] The improved outcome associated with CR was similar in patients who achieved CR before or after the first 6 months of therapy.[78]

Similarly, early relapse[82] and loss of CR[80] also confer a poor prognosis in MM.

Immunophenotypic and Molecular CR

The proportion of patients achieving CR has increased considerably through the introduction of novel agents as well as the use of high-dose therapy in younger patients. Therefore, more sensitive approaches, such as multiparameter flow cytometry and molecular techniques including allele-specific oligonucleotide polymerase chain reaction (PCR), are needed to evaluate residual MM cells in the BM. Molecular approaches seem to be more sensitive than multiparameter flow cytometry. However, immunophenotyping is less time consuming and applicable to a greater proportion of patients with MM.

Persistent minimal residual disease (MRD) in patients that achieved CR after auto-SCT was associated with impaired TTP and OS,[83] when compared with patients who achieved immunophenotypic CR. Especially patients with immunophenotypic CR and standard-risk cytogenetics had a very good outcome (3-year TTP: 94% and 3-year OS 100%), whereas the worst outcome was for patients with both persistent MRD and high-risk disease (3-year TTP: 0% and 3-year OS 32%).

Similar results were observed in the MRC MM IX trial. Presence of MRD was associated with a significant inferior outcome in terms of PFS and OS in the intensive pathway, and there was a trend toward inferior PFS for patients treated in the nonintensive pathway.[84] In the intensive pathway, the combination of cytogenetic risk group with MRD status provided a very powerful discriminator of outcome in patients receiving intensive treatment with high-dose therapy (median PFS for favorable cytogenetics: 44.2 and 33.7 months for MRD− and MRD+, respectively; median PFS for adverse cytogenetics: 15.7 and 8.7 months for MRD− and MRD+, respectively).[84]

Also in elderly patients achieving immunophenotypic CR after novel agent–containing induction therapy translates into superior PFS.[85] Patients in stringent CR without persistent MM tumor cells had a significantly improved PFS when compared with those patients in stringent CR with MRD.[85]

Molecular CR is rarely seen after auto-SCT; however, after bortezomib, thalidomide, dexamethasone (VTD) consolidation following auto-SCT, several patients achieved a persistent molecular remission determined by PCR. These patients had no clinical or molecular relapse after a median molecular remission duration of 27 months.[86] Also after allogeneic SCT (allo-SCT), molecular CR can be achieved. Molecular CR, and especially sustained molecular CR, confers prolonged PFS and OS following allo-SCT.[87]

PET/CT and MRI

The incorporation of several imaging techniques during follow-up has the potential to improve the definition of response. Importantly, MRD-negative patients by flow cytometry who are still immunofixation positive may partly represent patients who will ultimately achieve CR (long half-life of some M proteins), whereas in other patients this MRD assessment may fail to identify the presence of focal lesions or EM sites of active disease (false-negative results).[84] In this respect, PET/CT or MRI may be complementary techniques in the evaluation of MRD.

PET/CT

Persistence of FDG uptake after induction or after auto-SCT was associated with inferior PFS and OS.[58] Importantly, 23% of the patients who achieved CR were still

PET-positive, which conferred an inferior prognosis.[58] Also FDG suppression before transplantation in patients enrolled in TT3 conferred a survival benefit.[59] Furthermore, persistence of more than 3 focal lesions at day 7 after the start of induction therapy was associated with poor survival in TT3B.[64]

MRI

Walker and colleagues[61] showed that resolution of lesions, determined by MRI, after therapy is predictive of superior prognosis. Similarly, the Heidelberg group showed that the number of focal lesions after auto-SCT is associated with both PFS and OS.[62] Altogether this indicates that persistence of MRI lesions identifies a group of patients with an inferior response to therapy and that these residual focal lesions may represent the source of relapse.[62]

MODELS COMBINING PATIENT AND DISEASE CHARACTERISTICS

Because individual prognostic factors do not capture the full heterogeneity in outcome, several models have combined different patient and disease characteristics to improve risk stratification in MM. In this section, the authors describe several models that are frequently used in clinical practice.

Durie-Salmon Classification

The factors included in the Durie-Salmon classification include hemoglobin level, serum calcium level, number of bone lesions, as well as type and level of M protein (**Table 3**).[88] In addition, patients are grouped according to presence (B) or absence (A) of serum creatinine levels of 2 mg/dL or greater (see **Table 3**). This staging system reflects tumor mass and predicts outcome after standard-dose chemotherapy, but it has less prognostic value after high-dose therapy and with use of novel agents.[89]

ISS

Based on serum albumin and beta-2 microglobulin levels, 3 categories of patients can be defined with different OS (**Table 4**).[66] In this model, beta-2 microglobulin reflects

Table 3 Durie-Salmon staging system	
Stage	**Criteria**
I	*All of the following* • Hb >10 g/dL • Serum calcium: normal (≤12 mg/dL) • Skeletal survey: normal or solitary bone plasmacytoma only • Serum M-protein level: <50 g/L if IgG; <30 g/L if IgA • Urine light-chain M-component <4 g/24 h
II	Fitting neither stage I nor stage III
III	*One or more of the following* • Hb <8.5 g/dL • Serum calcium >12 mg/dL • Skeletal survey: 3 or more lytic bone lesions • Serum M-protein level: >70 g/L if IgG; >50 g/L if IgA • Urine light-chain M component >12 g/24 h
A	• Serum creatinine <2.0 mg/dL (<177 μM)
B	• Serum creatinine ≥2.0 mg/dL (≥177 μM)

Abbreviation: Hb, hemoglobin.

| Table 4 | |
| ISS criteria | |
Stage	Criteria
ISS I	Albumin ≥35 g/L and beta-2-microglobulin <3.5 mg/L
ISS II	Not stage I or III (beta-2-microglobulin <3.5 mg/L and albumin <35 g/L or beta-2-microglobulin between 3.5 and 5.5 mg/L irrespective of albumin level)
ISS III	Beta-2 microglobulin ≥5.5 mg/L

both tumor burden and renal function. Reduced albumin in patients with MM may reflect both the general performance status of patients as well as the effect of interleukin-6, produced by the BM microenvironment, on the liver. The ISS system has prognostic value for both younger and elderly patients and after high-dose therapy as well as standard-dose therapy.[66]

The study that constructed the ISS included patients treated up to 2002, which indicates that only few patients received novel agents. However, a recent study showed that the ISS system has also prognostic value in MM patients treated with novel agents,[67] indicating that the novel agents cannot fully overcome the negative prognostic impact of high-risk ISS.

Mayo Stratification of Myeloma and Risk-Adapted Therapy

The Mayo Stratification of Myeloma and Risk-Adapted Therapy (mSMART) criteria use a combination of metaphase cytogenetics, FISH, and PCLI and recently also GEP as tools to identify 3 risk categories (standard risk, intermediate risk, and high risk) for prognostication of patients with newly diagnosed MM (**Table 5**).[29] This model retains its prognostic value since the introduction of the novel agents.[90] Based on this model, patients can be treated with different therapeutic approaches.[29] However, this risk-adapted therapy has not been validated in prospective studies.

ISS and FISH

The combination of ISS score with information on the presence of high-risk genetic lesions by FISH results in a model that reflects tumor mass, patient condition, as well as intrinsic plasma cell characteristics. Several studies have shown that this model improves the prediction of patient outcomes in MM.

Avet-Loiseau and colleagues[9] showed that the presence of t(4;14) and/or del(17p), defined by FISH, separates 2 groups of patients with different EFS and OS within each ISS stage.

Similarly, a retrospective analysis of international studies showed that combining the presence of t(4;14) and del(17p) with ISS stage significantly improved the prognostic assessment in terms of both PFS and OS.[7] Within the 3 different groups of

| Table 5 | | |
| mSMART criteria | | |
High Risk	Intermediate Risk	Standard Risk
• FISH: del(17p), t(14;16), t(14;20) • GEP: high-risk signature	• FISH: t(4;14) • Cytogenetic del(13) • Hypodiploidy • PCLI ≥3%	*All others including* • FISH: t(11;14), t(6;14)

Data from Mikhael JR, Dingli D, Roy V, et al. Management of newly diagnosed symptomatic multiple myeloma: updated Mayo Stratification of Myeloma and Risk-Adapted Therapy (mSMART) consensus guidelines 2013. Mayo Clin Proc 2013;88(4):360–76.

patients there was also a strong prognostic impact of age (<65 years and ≥65 years) and use of high-dose therapy with autologous stem cell rescue.[7]

Neben and colleagues[8] also combined the ISS score with the presence or absence of t(4;14)/del(17p) defined by FISH. The median PFS after autologous SCT (after VAD, thalidomide, adriamycin, dexamethasone (TAD), or PAD induction) were 2.7, 2.0 and 1.2 years for the favorable-risk group (ISS I and no high-risk aberrations), intermediate-risk group (ISS I and high-risk aberrations or ISS II/III without high-risk abnormalities), and poor-risk group (ISS II/III and presence of high-risk aberrations), respectively. The 5-year OS for the favorable, intermediate, and poor prognostic groups were 72%, 62%, and 41%, respectively.[8] The combination of ISS and FISH predicted PFS and OS much better than ISS alone.[8] Also in the Hovon-65/GMMG-HD4 combination of ISS and high-risk aberrations by FISH (del[17p], t[4;14], or amp [1q21] [>3 copies]), resulted in a robust model predicting survival in newly diagnosed MM.[16]

Boyd and colleagues[12] also combined ISS and the presence of 0, 1, or greater than 1 adverse genetic lesions (t[4;14], t[14;16], t[14;20], del[17p], or amp[1q21]) as defined by FISH in the Myeloma IX trial. The median PFS and OS in the ultrahigh risk group, defined by ISS II or III plus greater than 1 adverse genetic lesion, was only 9.9 months and 19.4 months, respectively. The favorable-risk group had a median OS of 67.8 months.

ISS, FISH, AND FAILURE TO ACHIEVE CR AFTER INDUCTION THERAPY

Salwender and colleagues[91] performed a retrospective analysis of several European studies that evaluated a bortezomib-based induction regimen followed by single or double auto-SCT. Based on the presence or absence of ISS stage III, t(4;14) or del(17p) by FISH, and CR after induction therapy, 4 groups of patients with different risks of progression and/or death were identified. Patients with ISS stage I or II, no adverse cytogenetic abnormalities, and CR after induction (13% of all patients) had a median PFS of 61 months, whereas patients with ISS stage III plus the presence of high-risk cytogenetics and without CR after induction (3%) had a median PFS of only 26 months. The median PFS was 56 and 36 months for patients with 1 or 2 risk factors, respectively.[91] OS at 5 years was 84%, 81%, 56%, and 33% for patients with 0, 1, 2, or 3 adverse variables, respectively.[91]

ISS and LDH

Within each ISS subgroup, the presence of high LDH is associated with a worse median OS.[52]

ISS, LDH, and FISH

A recent retrospective analysis of 4 phase 3 studies, which evaluated novel agent-based induction and auto-SCT, showed that combining ISS stage, LDH, and FISH identifies a population (5%–8% of total population) at very high risk of myeloma progression-related death (JCO Moreau, unpublished, 2014). Patients with ISS stage III, elevated LDH, and t(4;14) or del(17p) have a 2-year OS of only 54.6% (JCO Moreau, unpublished, 2014).

CONCLUDING REMARKS AND FUTURE PERSPECTIVES

Risk stratification in MM is important to predict survival from diagnosis and to define a treatment strategy.[89] In addition, prognostic classification is also useful to compare different trial populations.[92] Before the start of therapy, several variables reflecting the biology of the MM clone and tumor burden as well as patient characteristics are important determinants of outcome (**Fig. 1**). Furthermore, the quality of response following therapy has prognostic value; especially achieving MRD negativity, as determined by immunophenotypic analysis or molecular techniques, predicts for a prolonged survival (see **Fig. 1**).

Identification of cytogenetic abnormalities by FISH and the ISS staging system are currently the most important and widely available prognostic factors in MM. The International Myeloma Working Group (IMWG) consensus panel on FISH recommends to test for the presence of del(17p), t(4;14), and t(14;16).[89] However, testing for chromosome 1 abnormalities is also strongly recommended by the European Myeloma Network.[93] An extended panel, which may be incorporated in clinical trials, includes testing for t(11;14), t(14;20), del(13q), and ploidy status.[93]

The combination of independent prognostic factors provides greater prognostic information. In this respect, the IMWG recently recommended to use the combination of FISH and ISS stage for risk stratification in MM.[94] High-risk MM was defined by ISS II/III and the presence of del(17p) or t(4;14), whereas low-risk disease was defined by ISS I/II, absence of adverse cytogenetic abnormalities (t[4;14], del[17p], or ampl[1q21]), and age less than 55 years.[94] However, other features, such as renal failure, LDH, plasma cell proliferative rate, and presence of EM disease, may be helpful in certain circumstances.[89] Furthermore, GEP is emerging as a prognostic tool to further improve risk stratification. However, further evaluation of this technique is warranted. Other new approaches that hold promise to predict survival include analysis of microRNA expression profiles[95,96] and evaluation of methylation and splicing patterns.

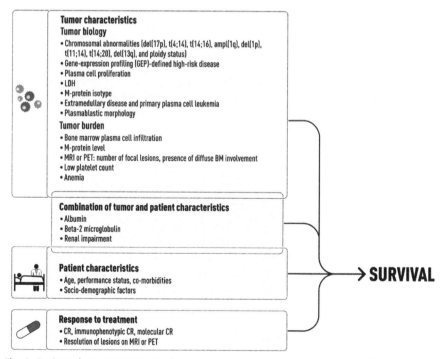

Fig. 1. Patient characteristics as well as variables reflecting tumor burden and tumor biology have prognostic value in MM. Also response to therapy is an important prognostic factor.

Importantly, high-risk features will change in the future with the introduction of next-generation novel agents and new treatment strategies.[89]

The use of risk stratification to determine the choice of therapy remains unproven because risk-adapted strategies have not been prospectively validated. Therefore, clinical trials should be designed in which high-risk patients are offered an intensive treatment approach to achieve long-term disease control. Bortezomib has a clear impact on the prognosis of high-risk patients and should be part of the treatment regimen of this subgroup.[97] One of the strategies that may be explored in high-risk MM is double auto-SCT, because a retrospective analysis recently demonstrated that patients with high-risk cytogenetics and treated with bortezomib-based induction regimens may benefit from double auto-SCT compared with single transplant.[91] Given the very poor outcome using the standard therapeutic approaches, younger patients with high-risk disease may also be offered allo-SCT within the context of clinical trials. Kröger and colleagues[87] demonstrated that up-front auto-allo tandem SCT overcomes the negative prognostic value of del(17p) and t(4;14). Similarly, a retrospective analysis from France showed that after allo-SCT, del(17p) and t(4;14) had no impact on outcome.[98] Clinical trials should also evaluate next-generation novel agents with new mechanisms of action including monoclonal antibodies, such as daratumumab and elotuzumab, BH3 mimetics, and inhibitors of histone deacetylase, Akt, MEK, and kinesin spindle protein.[99,100] MRD assessment and serial PET examinations could further help clinicians to individualize treatment intensity and duration.

In contrast, standard-risk patients could be offered a sequential therapy approach.[101] This approach may prevent overtreatment and reduce treatment-related toxicity of low-risk patients. However, this may also lead to undertreatment of patients and, thereby, inferior outcomes.[94] Very-good-risk patients are currently not well defined. It will be important to define these patients by using studies with long-term follow-up, so that they can possibly be offered less toxic treatment approaches, also in the context of clinical trials.

In addition to better risk stratification, an important challenge will be the development of biomarkers predictive for the efficacy of novel therapeutics. This development will contribute to the selection of an effective therapy for different subsets of patients. For example, analysis of cereblon expression may be useful to predict the outcome of treatment with immunomodulatory drugs[102,103]; expression of certain genes (including genes reflecting nuclear factor–kappa-B activity and protein biosynthesis) predicts the response to bortezomib[104]; the response to ARRY-520 is higher in patients with low α-1 acid glycoprotein levels[105]; patients with CD56-positive tumors may benefit from the antibody-drug conjugate lorvotuzumab mertansine[106]; vemurafenib has anti-MM activity in patients with BRAF V600E mutation.[107,108] Another important development is a better understanding of the genetic background of patients by using SNP arrays, which may help identify patients with a higher probability of developing toxicities, including drug-induced peripheral neuropathy,[109] bisphosphonate-induced osteonecrosis of the jaw,[110] or venous thromboembolism.[111] Future studies should incorporate analysis of biomarker components that can predict the safety and effectiveness of novel drugs. Altogether these developments will contribute to the development of personalized therapy in MM, which is hoped to be more effective and better tolerated.

REFERENCES

1. Kyle RA, Gertz MA, Witzig TE, et al. Review of 1027 patients with newly diagnosed multiple myeloma. Mayo Clin Proc 2003;78(1):21–33.

2. Dimopoulos MA, Terpos E, Chanan-Khan A, et al. Renal impairment in patients with multiple myeloma: a consensus statement on behalf of the International Myeloma Working Group. J Clin Oncol 2010;28(33):4976–84.
3. Bringhen S, Mateos MV, Zweegman S, et al. Age and organ damage correlate with poor survival in myeloma patients: meta-analysis of 1435 individual patient data from 4 randomized trials. Haematologica 2013;98(6):980–7.
4. Palumbo A, Anderson K. Multiple myeloma. N Engl J Med 2011;364(11): 1046–60.
5. Dimopoulos M, Terpos E, Comenzo RL, et al. International Myeloma Working Group consensus statement and guidelines regarding the current role of imaging techniques in the diagnosis and monitoring of multiple Myeloma. Leukemia 2009;23(9):1545–56.
6. Munshi NC, vet-Loiseau H. Genomics in multiple myeloma. Clin Cancer Res 2011;17(6):1234–42.
7. vet-Loiseau H, Durie BG, Cavo M, et al. Combining fluorescent in situ hybridization data with ISS staging improves risk assessment in myeloma: an International Myeloma Working Group collaborative project. Leukemia 2013;27(3): 711–7.
8. Neben K, Jauch A, Bertsch U, et al. Combining information regarding chromosomal aberrations t(4;14) and del(17p13) with the International Staging System classification allows stratification of myeloma patients undergoing autologous stem cell transplantation. Haematologica 2010;95(7):1150–7.
9. Avet-Loiseau H, Attal M, Moreau P, et al. Genetic abnormalities and survival in multiple myeloma: the experience of the Intergroupe Francophone du Myelome. Blood 2007;109(8):3489–95.
10. Chiecchio L, Protheroe RK, Ibrahim AH, et al. Deletion of chromosome 13 detected by conventional cytogenetics is a critical prognostic factor in myeloma. Leukemia 2006;20(9):1610–7.
11. Melchor L, Boyle EM, Brioli A, et al. Co-existent hyperdiploidy does not abrogate the poor prognosis associated with adverse cytogenetics in myeloma. Blood 2013;122(21):529.
12. Boyd KD, Ross FM, Chiecchio L, et al. A novel prognostic model in myeloma based on co-segregating adverse FISH lesions and the ISS: analysis of patients treated in the MRC Myeloma IX trial. Leukemia 2012;26(2):349–55.
13. Moreau P, Facon T, Leleu X, et al. Recurrent 14q32 translocations determine the prognosis of multiple myeloma, especially in patients receiving intensive chemotherapy. Blood 2002;100(5):1579–83.
14. Gertz MA, Lacy MQ, Dispenzieri A, et al. Clinical implications of t(11;14)(q13;q32), t(4;14)(p16.3;q32), and -17p13 in myeloma patients treated with high-dose therapy. Blood 2005;106(8):2837–40.
15. Fonseca R, Blood E, Rue M, et al. Clinical and biologic implications of recurrent genomic aberrations in myeloma. Blood 2003;101(11):4569–75.
16. Neben K, Lokhorst HM, Jauch A, et al. Administration of bortezomib before and after autologous stem cell transplantation improves outcome in multiple myeloma patients with deletion 17p. Blood 2012;119(4):940–8.
17. Jaksic W, Trudel S, Chang H, et al. Clinical outcomes in t(4;14) multiple myeloma: a chemotherapy-sensitive disease characterized by rapid relapse and alkylating agent resistance. J Clin Oncol 2005;23(28):7069–73.
18. vet-Loiseau H, Leleu X, Roussel M, et al. Bortezomib plus dexamethasone induction improves outcome of patients with t(4;14) myeloma but not outcome of patients with del(17p). J Clin Oncol 2010;28(30):4630–4.

19. vet-Loiseau H, Hulin C, Campion L, et al. Chromosomal abnormalities are major prognostic factors in elderly patients with multiple myeloma: the intergroupe francophone du myelome experience. J Clin Oncol 2013;31(22):2806–9.

20. San Miguel JF, Schlag R, Khuageva NK, et al. Bortezomib plus melphalan and prednisone for initial treatment of multiple myeloma. N Engl J Med 2008;359(9): 906–17.

21. Barlogie B, Anaissie E, van RF, et al. Incorporating bortezomib into upfront treatment for multiple myeloma: early results of total therapy 3. Br J Haematol 2007; 138(2):176–85.

22. Cavo M, Tacchetti P, Patriarca F, et al. Bortezomib with thalidomide plus dexamethasone compared with thalidomide plus dexamethasone as induction therapy before, and consolidation therapy after, double autologous stem-cell transplantation in newly diagnosed multiple myeloma: a randomised phase 3 study. Lancet 2010;376(9758):2075–85.

23. Sonneveld P, Schmidt-Wolf IG, van der HB, et al. Bortezomib induction and maintenance treatment in patients with newly diagnosed multiple myeloma: results of the randomized phase III HOVON-65/GMMG-HD4 trial. J Clin Oncol 2012;30(24):2946–55.

24. vet-Loiseau H, Malard F, Campion L, et al. Translocation t(14;16) and multiple myeloma: is it really an independent prognostic factor? Blood 2011;117(6): 2009–11.

25. Fonseca R, Blood EA, Oken MM, et al. Myeloma and the t(11;14)(q13;q32); evidence for a biologically defined unique subset of patients. Blood 2002;99(10): 3735–41.

26. Zojer N, Konigsberg R, Ackermann J, et al. Deletion of 13q14 remains an independent adverse prognostic variable in multiple myeloma despite its frequent detection by interphase fluorescence in situ hybridization. Blood 2000;95(6): 1925–30.

27. Facon T, vet-Loiseau H, Guillerm G, et al. Chromosome 13 abnormalities identified by FISH analysis and serum beta2-microglobulin produce a powerful myeloma staging system for patients receiving high-dose therapy. Blood 2001;97(6):1566–71.

28. Walker BA, Leone PE, Chiecchio L, et al. A compendium of myeloma-associated chromosomal copy number abnormalities and their prognostic value. Blood 2010;116(15):e56–65.

29. Mikhael JR, Dingli D, Roy V, et al. Management of newly diagnosed symptomatic multiple myeloma: updated Mayo Stratification of Myeloma and Risk-Adapted Therapy (mSMART) consensus guidelines 2013. Mayo Clin Proc 2013;88(4): 360–76.

30. Shaughnessy JD, Zhou Y, Haessler J, et al. TP53 deletion is not an adverse feature in multiple myeloma treated with total therapy 3. Br J Haematol 2009; 147(3):347–51.

31. Chang H, Qi X, Jiang A, et al. 1p21 deletions are strongly associated with 1q21 gains and are an independent adverse prognostic factor for the outcome of high-dose chemotherapy in patients with multiple myeloma. Bone Marrow Transplant 2010;45(1):117–21.

32. Avet-Loiseau H, Li C, Magrangeas F, et al. Prognostic significance of copy-number alterations in multiple myeloma. J Clin Oncol 2009;27(27):4585–90.

33. Carrasco DR, Tonon G, Huang Y, et al. High-resolution genomic profiles define distinct clinico-pathogenetic subgroups of multiple myeloma patients. Cancer Cell 2006;9(4):313–25.

34. Chng WJ, Kumar S, Vanwier S, et al. Molecular dissection of hyperdiploid multiple myeloma by gene expression profiling. Cancer Res 2007;67(7):2982–9.
35. Kumar S, Fonseca R, Ketterling RP, et al. Trisomies in multiple myeloma: impact on survival in patients with high-risk cytogenetics. Blood 2012; 119(9):2100–5.
36. Broyl A, Hose D, Lokhorst H, et al. Gene expression profiling for molecular classification of multiple myeloma in newly diagnosed patients. Blood 2010;116(14): 2543–53.
37. Zhan F, Huang Y, Colla S, et al. The molecular classification of multiple myeloma. Blood 2006;108(6):2020–8.
38. Bergsagel PL, Kuehl WM, Zhan F, et al. Cyclin D dysregulation: an early and unifying pathogenic event in multiple myeloma. Blood 2005;106(1):296–303.
39. Shaughnessy JD Jr, Zhan F, Burington BE, et al. A validated gene expression model of high-risk multiple myeloma is defined by deregulated expression of genes mapping to chromosome 1. Blood 2007;109(6):2276–84.
40. Shaughnessy JD Jr, Qu P, Usmani S, et al. Pharmacogenomics of bortezomib test-dosing identifies hyperexpression of proteasome genes, especially PSMD4, as novel high-risk feature in myeloma treated with Total Therapy 3. Blood 2011;118(13):3512–24.
41. Kuiper R, Broyl A, de KY, et al. A gene expression signature for high-risk multiple myeloma. Leukemia 2012;26(11):2406–13.
42. Decaux O, Lode L, Magrangeas F, et al. Prediction of survival in multiple myeloma based on gene expression profiles reveals cell cycle and chromosomal instability signatures in high-risk patients and hyperdiploid signatures in low-risk patients: a study of the Intergroupe Francophone du Myelome. J Clin Oncol 2008;26(29):4798–805.
43. Dickens NJ, Walker BA, Leone PE, et al. Homozygous deletion mapping in myeloma samples identifies genes and an expression signature relevant to pathogenesis and outcome. Clin Cancer Res 2010;16(6):1856–64.
44. Larsen JT, Chee CE, Lust JA, et al. Reduction in plasma cell proliferation after initial therapy in newly diagnosed multiple myeloma measures treatment response and predicts improved survival. Blood 2011;118(10):2702–7.
45. Paiva B, Vidriales MB, Montalban MA, et al. Multiparameter flow cytometry evaluation of plasma cell DNA content and proliferation in 595 transplant-eligible patients with myeloma included in the Spanish GEM2000 and GEM2005<65y trials. Am J Pathol 2012;181(5):1870–8.
46. Alexandrakis MG, Passam FH, Kyriakou DS, et al. Ki-67 proliferation index: correlation with prognostic parameters and outcome in multiple myeloma. Am J Clin Oncol 2004;27(1):8–13.
47. Hose D, Reme T, Hielscher T, et al. Proliferation is a central independent prognostic factor and target for personalized and risk-adapted treatment in multiple myeloma. Haematologica 2011;96(1):87–95.
48. Barlogie B, Smallwood L, Smith T, et al. High serum levels of lactic dehydrogenase identify a high-grade lymphoma-like myeloma. Ann Intern Med 1989; 110(7):521–5.
49. Dimopoulos MA, Barlogie B, Smith TL, et al. High serum lactate dehydrogenase level as a marker for drug resistance and short survival in multiple myeloma. Ann Intern Med 1991;115(12):931–5.
50. Suguro M, Kanda Y, Yamamoto R, et al. High serum lactate dehydrogenase level predicts short survival after vincristine-doxorubicin-dexamethasone (VAD) salvage for refractory multiple myeloma. Am J Hematol 2000;65(2):132–5.

51. Anagnostopoulos A, Gika D, Symeonidis A, et al. Multiple myeloma in elderly patients: prognostic factors and outcome. Eur J Haematol 2005;75(5):370–5.
52. Terpos E, Katodritou E, Roussou M, et al. High serum lactate dehydrogenase adds prognostic value to the international myeloma staging system even in the era of novel agents. Eur J Haematol 2010;85(2):114–9.
53. Eleftherakis-Papapiakovou E, Kastritis E, Roussou M, et al. Renal impairment is not an independent adverse prognostic factor in patients with multiple myeloma treated upfront with novel agent-based regimens. Leuk Lymphoma 2011;52(12): 2299–303.
54. Pandey S, Kyle RA. Unusual myelomas: a review of IgD and IgE variants. Oncology (Williston Park) 2013;27(8):798–803.
55. Kim MK, Suh C, Lee DH, et al. Immunoglobulin D multiple myeloma: response to therapy, survival, and prognostic factors in 75 patients. Ann Oncol 2011;22(2): 411–6.
56. Usmani SZ, Heuck C, Mitchell A, et al. Extramedullary disease portends poor prognosis in multiple myeloma and is over-represented in high-risk disease even in the era of novel agents. Haematologica 2012;97(11):1761–7.
57. Blade J, de Larrea CF, Rosinol L. Extramedullary involvement in multiple myeloma. Haematologica 2012;97(11):1618–9.
58. Zamagni E, Patriarca F, Nanni C, et al. Prognostic relevance of 18-F FDG PET/CT in newly diagnosed multiple myeloma patients treated with up-front autologous transplantation. Blood 2011;118(23):5989–95.
59. Bartel TB, Haessler J, Brown TL, et al. F18-fluorodeoxyglucose positron emission tomography in the context of other imaging techniques and prognostic factors in multiple myeloma. Blood 2009;114(10):2068–76.
60. van de Donk NW, Lokhorst HM, Anderson KC, et al. How I treat plasma cell leukemia. Blood 2012;120(12):2376–89.
61. Walker R, Barlogie B, Haessler J, et al. Magnetic resonance imaging in multiple myeloma: diagnostic and clinical implications. J Clin Oncol 2007;25(9):1121–8.
62. Hillengass J, Ayyaz S, Kilk K, et al. Changes in magnetic resonance imaging before and after autologous stem cell transplantation correlate with response and survival in multiple myeloma. Haematologica 2012;97(11):1757–60.
63. Moulopoulos LA, Gika D, Anagnostopoulos A, et al. Prognostic significance of magnetic resonance imaging of bone marrow in previously untreated patients with multiple myeloma. Ann Oncol 2005;16(11):1824–8.
64. Usmani SZ, Mitchell A, Waheed S, et al. Prognostic implications of serial 18-fluoro-deoxyglucose emission tomography in multiple myeloma treated with total therapy 3. Blood 2013;121(10):1819–23.
65. Waheed S, Mitchell A, Usmani S, et al. Standard and novel imaging methods for multiple myeloma: correlates with prognostic laboratory variables including gene expression profiling data. Haematologica 2013;98(1):71–8.
66. Greipp PR, San MJ, Durie BG, et al. International staging system for multiple myeloma. J Clin Oncol 2005;23(15):3412–20.
67. Kastritis E, Zervas K, Symeonidis A, et al. Improved survival of patients with multiple myeloma after the introduction of novel agents and the applicability of the International Staging System (ISS): an analysis of the Greek Myeloma Study Group (GMSG). Leukemia 2009;23(6):1152–7.
68. Greipp PR, Leong T, Bennett JM, et al. Plasmablastic morphology–an independent prognostic factor with clinical and laboratory correlates: Eastern Cooperative Oncology Group (ECOG) myeloma trial E9486 report by the ECOG Myeloma Laboratory Group. Blood 1998;91(7):2501–7.

69. Bringhen S, Evangelista A, Offidani M, et al. A simple score, based on geriatric assessment, improves prediction of survival, and risk of serious adverse events in elderly newly diagnosed multiple myeloma patients. Blood 2013;122(21):687.

70. Palumbo A, Rajkumar SV, San Miguel JF, et al. International Myeloma Working Group Consensus statement for the management, treatment, and supportive care of patients with myeloma not eligible for standard autologous stem-cell transplantation. J Clin Oncol 2014;32(6):587–600.

71. Al-Hamadani M, Go RS. Long-term (10 years or more) survivors of multiple myeloma: a population-based analysis of the US National Cancer Data Base. Blood 2013;122(21):760.

72. Scheid C, Sonneveld P, Schmidt-Wolf IG, et al. Bortezomib before and after autologous stem cell transplantation overcomes the negative prognostic impact of renal impairment in newly diagnosed multiple myeloma: a Subgroup Analysis From the HOVON-65/GMMG-HD4 Trial. Haematologica 2014;99(1):148–54.

73. Roussou M, Kastritis E, Christoulas D, et al. Reversibility of renal failure in newly diagnosed patients with multiple myeloma and the role of novel agents. Leuk Res 2010;34(10):1395–7.

74. Dimopoulos MA, Roussou M, Gkotzamanidou M, et al. The role of novel agents on the reversibility of renal impairment in newly diagnosed symptomatic patients with multiple myeloma. Leukemia 2013;27(2):423–9.

75. Dimopoulos MA, Richardson PG, Schlag R, et al. VMP (bortezomib, melphalan, and prednisone) is active and well tolerated in newly diagnosed patients with multiple myeloma with moderately impaired renal function, and results in reversal of renal impairment: cohort analysis of the phase III VISTA study. J Clin Oncol 2009;27(36):6086–93.

76. Ludwig H, Adam Z, Hajek R, et al. Light chain-induced acute renal failure can be reversed by bortezomib-doxorubicin-dexamethasone in multiple myeloma: results of a phase II study. J Clin Oncol 2010;28(30):4635–41.

77. Dimopoulos M, Alegre A, Stadtmauer EA, et al. The efficacy and safety of lenalidomide plus dexamethasone in relapsed and/or refractory multiple myeloma patients with impaired renal function. Cancer 2010;116(16):3807–14.

78. Gay F, Larocca A, Wijermans P, et al. Complete response correlates with long-term progression-free and overall survival in elderly myeloma treated with novel agents: analysis of 1175 patients. Blood 2011;117(11):3025–31.

79. van de Velde HJ, Liu X, Chen G, et al. Complete response correlates with long-term survival and progression-free survival in high-dose therapy in multiple myeloma. Haematologica 2007;92(10):1399–406.

80. Hoering A, Crowley J, Shaughnessy JD Jr, et al. Complete remission in multiple myeloma examined as time-dependent variable in terms of both onset and duration in Total Therapy protocols. Blood 2009;114(7):1299–305.

81. Martinez-Lopez J, Blade J, Mateos MV, et al. Long-term prognostic significance of response in multiple myeloma after stem cell transplantation. Blood 2011;118(3):529–34.

82. Kumar S, Mahmood ST, Lacy MQ, et al. Impact of early relapse after auto-SCT for multiple myeloma. Bone Marrow Transplant 2008;42(6):413–20.

83. Paiva B, Gutierrez NC, Rosinol L, et al. High-risk cytogenetics and persistent minimal residual disease by multiparameter flow cytometry predict unsustained complete response after autologous stem cell transplantation in multiple myeloma. Blood 2012;119(3):687–91.

84. Rawstron AC, Child JA, de Tute RM, et al. Minimal residual disease assessed by multiparameter flow cytometry in multiple myeloma: impact on outcome in

the Medical Research Council Myeloma IX Study. J Clin Oncol 2013;31(20): 2540–7.

85. Paiva B, Martinez-Lopez J, Vidriales MB, et al. Comparison of immunofixation, serum free light chain, and immunophenotyping for response evaluation and prognostication in multiple myeloma. J Clin Oncol 2011;29(12):1627–33.

86. Ladetto M, Pagliano G, Ferrero S, et al. Major tumor shrinking and persistent molecular remissions after consolidation with bortezomib, thalidomide, and dexamethasone in patients with autografted myeloma. J Clin Oncol 2010; 28(12):2077–84.

87. Kröger N, Badbaran A, Zabelina T, et al. Impact of high-risk cytogenetics and achievement of molecular remission on long-term freedom from disease after autologous-allogeneic tandem transplantation in patients with multiple myeloma. Biol Blood Marrow Transplant 2013;19(3):398–404.

88. Durie BG, Salmon SE. A clinical staging system for multiple myeloma. Correlation of measured myeloma cell mass with presenting clinical features, response to treatment, and survival. Cancer 1975;36(3):842–54.

89. Munshi NC, Anderson KC, Bergsagel PL, et al. Consensus recommendations for risk stratification in multiple myeloma: report of the International Myeloma Workshop Consensus Panel 2. Blood 2011;117(18):4696–700.

90. Kapoor P, Fonseca R, Rajkumar SV, et al. Evidence for cytogenetic and fluorescence in situ hybridization risk stratification of newly diagnosed multiple myeloma in the era of novel therapies. Mayo Clin Proc 2010;85(6):532–7.

91. Salwender H, Rosiñol L, Moreau P, et al. Double vs single autologous stem cell transplantation after bortezomib-based induction regimens for multiple myeloma: an integrated analysis of patient-level data from Phase European III Studies. Blood 2013;122(21):767.

92. Fonseca R, Bergsagel PL, Drach J, et al. International Myeloma Working Group molecular classification of multiple myeloma: spotlight review. Leukemia 2009; 23(12):2210–21.

93. Ross FM, vet-Loiseau H, Ameye G, et al. Report from the European Myeloma Network on interphase FISH in multiple myeloma and related disorders. Haematologica 2012;97(8):1272–7.

94. Chng WJ, Dispenzieri A, Chim CS, et al. IMWG consensus on risk stratification in multiple myeloma. Leukemia 2014;28(2):269–77.

95. Wu P, Agnelli L, Walker BA, et al. Improved risk stratification in myeloma using a microRNA-based classifier. Br J Haematol 2013;162(3):348–59.

96. Corthals SL, Sun SM, Kuiper R, et al. MicroRNA signatures characterize multiple myeloma patients. Leukemia 2011;25(11):1784–9.

97. Bergsagel PL, Mateos MV, Gutierrez NC, et al. Improving overall survival and overcoming adverse prognosis in the treatment of cytogenetically high-risk multiple myeloma. Blood 2013;121(6):884–92.

98. Roos-Weil D, Moreau P, vet-Loiseau H, et al. Impact of genetic abnormalities after allogeneic stem cell transplantation in multiple myeloma: a report of the Societe Francaise de Greffe de Moelle et de Therapie Cellulaire. Haematologica 2011;96(10):1504–11.

99. van de Donk NW, Kamps S, Mutis T, et al. Monoclonal antibody-based therapy as a new treatment strategy in multiple myeloma. Leukemia 2012;26(2): 199–213.

100. van de Donk NW, Lokhorst HM. New developments in the management and treatment of newly diagnosed and relapsed/refractory multiple myeloma patients. Expert Opin Pharmacother 2013;14(12):1569–73.

101. Rajkumar SV, Gahrton G, Bergsagel PL. Approach to the treatment of multiple myeloma: a clash of philosophies. Blood 2011;118(12):3205–11.
102. Broyl A, Kuiper R, van DM, et al. High cereblon expression is associated with better survival in patients with newly diagnosed multiple myeloma treated with thalidomide maintenance. Blood 2013;121(4):624–7.
103. Schuster SR, Kortuem KM, Zhu YX, et al. The clinical significance of cereblon expression in multiple myeloma. Leuk Res 2014;38(1):23–8.
104. Mulligan G, Mitsiades C, Bryant B, et al. Gene expression profiling and correlation with outcome in clinical trials of the proteasome inhibitor bortezomib. Blood 2007;109(8):3177–88.
105. Shah JJ, Zonder J, Bensinger WI, et al. Prolonged survival and improved response rates with ARRY-520 in relapsed/refractory multiple myeloma (RRMM) patients with low α-1 acid glycoprotein (AAG) levels: results from a Phase 2 Study. Blood 2013;122(21):285.
106. Berdeja JG. Lorvotuzumab mertansine: antibody-drug-conjugate for CD56(+) multiple myeloma. Front Biosci (Landmark Ed) 2014;19:163–70.
107. Andrulis M, Lehners N, Capper D, et al. Targeting the BRAF V600E mutation in multiple myeloma. Cancer Discov 2013;3(8):862–9.
108. Gonen M, Redling K, Lendvai N, et al. Pilot study to evaluate the prevalence of actionable oncogenic mutations in patients with relapsed refractory multiple myeloma. Blood 2013;122(21):755.
109. Broyl A, Corthals SL, Jongen JL, et al. Mechanisms of peripheral neuropathy associated with bortezomib and vincristine in patients with newly diagnosed multiple myeloma: a prospective analysis of data from the HOVON-65/GMMG-HD4 trial. Lancet Oncol 2010;11(11):1057–65.
110. Sarasquete ME, Garcia-Sanz R, Marin L, et al. Bisphosphonate-related osteonecrosis of the jaw is associated with polymorphisms of the cytochrome P450 CYP2C8 in multiple myeloma: a genome-wide single nucleotide polymorphism analysis. Blood 2008;112(7):2709–12.
111. Johnson DC, Corthals S, Ramos C, et al. Genetic associations with thalidomide mediated venous thrombotic events in myeloma identified using targeted genotyping. Blood 2008;112(13):4924–34.
112. Kyle RA, Durie BG, Rajkumar SV, et al. Monoclonal gammopathy of undetermined significance (MGUS) and smoldering (asymptomatic) multiple myeloma: IMWG consensus perspectives risk factors for progression and guidelines for monitoring and management. Leukemia 2010;24(6):1121–7.
113. Kyle RA, Rajkumar SV. Criteria for diagnosis, staging, risk stratification and response assessment of multiple myeloma. Leukemia 2009;23(1):3–9.

Treatment of Transplant-Eligible Patients with Multiple Myeloma in 2014

 CrossMark

Heather Landau, MD[a,b], Sergio Giralt, MD[a,b],*

KEYWORDS

- Stem cell transplantation • Melphalan • Corticosteroids • Toxicity • Dexamethasone

KEY POINTS

- Induction regimens containing a proteasome inhibitor and/or immunomodulatory agent with dexamethasone result in rapid disease control before autologous stem cell transplantation (ASCT).
- ASCT followed by consolidation and/or maintenance further improves depth of response following effective induction.
- Overall survival of transplant-eligible patients has been extended with modern therapeutic strategies.
- The optimal timing of ASCT and methods to prevent relapse following ASCT are under active investigation.
- Different patient populations may benefit differentially from currently available treatments.

INTRODUCTION

High-dose melphalan therapy (HDT) with autologous stem cell transplant (ASCT) has been an integral component of myeloma therapy for close to 3 decades after McElwain and Powles demonstrated the clinical relevance of melphalan dose and disease response in patients with relapsed and refractory disease.[1] These results led to the exploration of HDT-ASCT as consolidation of initial remission in newly diagnosed multiple myeloma (MM). Compared with conventional chemotherapy, HDT and ASCT were associated with improved outcomes including event-free, progression-free (PFS), and overall survival (OS).[2–8] Depth of response, particularly achievement of a complete response (CR), was associated with longer PFS and OS in MM and was likely responsible for the initial success of HDT and SCT.[9]

Novel induction regimens incorporating proteasome inhibitors (bortezomib and carfilzomib) and the immunomodulatory drugs (IMIDs) (thalidomide and lenalidomide)

[a] Adult BMT Service, Memorial Sloan Kettering Cancer Center, 1275 York Avenue, New York, NY 10065, USA; [b] Weill Cornell Medical College, New York, NY 10065, USA
* Corresponding author. Adult BMT Service, Memorial Sloan Kettering Cancer Center, 1275 York Avenue, New York, NY 10065.
E-mail address: sagiralt@gmail.com

Hematol Oncol Clin N Am 28 (2014) 815–827
http://dx.doi.org/10.1016/j.hoc.2014.06.004
0889-8588/14/$ – see front matter © 2014 Elsevier Inc. All rights reserved.

have demonstrated very high CR rates that compare to those produced with HDT and ASCT.[10] Proteasome inhibitors and IMIDs have changed the context in which patients are receiving HDT and ASCT. Ongoing studies are investigating in transplant-eligible patients whether HDT is required early in the course of the disease or can be used as salvage therapy.[11,12] In patients who received alkylator-based induction, early ASCT was associated with better quality-of-life (QOL) parameters such as time without symptoms and therapy-related toxicity.[2] As myeloma therapy evolves to include post-ASCT consolidation and maintenance, it will be important to incorporate QOL measurements into the current studies. Herein the authors describe the treatment of newly diagnosed transplant-eligible MM patients based on currently available data and highlight important studies that will instruct us as the field continues to move forward.

DEFINING AN OPTIMAL INDUCTION REGIMEN

Response before SCT has been shown to improve outcomes, but the optimal type and duration of induction has not been well defined.[13] In responding patients, treatment with a fixed number of induction cycles or treatment until best response is the common strategy. Randomized trials comparing conventional chemotherapy with a regimen that contains thalidomide, lenalidomide, and/or bortezomib along with corticosteroids have established that induction with an IMID, proteasome inhibitor, or both is the standard of care.[14-17] Deeper and quicker responses are typically achieved with 3-drug regimens such as thalidomide-bortezomib-dexamethasone, cyclophosphamide-bortezomib-dexamethasone, bortezomib-adriamycin-dexamethasone, or lenalidomide-bortezomib-dexamethasone versus 2-drug regimens, thalidomide-dexamethasone, lenalidomide-dexamethasone, or bortezomib-dexamethasone (VD), although the impact on OS has not been established (**Table 1**).[15-21] Attempts to increase to a 4-drug regimen are associated with increased toxicity and no clear advantage over 3-drug regimens.[22]

Notably few randomized studies comparing modern induction regimens have been performed to date; and lenalidomide-based combinations have not been compared with either bortezomib- or thalidomide-based combinations. A trial of VD versus reduced-dose bortezomib-thalidomide-dexamethasone (VTD) as induction pre-SCT conducted by the Intergroupe Francophone du Myelome (IFM) did not suggest a benefit of the 3-drug combination over the 2-drug combination in terms of the frequency of CR after 4 cycles (13% and 12%, $P = .74$), which was their primary end point.[23] However, higher very good partial response (VGPR) rates were noted with VTD compared with VD both before (49% vs 36%, $P = .05$) and after SCT (74% vs 58%, $P = .02$). In addition,

Table 1				
Response and toxicity to selected induction regimens				
Reference	Regimen	[a]ORR (%)	[a]CR (%)	Common Toxicities
15	VD	79	15	PN, GI toxicity, low PLTs
16	TD	79	11	Constipation, sedation, PN
21	[b]Ld	70	4	VTE, neutropenia
16	VTD	93	31	PN, GI toxicity, infection
19	RVD	74	6	PN, myelosuppression
18	VCD	96	46	Myelosuppression

Abbreviations: GI, gastrointestinal; PLT, platelet; PN, peripheral neuropathy; VTE, venous thromboembolism.

[a] Response rates following 4 cycles (unless otherwise indicated).
[b] Best response.

lower doses of bortezomib and thalidomide in the 3-drug combination translated into less grade 2 or higher neuropathy compared with the 2-drug regimen (14% and 34%, $P = .001$). A randomized phase II study examined the efficacy and tolerability of bortezomib-dexamethasone combined with lenalidomide (VDR) or cyclophosphamide (VDC) as well as the 4-drug regimen bortezomib-dexamethasone-cyclophosphamide-lenalidomide (VDCR).[22] After an interim analysis, VDC was modified (VDC-mod) to include 3 rather than 2 doses of cyclophosphamide based on results from a phase II trial investigating the same regimen.[24] After 4 cycles, 33%, 32%, and 41% of patients receiving VDCR, VDR, or VDC-mod achieved VGPR or better, respectively. VDCR was associated with more toxicity leading the investigators to conclude that the VDR and VDC-mod regimens should be evaluated further.[22] Ongoing randomized studies include the large randomized Southwest Oncology Group trial of lenalidomide and dexamethasone with or without bortezomib as initial therapy for untreated MM patients.[25] The results of this trial will be instructive with respect to rate and depth of response as well as safety profiles. Indeed lenalidomide-dexamethasone has the benefit of being an oral regimen and is well tolerated.[21]

Newer combinations include MLN-9708 (ixazomib), an oral proteasome inhibitor in combination with lenalidomide-dexamethasone, which is an entirely oral 3-drug regimen.[26] Preliminary data were presented at the American Society of Hematology meeting in December 2013 and suggested promising activity in 64 previously untreated patients with an overall response rate of 93%, including 67% with at least a VGPR. On this study, SCT-eligible patients underwent stem cell collection after 4 cycles of induction without difficulty (Paul G. Richardson, unpublished data, 2013). Carfilzomib, a second generation proteasome inhibitor, has also been combined with lenalidomide-dexamethasone (CRD), and in 53 newly diagnosed patients with MM, 38% achieved at least a near CR (nCR) after 4 cycles.[27] Stem cells were successfully collected in 34 of 35 patients but only 7 patients chose to undergo SCT after initial induction. The favorable toxicity profile of CRD, particularly the lack of neuropathy, allowed prolonged administration with deeper responses over time. However, carfilzomib is administered intravenously on days 1, 2, 8, 9, 15, and 16, which can be burdensome to patients.

Most but not all studies indicate that achieving CR is a surrogate for OS, although a patient's risk category is likely to play a role.[28,29] Patients with low-risk disease may not require CR for prolonged survival, whereas the goal for patients with high-risk disease is not only to achieve but sustain a CR.[30–33] With the exception of using bortezomib-based treatment of patients with the t (4;14) abnormality, there is not sufficient data to support using specific therapy for patients in different risk groups.[33] As molecular techniques evolve, the goal is to individualize therapy based on predictive markers that provide insight into the likelihood of response and/or toxicity to certain drugs or regimens.

ROLE OF HDT AND SCT

Based on superior outcomes when compared to conventional alkylator-based therapy, HDT and ASCT has become the standard approach to maximize response following an initial response to induction therapy.[2–8] The unprecedented responses to initial therapy with IMIDs and proteasome inhibitors, especially in combination, have called into question the role of HDT and SCT in MM. Yet, even in the context of modern induction regimens where more than 90% respond, the quality of response continues to improve following HDT and PFS approaches or exceeds 3 years.[15,16] Palumbo and colleagues[34] have presented the preliminary results of a prospective phase III trial that randomized 402 patients to consolidation with oral melphalan-prednisone-lenalidomide (MPR) versus HDT after 4 cycles of induction with lenalidomide-dexamethasone (LD). With relatively short follow-up of 26 months, there is a significant PFS benefit for patients randomized to transplant compared with those who received MPR with 73% versus 54% (HR 0.506, P = .0002) PFS at 2 years, but no difference in OS. Similarly, following 4 cycles of LD induction, 195 patients randomized to HDT and SCT had longer PFS compared with 194 patients randomized to consolidation with cyclophosphamide-lenalidomide-dexamethasone (CRD) with respective 3 years PFS 60% versus 38% (HR 0.62, P = .003).[35] After median follow-up of 31 months, there was no difference in OS. In contrast, among 53 newly diagnosed MM patients who received lenalidomide-bortezomib-dexamethasone (RVD) as initial therapy and had not progressed, a post-hoc landmark analysis at 1 year following treatment initiation showed no difference in PFS according to whether or not patients chose to pursue HDT and SCT (P = .38) after at least 4 cycles of induction.[19] The retrospective nature of the latter experience does not allow for conclusions to be drawn but has led to the Intergroup Francophone du Myeloma-Dana-Farber Cancer Institute (IFM-DFCI) study of RVD with or without HDT and SCT.[36]

Two studies have suggested that 2 courses of high-dose melphalan are superior to a single SCT, but the benefit appears to be limited to patients who had not achieved VGPR after the first transplant.[37,38] Neither of these studies included induction therapies with either an IMID or proteasome inhibitor and therefore, may not be relevant today. More recently, patients who received bortezomib-based induction therapy and either single or double SCT on European phase III trials were analyzed. In comparison with patients for whom a single SCT was planned by study design, those who were assigned to receive tandem SCT had significantly longer PFS (median: 38 vs 50 months, P<.001) and OS (5-year estimates: 63% vs 75%, P = .002).[29] From this dataset, the benefit of tandem ASCT was greatest for patients with high-risk cytogenetics defined as t (4;14) and/or del 17p and also for those who had not attained CR following bortezomib-based induction. These data need to be confirmed by prospective, randomized phase III studies that are currently ongoing.[39]

Fermand and colleagues[2] reported in 1998 that patients who receive ASCT as consolidation of initial remission have similar survival to those who were assigned to transplant at the time of relapse. However, early ASCT was associated with more time without symptoms, less therapy-related toxicity, and better QOL parameters, favoring this approach. With more effective induction therapies that are relatively well tolerated, many patients and physicians have deferred HDT with ASCT.[21,27,40] A landmark analysis of the E4A03 trial that compared lenalidomide-low-dose dexamethasone with lenalidomide-high-dose dexamethasone included patients who completed 4 cycles of induction therapy. Patients who elected to receive HDT at that time (N = 90) had an estimated 3-year OS of 92% versus 79% for those who continued on primary therapy (N = 248).[21] In an attempt to abrogate the selection bias inherent in this comparison, Siegel and colleagues[40] analyzed the data according to age and found that early ASCT was associated with better outcomes in all age groups. The Mayo group recently published their experience on 290 newly diagnosed patients with MM who received induction therapy with either thalidomide-dexamethasone or lenalidomide-dexamethasone and had stem cells collected.[41] One hundred seventy-eight patients who underwent HDT and ASCT within 12 months of diagnosis made up the early ASCT group; their outcomes including response rates, time to progression (TTP), and OS were no different than the outcomes of the 112 patients who made up the delayed ASCT group. However, the retrospective nature of these data and lack of QOL measurements, again limit the utility of these findings.

Indeed the results from the Intergroup Francophone du Myeloma-Dana-Farber Cancer Institute (IFM-DFCI) study of RVD with or without HDT and ASCT as well as others using lenalidomide-dexamethasone as induction followed by early versus delayed ASCT are eagerly awaited.[36,42,43]

Although the timing of HDT and ASCT remains an area of active debate and investigation, patients who are eligible and responding to initial therapy should have stem cells mobilized and collected after 3 to 6 cycles of therapy. Prolonged therapy, especially with lenalidomide increases the risk of insufficient collection.[44] Age also appears to be a strong predictor of inadequate collection, but age in and of itself does not define eligibility for transplant that is more dependent on comorbidities and performance status. Although phase III trials restricted enrollment to patients aged less than 65 years, retrospective studies suggest that selected patients even in the 8th decade of life may benefit from ASCT with a similarly low risk of treatment toxicity and equivalent remission rates and PFS as seen in younger patients.[45–49]

PREVENTING RELAPSE

Despite effective induction and HDT, myeloma recurrence occurs almost universally in patients who do not receive post-transplantation therapy. A defined course of often intensive treatment designed to maximize the depth of response after SCT is considered "consolidation" therapy, whereas "maintenance" typically includes a planned treatment that should be effective, well-tolerated with manageable toxicities, simple to administer, and can be given for an extended period of time. Both strategies have been used to improve outcomes after a single or tandem ASCT and in general deepen responses with variable effect on time-to-event data.

The benefits of consolidation were reported by Ladetto and colleagues[50] who showed that 4 cycles of VTD consolidation following tandem ASCT in patients with MM who achieved at least a VGPR (N = 39) increased the frequency of CR from 15% to 49% and molecular remissions from 3% to 18%. Phase III data included 480 newly diagnosed MM patients who received induction with VTD or TD, that was followed by tandem ASCT and 2 cycles of VTD or TD consolidation according to the induction arm.[51] Although CR rates were not statistically different in the VTD versus TD arms following HDT, the CR rate was 61% after VTD and 47% after TD consolidation (P = .012). To date, PFS but not OS is longer in the VTD arm. A retrospective study examined the outcomes of newly diagnosed MM patients who received either VTD followed by single SCT (N = 96) or the same induction, a single ASCT, and 2 cycles of VTD consolidation (N = 121).[52] Similar to the phase III trial, an increased proportion of patients who received VTD consolidation achieved CR (52% vs 30%, P = .001); longer TTP (estimated 4-year TTP 62% vs 29%, P = .005) was also evident in patients receiving consolidation. The Nordic Myeloma Study Group randomized 370 bortezomib-naïve patients to 20 weekly doses of bortezomib or no consolidation at 3 months post-transplantation.[53] Again, response rates improved in patients who received consolidation with 71% versus 57% (P<.01) achieving at least VGPR and PFS was extended (27 vs 20 months, P = .05), but the advantage was only seen in patients with less VGPR rates after ASCT. There was no difference in OS between the groups.

Several studies have examined the role of different types of maintenance including interferon-α, glucocorticoids, and low-dose melphalan to improve response and outcome.[54] However, these agents had limited efficacy and tolerability. Thalidomide maintenance after HDT and ASCT improved the quality of response and increased PFS in 6 studies and OS in 3 of them.[55] However, thalidomide maintenance has been limited by toxicity, namely neuropathy and fatigue, which have made it difficult for physicians and patients to adopt. Lenalidomide has a more favorable side-effect profile and was a logical candidate drug to study as posttransplantation maintenance therapy. Two phase III trials examining the role of lenalidomide maintenance following SCT in newly diagnosed MM patients have been performed and reported.[56,57] The CALGB 100104 study examined 462 MM patients who were randomized to lenalidomide or placebo without consolidation until disease progression.[56] A significant increase in TTP was seen for patients in the lenalidomide arm compared with those receiving placebo (46 vs 27 months, $P<.0001$). With a median follow-up of 34 months, 3-year OS was 88% for patients receiving lenalidomide and 80% for those receiving placebo ($P = .028$). All patients benefitted from lenalidomide maintenance regardless of remission status or prior exposure to IMID therapy; there was evidence that induction therapy with lenalidomide was associated with improved OS in the group that received lenalidomide maintenance ($P = .03$). An updated analysis was performed at 48 months of follow-up and shows that despite cross-over of 71% of placebo patients, the risk of death on lenalidomide maintenance (20%) is lower than on placebo (30%) (hazard ratio [HR] 0.61, $P = .008$).[58] The IFM 2005-02 trial reported on 614 patients who were randomized to lenalidomide or placebo after single (79%) or tandem (21%) and 2 cycles of lenalidomide consolidation (25 mg $\times$ 21 days).[57] Similar to the CALGB study, lenalidomide improved median PFS (41 months vs 23 months) compared with placebo (HR 0.50, $P<.001$). However, the 5-year post-randomization OS is similar (68% vs 67%, HR 1) due to a shorter median OS after the first progression in the lenalidomide group (29 months) versus those who received placebo (48 months) ($P<.0001$).[59] In both studies a higher incidence of secondary primary malignancies (SPMs) in the lenalidomide arm was detected (**Table 2**). Yet analysis of CALGB 100104 showed that despite a higher cumulative incidence risk (CIR) of developing a second primary malignancy (SPM) in the lenalidomide arm ($P = .03$), the CIR of progression ($P = .001$) or death ($P = .002$) is higher for placebo.[58] One major difference between the CALGB study and the IFM study is that maintenance lenalidomide was continued in the US study, whereas it was stopped at a median of 2 years due to concerns regarding SPM.[59] The benefit of prolonged lenalidomide maintenance on PFS and more recently OS has been shown by the Italian group in both transplant-eligible and transplant-ineligible patients.[60,61]

Bortezomib maintenance has also recently been shown to reduce the risk of death after ASCT.[62] Sonneveld and colleagues[17] reported the outcomes of the HOVON-65/GMMG-HD4 including 827 patients randomized to receive bortezomib during induction in combination with doxorubicin and dexamethasone (PAD), followed by post-ASCT bortezomib every other week for 2 years or thalidomide during induction and posttransplantation and showed superior PFS and OS for the

Table 2 Lenalidomide maintenance (vs placebo) following ASCT		
	CALGB 100104[56,58]	IFM 2005-02[57,59]
N	460	614
Initial dosing	10 mg (5–15 mg)	10 mg (5–15 mg)
Duration	Until progression	24 mos
TTP/PFS	TTP: 46 vs 27 mos ($P<.001$)	PFS: 41 vs 23 mos ($P<.001$)
OS	3 y OS: 88% vs 80% ($P = .028$)	5 y OS: 68% vs 67%
SPM total	18 vs 6 cases	23 vs 8 cases
Hematologic malignancy	8 vs 1	13 vs 4
Solid tumors	10 vs 5	10 vs 4

bortezomib-based therapy. Whether the presence of bortezomib in induction or maintenance therapy had the greatest effect on PFS and OS cannot be discerned from that study. A landmark analysis from the start of maintenance shows that the OS was superior for the PAD arm (HR 0.71, $P = .035$), despite no difference in PFS, which is difficult to interpret.[62] There was no increase in the incidence of SPM in patients who received bortezomib.

The role of allogeneic SCT remains controversial due to high treatment-related mortality and the risk of graft versus host disease even with nonmyeloablative regimens. The European Group for Blood and Marrow Transplantation Non-Myeloablative Allogeneic stem cell transplantation in MM 2000 study compared tandem ASCT and reduced intensity conditioning (RIC) allogeneic transplantation to ASCT (single or tandem optional) alone in 357 patients who were biologically randomized based on the availability of an Human Leukocyte Antigen (HLA)-identical sibling. At a median of 96 months of follow-up, PFS and OS were 22% and 49% versus 12% ($P = .027$) and 36% ($P = .030$) with ASCT/RIC allogeneic SCT and ASCT, respectively.[63] The largest study including 625 patients performed through the Blood and Marrow Clinical Trials Network biologically assigned patients to tandem ASCT or RIC allogeneic and showed that at 36 months of follow-up there was no difference in PFS or OS.[64] In an exploratory analysis of high-risk patients (defined by B2-microglobulin >4 mg/L or deletion chromosome 13 by metaphase cytogenetics), there was a trend toward favorable OS that may or may not be appreciated with longer follow-up. Two other prospective studies, from the HOVON and Italian Study groups, with somewhat different trial designs have failed to conclusively show a benefit for allogeneic SCT in the upfront treatment of MM despite some suggestion of a better outcome with RIC allogeneic SCT in the Italian study.[65,66] However, the tandem ASCT arm of that study has a curiously short survival (median 48 months). Recent registry data assessing the role of allogeneic SCT in more than 1200 patients with MM reported 5-year PFS and OS of 14% and 29%, respectively with older age, longer interval from diagnosis to transplantation, and unrelated donor grafts adversely affecting OS.[67] Therefore, allogeneic SCT as part of frontline therapy for MM remains experimental but should continue to be explored in the context of clinical trials for young patients, with International Staging System (ISS) II and III disease associated with t (4;14) or del 17p in whom median OS is only 2 years (**Table 3**).[33]

SUMMARY AND FUTURE DIRECTIONS

- The best available strategy to achieve high CR rates and prolong PFS seems to be induction with 3-drug bortezomib-based combinations followed by autologous SCT with bortezomib or IMID-based consolidation and lenalidomide maintenance.

Table 3
Risk stratification in MM and OS

	High-Risk	Standard-Risk	Low-Risk
	ISS II/III and t (4;14) or del 17p	Others	Age <55, ISS I/II and absence of t (4;14), del 17p or gain 1q21
Frequency	20%	60%	20%
Median OS	2 y	7 y	>10 y

Adapted from Chng WJ, Dispenzieri A, Chim CS, et al. IMWG consensus on risk stratification in multiple myeloma. Leukemia 2014;28(2):273.

- However, the best timing of ASCT in the era of effective therapies represents an area of active debate and major interest.
- Until the final results of ongoing clinical trials comparing early versus late ASCT plus novel agents become available, ASCT up-front should be considered the preferred approach for patients who are transplant eligible.
- RCTs evaluating 2- versus 3-drug induction regimens are ongoing; based on currently available data the authors favor bortezomib-based triple drug induction for most ASCT-eligible patients especially those who require a rapid response (symptomatic bone disease or renal failure) but consider lenalidomide and dexamethasone for patients with low-risk, clinically asymptomatic disease who prefer oral therapy.
- Whether a second transplant versus consolidation or maintenance therapy alone will be most effective to prevent relapse remains unknown but is being addressed.
- In most patients, the authors are offering lenalidomide maintenance while educating patients about the risk of SPM, which has to be considered in the context of the risk of progression and death due to MM.

Despite the improvement in outcomes with effective new therapies, nearly all patients relapse as the result of clonal heterogeneity and genomic instability causing the selection of more aggressive subclones responsible for drug resistance and death from disease.[68] Drug resistance may be different in different risk groups that to date have largely been defined by cytogenetics and gene-expression profiling; but resistance is also influenced by the bone marrow microenvironment.[33,69,70] Minimal residual disease (MRD) is being studied by a variety of methods and may be informative to not only understand how depth of response influences outcomes but also to better characterize residual disease. A better understanding of immune regulation throughout a course of treatment and particularly in the MRD setting may be of particular value to optimize immune-based regimens, which are currently being studied. Ongoing participation in well-designed clinical trials is essential to tease out how to minimize toxicity from therapy and develop "risk-stratified" treatment approaches.

REFERENCES

1. McElwain TJ, Powles RL. High-dose intravenous melphalan for plasma-cell leukaemia and myeloma. Lancet 1983;2(8354):822–4.
2. Fermand JP, Ravaud P, Chevret S, et al. High-dose therapy and autologous peripheral blood stem cell transplantation in multiple myeloma: up-front or rescue treatment? Results of a multicenter sequential randomized clinical trial. Blood 1998;92(9):3131–6.
3. Child JA, Morgan GJ, Davies FE, et al. High-dose chemotherapy with hematopoietic stem-cell rescue for multiple myeloma. N Engl J Med 2003;348(19):1875–83.
4. Blade J, et al. High-dose therapy intensification compared with continued standard chemotherapy in multiple myeloma patients responding to the initial chemotherapy: long-term results from a prospective randomized trial from the Spanish cooperative group PETHEMA. Blood 2005;106(12):3755–9.
5. Fermand JP, Katsahian S, Divine M, et al. High-dose therapy and autologous blood stem-cell transplantation compared with conventional treatment in myeloma patients aged 55 to 65 years: long-term results of a randomized control trial from the Group Myelome-Autogreffe. J Clin Oncol 2005;23(36):9227–33.

6. Attal M, Harousseau JL, Stoppa AM, et al. A prospective, randomized trial of autologous bone marrow transplantation and chemotherapy in multiple myeloma. Intergroupe Francais du Myelome. N Engl J Med 1996;335(2):91–7.
7. Barlogie B, Jagannath S, Vesole DH, et al. Superiority of tandem autologous transplantation over standard therapy for previously untreated multiple myeloma. Blood 1997;89(3):789–93.
8. Lenhoff S, Hjorth M, Holmberg E, et al. Impact on survival of high-dose therapy with autologous stem cell support in patients younger than 60 years with newly diagnosed multiple myeloma: a population-based study. Nordic Myeloma Study Group. Blood 2000;95(1):7–11.
9. Alexanian R, Weber D, Giralt S, et al. Impact of complete remission with intensive therapy in patients with responsive multiple myeloma. Bone Marrow Transplant 2001;27(10):1037–43.
10. Richardson PG, Mitsiades C, Schlossman R, et al. New drugs for myeloma. Oncologist 2007;12(6):664–89.
11. Randomized trial of lenalidomide, bortezomib and dexamethasone vs high-dose treatment with SCT in MM patients up to age 65 (DFCI 10-106) (IFM DFCI 2009). Available at: http://clinicaltrials.gov/show/NCT01208662. Accessed July 17, 2014.
12. Study to compare VMP with HDM followed by VRD consolidation and lenalidomide maintenance in newly diagnosed multiple myeloma (EMN 2) (H095). Available at: http://clinicaltrials.gov/show/NCT01208766. Accessed July 17, 2014.
13. Alvares CL, Davies FE, Horton C, et al. Long-term outcomes of previously untreated myeloma patients: responses to induction chemotherapy and high-dose melphalan incorporated within a risk stratification model can help to direct the use of novel treatments. Br J Haematol 2005;129(5):607–14.
14. Lokhorst HM, van der Holt B, Zweegman S, et al. A randomized phase 3 study on the effect of thalidomide combined with adriamycin, dexamethasone, and high-dose melphalan, followed by thalidomide maintenance in patients with multiple myeloma. Blood 2010;115(6):1113–20.
15. Harousseau JL, Attal M, Avet-Loiseau H, et al. Bortezomib plus dexamethasone is superior to vincristine plus doxorubicin plus dexamethasone as induction treatment prior to autologous stem-cell transplantation in newly diagnosed multiple myeloma: results of the IFM 2005-01 phase III trial. J Clin Oncol 2010; 28(30):4621–9.
16. Cavo M, Tacchetti P, Patriarca F, et al. Bortezomib with thalidomide plus dexamethasone compared with thalidomide plus dexamethasone as induction therapy before, and consolidation therapy after, double autologous stem-cell transplantation in newly diagnosed multiple myeloma: a randomised phase 3 study. Lancet 2010;376(9758):2075–85.
17. Sonneveld P, Schmidt-Wolf IG, van der Holt B, et al. Bortezomib induction and maintenance treatment in patients with newly diagnosed multiple myeloma: results of the randomized phase III HOVON-65/GMMG-HD4 trial. J Clin Oncol 2012;30(24):2946–55.
18. Reeder CB, Reece DE, Kukreti V, et al. Once- versus twice-weekly bortezomib induction therapy with CyBorD in newly diagnosed multiple myeloma. Blood 2010;115(16):3416–7.
19. Richardson PG, Weller E, Lonial S, et al. Lenalidomide, bortezomib, and dexamethasone combination therapy in patients with newly diagnosed multiple myeloma. Blood 2010;116(5):679–86.

20. Rajkumar SV, Rosinol L, Hussein M, et al. Multicenter, randomized, double-blind, placebo-controlled study of thalidomide plus dexamethasone compared with dexamethasone as initial therapy for newly diagnosed multiple myeloma. J Clin Oncol 2008;26(13):2171–7.

21. Rajkumar SV, Jacobus S, Callander NS, et al. Lenalidomide plus high-dose dexamethasone versus lenalidomide plus low-dose dexamethasone as initial therapy for newly diagnosed multiple myeloma: an open-label randomised controlled trial. Lancet Oncol 2010;11(1):29–37.

22. Kumar S, Flinn I, Richardson PG, et al. Randomized, multicenter, phase 2 study (EVOLUTION) of combinations of bortezomib, dexamethasone, cyclophosphamide, and lenalidomide in previously untreated multiple myeloma. Blood 2012;119(19):4375–82.

23. Moreau P, Avet-Loiseau H, Facon T, et al. Bortezomib plus dexamethasone versus reduced-dose bortezomib, thalidomide plus dexamethasone as induction treatment before autologous stem cell transplantation in newly diagnosed multiple myeloma. Blood 2011;118(22):5752–8 [quiz: 5982].

24. Reeder CB, Reece DE, Kukreti V, et al. Cyclophosphamide, bortezomib and dexamethasone induction for newly diagnosed multiple myeloma: high response rates in a phase II clinical trial. Leukemia 2009;23(7):1337–41.

25. Lenalidomide and dexamethasone with or without bortezomib in treating patients with previously untreated multiple myeloma.

26. Hofmeister CC, Rosenbaum CA, Htut M, et al. Twice-weekly oral MLN9708 (Ixazomib Citrate), an investigational proteasome inhibitor, in combination with lenalidomide (Len) and dexamethasone (Dex) in patients (Pts) with newly diagnosed multiple myeloma (MM): final phase 1 results and phase 2 data. Blood 2013;122(21):535.

27. Jakubowiak AJ, Dytfeld D, Griffith KA, et al. A phase 1/2 study of carfilzomib in combination with lenalidomide and low-dose dexamethasone as a frontline treatment for multiple myeloma. Blood 2012;120(9):1801–9.

28. Lahuerta JJ, Mateos MV, Martinez-Lopez J, et al. Influence of pre- and post-transplantation responses on outcome of patients with multiple myeloma: sequential improvement of response and achievement of complete response are associated with longer survival. J Clin Oncol 2008;26(35):5775–82.

29. Salwender H, Rosiñol L, Moreau P, et al. Double vs single autologous stem cell transplantation after bortezomib-based induction regimens for multiple myeloma: an integrated analysis of patient-level data from phase European III studies. Blood 2013;122(21):767.

30. Haessler J, Shaughnessy JD Jr, Zhan F, et al. Benefit of complete response in multiple myeloma limited to high-risk subgroup identified by gene expression profiling. Clin Cancer Res 2007;13(23):7073–9.

31. Hoering A, Crowley J, Shaughnessy JD Jr, et al. Complete remission in multiple myeloma examined as time-dependent variable in terms of both onset and duration in total therapy protocols. Blood 2009;114(7):1299–305.

32. Barlogie B, Anaissie E, Haessler J, et al. Complete remission sustained 3 years from treatment initiation is a powerful surrogate for extended survival in multiple myeloma. Cancer 2008;113(2):355–9.

33. Chng WJ, Dispenzieri A, Chim CS, et al. IMWG consensus on risk stratification in multiple myeloma. Leukemia 2014;28(2):269–77.

34. Palumbo A, Cavallo F, Hardan I, et al. Melphalan/Prednisone/Lenalidomide (MPR) versus high-dose melphalan and autologous transplantation (MEL200)

in newly diagnosed multiple myeloma (MM) patients <65 years: results of a randomized phase III study. Blood 2011;118(21):3069.

35. Gay F, Spencer A, Di Raimondo F, et al. A phase III study of ASCT vs cyclophosphamide-lenalidomide-dexamethasone and lenalidomide-prednisone maintenance vs lenalidomide alone in newly diagnosed myeloma patients. Blood 2013;122(21):763.

36. Randomized trial of lenalidomide, bortezomib, dexamethasone vs high-dose treatment with SCT in MM patients up to age 65 (DFCI 10-106). Available at: http://clinicaltrials.gov/show/NCT01208662. Accessed July 17, 2014.

37. Attal M, Harousseau JL, Facon T, et al. Single versus double autologous stem-cell transplantation for multiple myeloma. N Engl J Med 2003;349(26): 2495–502.

38. Cavo M, Tosi P, Zamagni E, et al. Prospective, randomized study of single compared with double autologous stem-cell transplantation for multiple myeloma: Bologna 96 clinical study. J Clin Oncol 2007;25(17):2434–41.

39. A trial of single autologous transplant with or without consolidation therapy versus tandem autologous transplant with lenalidomide maintenance for patients with multiplemyeloma (BMT CTN 0702). Available at: http://clinicaltrials.gov/show/NCT01109004. Accessed July 17, 2014.

40. Siegel DS, Jacobus S, Rajkumar SV, et al. Outcome with lenalidomide plus dexamethasone followed by early autologous stem cell transplantation in the ECOG E4A03 randomized clinical trial. Blood 2010;116(21):38.

41. Kumar SK, Lacy MQ, Dispenzieri A, et al. Early versus delayed autologous transplantation after immunomodulatory agents-based induction therapy in patients with newly diagnosed multiple myeloma. Cancer 2012;118(6):1585–92.

42. Lenalidomide and dexamethasone with/without stem cell transplant in patients with multiple myeloma. Available at: http://clinicaltrials.gov/show/NCT01731 886. Accessed July 17, 2014.

43. Lenalidomide (Revlimid) plus low-dose dexamethasone (ld × 4 cycles) then stem cell collection followed by randomization to continued Ld or stem cell transplantation (SCT) plus maintenance L. Available at: http://clinicaltrials.gov/show/NCT00807599. Accessed July 17, 2014.

44. Kumar S, Giralt S, Stadtmauer EA, et al. Mobilization in myeloma revisited: IMWG consensus perspectives on stem cell collection following initial therapy with thalidomide-, lenalidomide-, or bortezomib-containing regimens. Blood 2009;114(9):1729–35.

45. Qazilbash MH, Saliba RM, Hosing C, et al. Autologous stem cell transplantation is safe and feasible in elderly patients with multiple myeloma. Bone Marrow Transplant 2007;39(5):279–83.

46. O'Shea D, Giles C, Terpos E, et al. Predictive factors for survival in myeloma patients who undergo autologous stem cell transplantation: a single-centre experience in 211 patients. Bone Marrow Transplant 2006;37(8):731–7.

47. Kumar SK, Dingli D, Lacy MQ, et al. Autologous stem cell transplantation in patients of 70 years and older with multiple myeloma: Results from a matched pair analysis. Am J Hematol 2008;83(8):614–7.

48. El Cheikh J, Kfoury E, Calmels B, et al. Age at transplantation and outcome after autologous stem cell transplantation in elderly patients with multiple myeloma. Hematol Oncol Stem Cell Ther 2011;4(1):30–6.

49. Bashir Q, Shah N, Parmar S, et al. Feasibility of autologous hematopoietic stem cell transplant in patients aged >/=70 years with multiple myeloma. Leuk Lymphoma 2012;53(1):118–22.

50. Ladetto M, Pagliano G, Ferrero S, et al. Major tumor shrinking and persistent molecular remissions after consolidation with bortezomib, thalidomide, and dexamethasone in patients with autografted myeloma. J Clin Oncol 2010; 28(12):2077–84.

51. Cavo M, Pantani L, Petrucci MT, et al. Bortezomib-thalidomide-dexamethasone is superior to thalidomide-dexamethasone as consolidation therapy after autologous hematopoietic stem cell transplantation in patients with newly diagnosed multiple myeloma. Blood 2012;120(1):9–19.

52. Leleu X, Fouquet G, Hebraud B, et al. Consolidation with VTd significantly improves the complete remission rate and time to progression following VTd induction and single autologous stem cell transplantation in multiple myeloma. Leukemia 2013;27(11):2242–4.

53. Mellqvist UH, Gimsing P, Hjertner O, et al. Bortezomib consolidation after autologous stem cell transplantation in multiple myeloma: a Nordic Myeloma Study Group randomized phase 3 trial. Blood 2013;121(23):4647–54.

54. McCarthy PL. Part I: the role of maintenance therapy in patients with multiple myeloma undergoing autologous hematopoietic stem cell transplantation. J Natl Compr Canc Netw 2013;11(1):35–42.

55. Ludwig H, Durie BG, McCarthy P, et al. IMWG consensus on maintenance therapy in multiple myeloma. Blood 2012;119(13):3003–15.

56. McCarthy PL, Owzar K, Hofmeister CC, et al. Lenalidomide after stem-cell transplantation for multiple myeloma. N Engl J Med 2012;366(19):1770–81.

57. Attal M, Lauwers-Cances V, Marit G, et al. Lenalidomide maintenance after stem-cell transplantation for multiple myeloma. N Engl J Med 2012;366(19): 1782–91.

58. Shimizu K. Overview of the international myeloma workshop 2013 kyoto. Clin Lymphoma Myeloma Leuk 2014;14(1):2–4.

59. Lauwers-Cances V, Marit G, Caillot D, et al. Lenalidomide maintenance after stem-cell transplantation for multiple myeloma: follow-up analysis of the IFM 2005-02 trial. Blood 2013;122(21):406.

60. Cavallo F, Caravita T, Cavalli M, et al. Maintenance therapy with lenalidomide significantly improved survival of yong newly diagnosed multiple myeloma patients. Blood 2013;122(21):2089.

61. Palumbo A, Hajek R, Delforge M, et al. Continuous lenalidomide treatment for newly diagnosed multiple myeloma. N Engl J Med 2012;366(19): 1759–69.

62. Scheid C, van der Holt B, el Jarari L, et al. Bortezomib induction and maintenance treatment improves survival in patients with newly diagnosed multiple myeloma:extended follow-up of the HOVON-65/GMMG-HD4 trial. Blood 2013; 122(21):404.

63. Gahrton G, Iacobelli S, Björkstrand B, et al. Autologous/reduced-intensity allogeneic stem cell transplantation vs autologous transplantation in multiple myeloma: long-term results of the EBMT-NMAM2000 study. Blood 2013; 121(25):5055–63.

64. Krishnan A, Pasquini MC, Logan B, et al. Autologous haemopoietic stem-cell transplantation followed by allogeneic or autologous haemopoietic stem-cell transplantation in patients with multiple myeloma (BMT CTN 0102): a phase 3 biological assignment trial. Lancet Oncol 2011;12(13):1195–203.

65. Lokhorst HM, van der Holt B, Cornelissen JJ, et al. Donor versus no-donor comparison of newly diagnosed myeloma patients included in the HOVON-50 multiple myeloma study. Blood 2012;119(26):6219–25 [quiz: 6399].

66. Bruno B, Rotta M, Patriarca F, et al. A comparison of allografting with autografting for newly diagnosed myeloma. N Engl J Med 2007;356(11):1110–20.
67. Kumar S, Zhang MJ, Li P, et al. Trends in allogeneic stem cell transplantation for multiple myeloma: a CIBMTR analysis. Blood 2011;118(7):1979–88.
68. Keats JJ, Chesi M, Egan JB, et al. Clonal competition with alternating dominance in multiple myeloma. Blood 2012;120(5):1067–76.
69. Bergsagel PL, Mateos MV, Gutierrez NC, et al. Improving overall survival and overcoming adverse prognosis in the treatment of cytogenetically high-risk multiple myeloma. Blood 2013;121(6):884–92.
70. Palumbo A, Anderson K. Multiple myeloma. N Engl J Med 2011;364(11):1046–60.

Frontline Therapy for Patients with Multiple Myeloma not Eligible for Stem Cell Transplantation

Philippe Moreau, MD[a],*, Cyrille Hulin, MD[b], Thierry Facon, MD[c]

KEYWORDS

- Multiple myeloma • Elderly patients • Novel agents • Therapy

KEY POINTS

- Considerable progress has been recently made in the treatment of elderly patients with multiple myeloma (MM).
- In Europe the combination of thalidomide with melphalan and prednisone and of bortezomib with melphalan and prednisone are 2 standards of care for frontline therapy for elderly patients.
- In United States the combination of lenalidomide and dexamethasone is the preferred option in this setting.

INTRODUCTION

Multiple myeloma (MM) accounts for 1% of all cancers and approximately 13% of all hematologic malignancies.[1] Approximately 86,000 new cases of MM occur annually worldwide.[2] This malignant neoplasm affects primarily elderly patients with a median age at the time of diagnosis of about 70 years. Approximately two-thirds of patients are older than 65 years and one-third older than 75 years.[1] Patients older than 65 years, who represent most of the newly diagnosed symptomatic cases, are generally considered ineligible for autologous stem cell transplantation (ASCT).[3] During the past decade, considerable progress has been made in the treatment of MM. In the group of elderly patients, newer regimens and therapies that increase overall response and even complete remission rates have been evaluated in phase II and III trials.[3] Before the introduction of novel agents, combination chemotherapy with melphalan and prednisone (MP) had been the standard treatment approach for

[a] Hematology Department, UMR892, University Hospital, Place Ricordeau, Nantes 44093, France; [b] Hematology Department, University Hospital, Rue du Morvan, Nancy 54511, France; [c] Hematology Department, University Hospital, Avenue Lambret, Lille 59037, France
* Corresponding author.
E-mail address: philippe.moreau@chu-nantes.fr

Hematol Oncol Clin N Am 28 (2014) 829–838
http://dx.doi.org/10.1016/j.hoc.2014.06.002
0889-8588/14/$ – see front matter © 2014 Elsevier Inc. All rights reserved.

elderly myeloma patients since the 1960s.[4] The addition of thalidomide to this regimen (MPT) was the first step leading to survival improvement.[5] Subsequently, bortezomib was added to MP (VMP), and this VMP regimen also showed a survival benefit over MP.[6] These 2 regimens, MPT and VMP, are the most widely used combinations in Europe. In the United States, a melphalan-free regimen has been developed, combining lenalidomide and low-dose dexamethasone (Rd), and this has shown favorable results.[7] The Rd combination has recently been compared with MPT in a large international prospective randomized trial, and this regimen will become another standard of care in the near future.[8] This article focuses on more recent therapeutic approaches in older MM patients, not eligible for high-dose therapy and ASCT.

THALIDOMIDE-BASED REGIMENS
Thalidomide-Dexamethasone

Thalidomide combined with dexamethasone (TD) has been compared prospectively to high-dose dexamethasone (RD) and was superior in terms of partial response (63% vs 41%)[9] and time to progression (TTP) (22.6 vs 6.5 months),[10,11] but was found to be more toxic. Similarly, TD was superior to MP for responses, but progression-free survival (PFS) was similar, and overall survival (OS) was shorter.[10] Therefore, the TD regimen is not considered to be among the main options for the frontline therapy for elderly patients.

Melphalan-Prednisone-Thalidomide

Six randomized studies have compared MPT with MP alone. Despite differences in doses and schedules among the trials, better responses and PFS were reported with MPT in all of these.[5,12–16] The effect on OS varied across the studies, and only 2 trials showed a significant survival benefit.[5,13] In a meta-analysis of individual data from 1682 patients, MPT improved PFS by 5.4 months (median 20.3 vs 14.9 months, respectively) and OS by 6.6 months versus MP (median 39.3 vs 32.7 months, respectively).[17] The benefit of MPT has to be balanced against the increased risks of toxic effects. MPT is associated with higher risks of thromboembolism and peripheral neuropathy than MP, but these adverse events are manageable. The introduction of systematic anticoagulant prophylaxis has considerably reduced the rate of thromboembolism to less than 5%.[18] Similarly, improvements in the management of neuropathy have been observed. Prompt reduction of thalidomide dose is recommended as soon as symptoms occur. Discontinuation of the drug is necessary when paresthesia is accompanied by pain, motor deficit, or interference with daily functions.[18] Other thalidomide-related adverse events include cytopenia and fatigue.[18] The MPT regimen was approved by the European Medicines agency in 2008 and is considered one of the standards of care in elderly patients. This combination, oral and cost-effective, is recommended by United States and European guidelines, as well as the International Myeloma Working Group (IMWG).[3,19,20]

Cyclophosphamide-Thalidomide-Dexamethasone

An attenuated regimen of cyclophosphamide, thalidomide, and dexamethasone (CTD) has been prospectively compared with MP in a large randomized study (MRC IX) in the United Kingdom in 856 patients with newly diagnosed MM ineligible for ASCT.[21] The overall response rate was significantly higher with CTD than MP (63.8% vs 32.6%), with a complete response (CR) rate of 13.1% versus 2.4%. No differences in PFS and OS were observed between the 2 groups. Therefore, the CTD regimen, although oral and cost-effective, is not routinely recommended as part of frontline therapy in elderly patients.

BORTEZOMIB-BASED REGIMENS
Bortezomib-Melphalan-Prednisone

Preclinical trials have demonstrated in vitro synergy when bortezomib, the first proteasome inhibitor, is combined with melphalan.[22] The phase I/II study of VMP in 60 newly diagnosed elderly MM patients, which was reported in 2006 by the Spanish group PETHEMA, was conducted to identify the most appropriate dose of bortezomib in combination with the standard MP regimen (phase I) and to determine the efficacy of bortezomib + MP in terms of response rate (phase II).[23] The VMP response rate was 89%, including 32% immunofixation-negative CRs, and the median TTP with VMP was 27.2 months. The 1.3 mg/m^2 intravenous bortezomib dose level was selected, with a biweekly administration of the drug. These impressive preliminary results were the basis for the prospective, randomized phase III VISTA (Velcade as Initial Standard Therapy) trial comparing MP with VMP. Six hundred eighty-two patients 65 years of age or older, not transplant eligible, and with untreated MM were randomized to receive MP for nine 6-week cycles (n = 338) or the VMP combination (n = 344).[6] The total duration of treatment was 54 weeks in both arms of the study. Response rates were higher in the VMP arm (30% vs 4%); the median TTP was 24 months in the VMP arm versus 16.6 months in the MP arm; and with a median follow-up of 16 months, OS was also significantly in favor of the VMP arm. This improvement was also observed in patients older than 75 years. The final analysis was published in 2013 and confirmed that there was a 31% reduced risk of death with VMP versus MP, which was maintained after a median follow-up of 5 years and despite substantial use of novel-agent–based salvage therapies.[24] VMP, although manageable, was more toxic than MP with a discontinuation rate of 34%. The most frequent grade 3 to 4 toxicities were neutropenia (40%), thrombocytopenia (37%), peripheral neuropathy (17%), and infections (10%). The efficacy results led to the approval of the VMP combination by the European authorities in 2008, and this regimen is also considered one of the standards of care in the frontline treatment of elderly patients and is currently recommended in United States and European guidelines, as well as in the IMWG consensus.[3,19,20]

VMP Modified

When the twice-per-week bortezomib administration schedule was reduced to once per week in 2 prospective trials conducted in Spain and Italy, the rate of grade 3 to 4 peripheral neuropathy was found to be significantly lower, 17% versus 8%, respectively, whereas efficacy was comparable with the 2 schedules.[25,26] In the Spanish trial, melphalan in the VMP regimen was substituted by thalidomide, and the combination of bortezomib-thalidomide-prednisone (VTP) was prospectively compared with VMP in 260 patients. This VTP regimen yielded similar response rates and survival outcomes as compared with VMP, but was associated with more serious adverse events and discontinuations.[25] A more intensive approach was used in the Italian trial in which VMP was compared with the 4-drug combination of VMP plus thalidomide (VMPT) in 511 patients and with a once-weekly bortezomib infusion. Maintenance with thalidomide and bortezomib (VT) was administered in the VMPT, but not in the VMP arm.[26,27] The VMPT-VT arm (nine 5-week cycles of VMPT followed by 2 years of VT maintenance) demonstrated better responses (38% CR vs 24%) and an improvement in 3-year PFS from 41% to 56% compared with VMP, but the efficacy advantage was mainly reported in fit patients aged 65 to 75 years old.[27] The updated results of this trial were recently published and have shown that the 5-year OS was greater with VMPT-VT (61%) than with VMP (51%; hazard ratio, 0.70; $P = .01$).[28] Despite positive results and recommendations from the IMWG,[3] this 4-drug induction regimen followed by 2 years of maintenance is not routinely used as part of frontline therapy in elderly patients.

Recently, bortezomib administered subcutaneously was shown to be as effective as the intravenous route of administration, with a reduced risk of peripheral neuropathy.[29] Therefore, subcutaneous bortezomib is now considered as a routine and feasible treatment of elderly patients and can be an option for prolonged therapy.[3,30]

Bortezomib-Cyclophosphamide-Dexamethasone, Bortezomib-Lenalidomide-Dexamethasone

Interesting results have been obtained when cyclophosphamide (VCD)[31–33] or lenalidomide (VRD)[34] were combined with bortezomib and RD, producing high-quality responses. Although VRD and VCD have not been evaluated in randomized phase III trials, these 2 regimens are commonly used in the United States in clinical practice on the basis of positive results from phase II studies.[35] VCD adds neither cost nor significant toxicity to the VD regimen, and the addition of cyclophosphamide allows for a weekly rather than twice weekly administration of bortezomib.[33] In a phase II randomized trial, VCD had similar activity compared with VRD.[31] Despite the lack of phase III data, these 2 regimens are recommended by the IMWG[3] and by the US guidelines.[19] VCD is the most cost-effective option.

LENALIDOMIDE-BASED REGIMENS
Lenalidomide–Low-dose Dexamethasone

Lenalidomide, an oral drug, is an analogue of thalidomide, which was designed to improve efficacy and tolerability over the parent drug. Lenalidomide has a safety profile that is distinct from that of thalidomide, with fewer neurologic symptoms but more myelosuppression. A phase III trial conducted by the ECOG (ECOG E4A03) assessed the safety and efficacy of lenalidomide plus high-dose RD versus lenalidomide plus low-dose dexamethasone (Rd) in 445 patients. The median age of the patient population was 66 years, and 233 patients were older than 65 years (up to 88 years).[7] Patients eligible for ASCT could discontinue therapy after 4 induction cycles. Patients treated with RD had a higher overall response rate (79% vs 68%) but a lower 1-year OS (87% vs 96%). For patients aged older than 65 years, the 1-year OS rate was 83% with RD and 94% with Rd. RD was associated with a higher incidence of grade 3 to 4 nonhematological adverse events when compared with Rd, particularly deep-vein thrombosis (26% vs 12%), infections (16% vs 9%), and fatigue (15% vs 9%). In routine practice, all patients treated with Rd require antithrombosis prophylaxis. Aspirin is adequate for most patients, but in patients who are at a higher risk of thrombosis, either low-molecular-weight heparin or Coumadin is needed. In the ECOG study Rd was associated with a reduction in the rates of discontinuation and of early death compared with RD. The 3-year OS rate with Rd in patients aged 70 years and older who did not receive ASCT was 70%,[7,35] which seems to be comparable to what is achieved with VMP or MPT. Therefore, the oral combination of Rd is widely used in the United States and is currently recommended by US guidelines,[19] and by the experts from IMWG,[3] but it is not approved in the Europe.

In the most remarkable recent study involving 1623 patients not eligible for transplantation (IFM07–01, MM020 trial), the combination of Rd administered until disease progression or intolerance (continued Rd) was compared with MPT administered for 12 cycles (72 weeks) or Rd administered for 18 cycles (72 weeks) (Rd18).[8] The trial revealed a significant benefit of continued Rd over Rd18 and MPT and a significant increase in OS over MPT. With a median follow-up of 37 months, the median PFS was 25.5 months for continued Rd compared with 20.7 months with Rd18 and 21.2 months for MPT (continued Rd vs MPT: $P = .0006$, continued Rd vs Rd18: $P = .0001$). Four-year OS was 59.4% for continued Rd, 55.7% for Rd18 and 51.4% for MPT (continued Rd vs MPT: $P = .017$, continued Rd vs Rd18: $P = .307$). Given the significant improvement in survival, the relatively acceptable toxicity, and the ease of administration of continued Rd, this combination will likely become a frequently used protocol and another standard of care in elderly patients in the near future.

Melphalan-Prednisone-Lenalidomide

The combination of melphalan, prednisone, and lenalidomide (MPR) has been investigated in a dose-escalating Phase I/II study,[36] which enrolled 54 patients (median age 71 years). They received 9 cycles of lenalidomide plus melphalan and prednisone every 6 weeks, followed by maintenance therapy with lenalidomide alone (10 mg/d, days 1–21, every month). The maximum tolerated dose was lenalidomide 10 mg/d for 21 days and melphalan 0.18 mg/kg for 4 days every 6 weeks. At this dose level, the overall response rate was 81%, including 24% of patients with immunofixation-negative CR. The 1-year event-free survival and OS rates were 92% and 100%, respectively. Overall, MPR was considered a promising first-line treatment of elderly patients, and these results formed the basis for an international randomized trial comparing MPR followed by lenalidomide maintenance (MPR-R) to MPR and MP (MM015 study).[37] MPR-R resulted in a higher overall response rate compared with MPR and MP (77% vs 68% vs 50%). Furthermore, MPR-R reduced the risk of disease progression by 60% compared with MP. The median PFS was 31 months in the MPR-R arm versus 14 and 13 months in the MPR and MP arms, respectively. The PFS benefit associated with MPR-R treatment was evidenced especially in patients aged 65 to 75 years of age. No difference was observed in terms of OS when comparing the 3 arms of the study. Lenalidomide maintenance was well tolerated with no evidence of cumulative toxicity and low rates of adverse events. The most frequent hematologic adverse events in the MPR-R arm were neutropenia (35%) and thrombocytopenia (11%). Infections were the most frequent nonhematologic adverse events (9%), whereas a low rate of deep-vein thrombosis was observed (1%) because patients received aspirin prophylaxis as part of the protocol. MPR-R is currently considered a reasonable option in elderly patients with de novo MM by the experts of the IMWG,[3] but the regimen is not approved in Europe and not widely used in the United States where Rd is the preferred option.

UNFIT PATIENTS

MM is a highly heterogeneous disease. Several patient and disease characteristics, such as serum albumin and beta-2 microglobulin levels, or cytogenetics, allow for the classification of patients into low- and high-risk groups, thereby providing important prognostic information. Some experts are even proposing the use of a risk-adapted strategy when planning frontline treatment.[35] In the elderly, this important issue is further complicated by the potential vulnerability of the patients, which is determined by frailty, comorbidity, and disability.[3,38] Frailty is characterized by the presence of greater than or equal to 3 elements (weakness, weight loss, low physical activity, poor endurance, and slow gait speed). Comorbidity is defined by the presence of greater than or equal to 2 concomitant, medically diagnosed diseases (including renal, pulmonary, hepatic, cardiac, gastrointestinal, bone marrow). Disability includes both physical and mental impairments and is defined by the degree of difficulty or dependency in carrying out common daily activities, including essential personal care, household tasks, and activities to maintain a suitable quality of life.[30,38] To date, despite the availability of different geriatric scales aimed at evaluating unfit patients, a definitive consensus has not yet been reached for the definition of this subgroup of elderly patients. Nevertheless, the importance of a personalized approach to therapy, based on a reduced intensity strategy or adequate dose reductions if required, is increasingly recognized, because unfit and frail patients are more susceptible to therapy-related adverse events resulting in a high frequency of treatment discontinuation. It has been proposed that, based on age, frailty, comorbidity, and disability, MM patients may be divided into specific groups, such as "full go", "slow go", or "very slow go or no go".[3] Fit patients (full go) may receive the full dose of novel-agent–based combinations, such as MPT, VMP, or Rd. On the other hand, dose-adaptations are required in unfit patients, and several dose-reduction guidelines have been proposed. Unfit patients should receive reduced-dose MPT or VMP or 2-drug combinations with bortezomib or reduced-dose Rd.[3,39] Indeed, in the randomized phase IIIb Upfront trial, which prospectively compared bortezomib-dexamethasone (VD), VTD, and VMP as frontline therapy in 502 transplant-ineligible patients in the US community practice setting, VD doublet therapy was as effective as VTD and VMP triplet therapy, and the discontinuation rate was lower with VD.[39] In this study, 48% of the patients (median age 73 years) had comorbidities at baseline, stressing the need for patient-adapted therapy, according to age, comorbidities, and frailty.

MAINTENANCE THERAPY

In almost all patients with MM, relapse of the disease after a maximal response to first-line therapy is inevitable, thus a treatment strategy to maintain disease control is necessary. The role of maintenance in the nontransplant setting has been investigated in several trials with all the novel agents, thalidomide, bortezomib, and lenalidomide.[3] Benefits in PFS have been seen with all of these; however, an OS advantage was only seen in the GIMEMA study discussed earlier, which compared VMPT followed by VT maintenance to VMP.[28] Because of the different regimens used during the initial phase of treatment, VMPT versus VMP, it is not possible to attribute the survival benefit exclusively to VT maintenance. Of note, in the MRC IX trial comparing thalidomide maintenance versus no maintenance, OS was decreased in the subgroup of patients with adverse cytogenetics who received thalidomide maintenance, raising the issue of clonal selection in high-risk disease.[40] All maintenance trials have defined the toxicity profile of novel agents in this setting.[3] Drug-related toxicity, especially neuropathy, associated with continuous thalidomide therapy may limit its long-term administration. Lenalidomide is better tolerated, although the higher risk of second primary malignancies, which has been observed with long-term lenalidomide administration, has to be borne in mind. Continuous treatment with bortezomib has the inconvenience of the need for intravenous administration, along with a slightly increased risk for peripheral neuropathy; however, the subcutaneous route of administration may be promising in the maintenance setting.[29] Taken together, because of limited data regarding a survival benefit for maintenance therapy, as well as toxicity issues, the routine use of maintenance in transplantation-ineligible patients is not yet recommended.[3,20] Future trials should carefully examine the outcome after progression, together with the optimal duration of maintenance (for a fixed duration or until progression/intolerance).

FUTURE DIRECTIONS

As mentioned earlier MPT, VMP, and Rd are the most frequently used regimens in the frontline therapy for elderly patients. Several other agents, such as carfilzomib, the second-in-class proteasome inhibitor (PI); ixazomib, an oral PI; elotuzumab, a monoclonal antibody targeting SLAMF7; or daratumumab, another CD38 monoclonal antibody, are currently or will soon be tested in phase III clinical trials, and it is expected that the results of these trials will drastically modify the standards of care in patients not eligible for ASCT.[41]

The VMP combination will be challenged by VMP plus daratumumab, or carfilzomib plus MP, whereas the Rd combination is currently being compared with Rd plus ixazomib, and Rd-elotuzumab and will also be challenged by Rd plus daratumumab.

A provocative approach is coming from the Spanish group, who has initiated a phase II randomized trial of lenalidomide plus VMP, administered either sequentially (9 cycles lenalidomide + 9 cycles VMP) or as 18 alternating cycles.[42] Despite a short follow-up, the preliminary results of this "total therapy" approach for elderly patients, which includes all available classes of therapeutic agents, are impressive with a 20-month PFS of 84% with the alternating regimen. The long-term follow-up of this trial could define another standard of care in the near future.

REFERENCES

1. Howlade N, Noone A, Krapcho M, et al. Seer cancer statistics review, 1975–2009 (vintage 2009 populations). Bethesda (MD): National Cancer Institute; 2012. based on November 2011 seer data submission, posted to the seer web site. Available at: http://seer.cancer.gov/csr/1975_2009_pops09/.
2. Beker N. Epidemiology of multiple myeloma. Recent Results Cancer Res 2011; 183:25–35.
3. Palumbo A, Rajkumar SV, San Miguel J, et al. International Myeloma Working Group consensus statement for the management, treatment, and supportive care of patients with myeloma not eligible for standard autologous stem-cell transplantation. J Clin Oncol 2014;32:587–600.
4. Myeloma Trialists' Collaborative Group. Combination chemotherapy versus melphalan and prednisone as treatment for multiple myeloma: an overview of 6633 patients from 27 randomized trials. J Clin Oncol 1998;16:3832–42.
5. Facon T, Mary JY, Hulin C, et al. Melphalan and prednisone plus thalidomide versus melphalan and prednisone alone or reduced-intensity autologous stem cell transplantation in elderly patients with multiple myeloma (IFM99-06): a randomised trial. Lancet 2007;370:1209–18.
6. San Miguel JF, Schlag R, Khuageva NK, et al. Bortezomib plus melphalan and prednisone for initial treatment of multiple myeloma. N Engl J Med 2008;359: 906–17.
7. Rajkumar SV, Jacobus S, Callander NS, et al. Lenalidomide plus high-dose dexamethasone versus lenalidomide plus low-dose dexamethasone as initial therapy for newly diagnosed multiple myeloma: an open-label randomised controlled trial. Lancet Oncol 2010;11:29–37.
8. Facon T, Dimopoulos MA, Dispenzieri A, et al. Initial phase 3 results of the First (Frontline Investigation of Lenalidomide + Dexamethasone Versus Standard Thalidomide) Trial (MM-020/IFM 07 01) in newly diagnosed multiple myeloma (NDMM) patients (Pts) ineligible for stem cell transplantation (SCT). Blood 2013; 122(21) [abstract: 2].

9. Rajkumar SV, Blood E, Vesole D, et al. Phase III clinical trial of thalidomide plus dexamethasone compared with dexamethasone alone in newly diagnosed multiple myeloma: a clinical trial coordinated by the Eastern Cooperative Oncology Group. J Clin Oncol 2006;24:431–6.

10. Rajkumar SV, Rosinol L, Hussein M, et al. A multicenter, randomized, double-blind, placebo-controlled study of thalidomide plus dexamethasone versus dexamethasone as initial therapy for newly diagnosed multiple myeloma. J Clin Oncol 2008;26:2171–7.

11. Ludwig H, Hajek R, Tothova E, et al. Thalidomide-dexamethasone compared with melphalan prednisolone in elderly patients with multiple myeloma. Blood 2009; 113:3435–42.

12. Palumbo A, Bringhen S, Liberati AM, et al. Oral melphalan, prednisone, and thalidomide in elderly patients with multiple myeloma: updated results of a randomized controlled trial. Blood 2008;112:107–14.

13. Hulin C, Facon T, Rodon P, et al. Efficacy of melphalan and prednisone plus thalidomide in patients older than 75 years with newly diagnosed multiple myeloma: IFM 01/01 trial. J Clin Oncol 2009;27:64–70.

14. Wijermans P, Schaafsma M, Termorshuizen F, et al. Phase III study of the value of thalidomide added to melphalan plus prednisone in elderly patients with newly diagnosed multiple myeloma: the HOVON 49 study. J Clin Oncol 2010;28: 3160–6.

15. Waage A, Gimsing P, Fayers P, et al. Melphalan and prednisone plus thalidomide or placebo in elderly patients with multiple myeloma. Blood 2010;116:1405–12.

16. Beksac M, Haznedar R, Firatli-Tuglular T, et al. Addition of thalidomide to oral melphalan/prednisone in patients with multiple myeloma not eligible for transplantation: results of a randomized trial from the Turkish Myeloma Study Group. Eur J Haematol 2011;86:16–22.

17. Fayers PM, Palumbo A, Hulin C, et al. Thalidomide for previously untreated elderly patients with multiple myeloma: meta-analysis of 1685 individual patient data from 6 randomized clinical trials. Blood 2011;118:1239–47.

18. Palumbo A, Waage A, Hulin C, et al. Safety of thalidomide in newly diagnosed elderly myeloma patients: a meta-analysis of data from individual patients in six randomized trials. Haematologica 2013;98:87–94.

19. National Comprehensive Cancer Network. NCCN Clinical Practice Guidelines in Oncology. Multiple myeloma. Version 2, 2014. Available at: www.nccn.org.

20. Moreau P, San Miguel J, Ludwig H, et al. Multiple myeloma: ESMO Clinical Practice Guidelines for diagnosis, treatment and follow-up. Ann Oncol 2013;21(Suppl 6): vi133–7.

21. Morgan GJ, Davies FE, Gregory WM, et al. Cyclophosphamide, thalidomide, and dexamethasone (CTD) as initial therapy for patients with multiple myeloma unsuitable for autologous transplantation. Blood 2011;118:1231–8.

22. Mitsiades N, Mitsiades CS, Richardson PG, et al. The proteasome inhibitor PS-341 markedly enhances sensitivity of multiple myeloma tumor cells to chemotherapeutic agents. Clin Cancer Res 2003;9:1136–44.

23. Mateos MV, Hernandez JM, Hernandez MT, et al. Bortezomib plus melphalan and prednisone in elderly untreated patients with multiple myeloma: results of a multicenter phase 1/2 study. Blood 2006;108:2165–72.

24. San Miguel JF, Schlag R, Khuageva NK, et al. Persistent overall survival benefit and no increased risk of second malignancies with bortezomib-melphalan-prednisone versus melphalan-prednisone in patients with previously untreated multiple myeloma. J Clin Oncol 2013;31:448–55.

25. Mateos MV, Oriol A, Martinez-Lopez J, et al. Bortezomib, melphalan, and prednisone versus bortezomib, thalidomide, and prednisone as induction therapy followed by maintenance treatment with bortezomib and thalidomide versus
bortezomib and prednisone in elderly patients with untreated multiple myeloma:
a randomised trial. Lancet Oncol 2010;11:934–41.

26. Bringhen S, Larocca A, Rossi D, et al. Efficacy and safety of once-weekly bortezomib in multiple myeloma patients. Blood 2010;116:4745–53.

27. Palumbo A, Bringhen S, Rossi D, et al. Bortezomib-melphalan-prednisone-thalidomide followed by maintenance with bortezomib-thalidomide compared with
bortezomib-melphalan-prednisone for initial treatment of multiple myeloma: a randomized controlled trial. J Clin Oncol 2010;28:5101–9.

28. Palumbo A, Bringhen S, Larocca A, et al. Bortezomib-melphalan-prednisone-
thalidomide followed by maintenance with bortezomib-thalidomide compared
with bortezomib-melphalan-prednisone for initial treatment of multiple myeloma: updated follow-up and improved survival. J Clin Oncol 2014;32:
634–40.

29. Moreau P, Pylypenko H, Grosicki S, et al. Subcutaneous versus intravenous
administration of bortezomib in patients with relapsed multiple myeloma: a randomised, phase 3, non-inferiority study. Lancet Oncol 2011;12:431–40.

30. Guglielmelli T, Antonio Palumbo A. Incorporating novel agents in the management of elderly myeloma patients. Curr Hematol Malig Rep 2013;8:261–9.

31. Kumar S, Flinn I, Richardson PG, et al. Randomized, multicenter, phase 2 study
(EVOLUTION) of combinations of bortezomib, dexamethasone, cyclophosphamide, and lenalidomide in previously untreated multiple myeloma. Blood 2012;
119:4375–82.

32. Reeder CB, Reece DE, Kukreti V, et al. Cyclophosphamide, bortezomib and
dexamethasone induction for newly diagnosed multiple myeloma: high response
rates in a phase II clinical trial. Leukemia 2009;23:1337–41.

33. Reeder CB, Reece DE, Kukreti V, et al. Once versus twice-weekly bortezomib induction therapy with CyBorD in newly diagnosed multiple myeloma. Blood 2010;
115:3416–7.

34. Richardson PG, Weller E, Lonial S, et al. Lenalidomide, bortezomib, and dexamethasone combination therapy in patients with newly diagnosed multiple myeloma.
Blood 2010;116:679–86.

35. Rajkumar SV. Initial treatment of multiple myeloma. Hematol Oncol 2013;
31(Suppl 1):33–7.

36. Palumbo A, Falco P, Corradini P, et al. Melphalan, prednisone, and lenalidomide
treatment for newly diagnosed myeloma: a report from the GIMEMA – Italian Multiple Myeloma Network. J Clin Oncol 2007;25:4459–65.

37. Palumbo A, Hajek R, Delforge M, et al. Continuous lenalidomide treatment for
newly diagnosed multiple myeloma. N Engl J Med 2012;366:1759–69.

38. Palumbo A, Bringhen S, Ludwig H, et al. Personalized therapy in multiple
myeloma according to patient age and vulnerability: a report of European
Myeloma Network (EMN). Blood 2011;118:4519–29.

39. Niesvizky R, Flinn IW, Rifkin R, et al. Efficacy and safety of three bortezomib-
based combinations in elderly, newly diagnosed multiple myeloma patients: results from all randomized patients in the community-based, phase 3b UPFRONT
study. Blood 2011;118 [abstract: 478].

40. Morgan GJ, Gregory WM, Davies FE, et al. The role of maintenance thalidomide
therapy in multiple myeloma: MRC Myeloma IX results and meta-analysis. Blood
2012;119:7–15.

41. Ocio E, Richardson PG, Rajkumar SV, et al. New drugs and novel mechanisms of action in multiple myeloma: a report from the International Myeloma Working Group (IMWG). Leukemia 2014;28:525–42.

42. Mateos MV, Martinez-Lopez J, Hernandez MT, et al. Comparison of sequential vs alternating administration of bortezomib, melphalan and prednisone (VMP) and lenalidomide plus dexamethasone (Rd) in elderly patients with newly diagnosed Multiple Myeloma (MM) patients: GEM2010MAS65 trial. Blood 2013;122(21):403 [abstract: ASH].

Maintenance Therapy for Multiple Myeloma

Philip L. McCarthy, MD[a], Antonio Palumbo, MD[b],*

KEYWORDS

- Multiple myeloma • Thalidomide • Lenalidomide • Bortezomib
- Transplant-ineligible • Transplant-eligible • Maintenance

KEY POINTS

- Maintenance therapy with novel agents prolonged remission duration in both transplant-ineligible and transplant-eligible patients with multiple myeloma.
- The appropriate maintenance strategy should be not only effective but also well tolerated.
- In transplant-ineligible patients, single-agent thalidomide or lenalidomide showed positive results after thalidomide-based and lenalidomide-based induction therapies, respectively. Bortezomib in association with thalidomide is also a valid strategy.
- In transplant-eligible patients, single-agent thalidomide resulted in improved progression-free survival (PFS) but was not well tolerated and in high-risk cytogenetic patients may lead to inferior survival, whereas bortezomib as part of induction and maintenance improves PFS in all patients and overall survival in patients with the del 17 cytogenetic abnormality and those who present in renal failure.
- In transplant-eligible patients, single-agent lenalidomide is effective as demonstrated in improved PFS and, in 2 of 3 studies, in improved OS.

INTRODUCTION

Multiple myeloma (MM) is a neoplasm typical of the elderly, with median age at diagnosis of 70 years, and approximately 65% of patients older than 65 years.[1] Many advances have been made thanks to the use of autologous hematopoietic stem cell transplantation (AHSCT) and the introduction of the immunomodulatory drugs and the proteasome inhibitors. Incorporation of novel agents into induction has resulted in improved overall survival (OS) over the past decade.[2,3] Indeed, in a large group of

Authorship: P. L. McCarthy and A. Palumbo collected the data and wrote the article.
Conflicts of interest: Dr P. L. McCarthy has served on advisory boards and consulted for Celgene, Janssen, Millenium, and Onyx. Dr A. Palumbo has received honoraria and consultancy fees from Celgene, Janssen-Cilag, Bristol-Myers Squibb, Millennium, Merck, and Onyx.
[a] Department of Medicine, Blood and Marrow Transplant Program, Roswell Park Cancer Institute, State University of New York at Buffalo, Elm and Carlton Streets, Buffalo, NY 14263, USA;
[b] Myeloma Unit, Division of Hematology, Azienda Ospedaliero-Universitaria Città della Salute e della Scienza di Torino, University of Torino, Via Genova 3, Torino 10126, Italy
* Corresponding author.
E-mail address: appalumbo@yahoo.com

Hematol Oncol Clin N Am 28 (2014) 839–859
http://dx.doi.org/10.1016/j.hoc.2014.06.006
0889-8588/14/$ – see front matter © 2014 Elsevier Inc. All rights reserved.

2981 patients with newly diagnosed MM, OS significantly improved from 29.9 to 44.8 months in patients diagnosed in the last decade (P<.001).[3] The agents that have most impacted on progression-free survival (PFS) and OS are thalidomide,[4,5] lenalidomide,[6,7] and bortezomib.[8–11] The alkylating agent cyclophosphamide, in combination with bortezomib and dexamethasone generated comparable deep responses to bortezomib, lenalidomide, and dexamethasone in a phase 2 study.[12] These combination induction regimens improve the overall response and the depth of response by increasing the percentage of patients achieving complete responses (CR). Many MM patients will have disease progression or relapse and die of MM within 10 years of the initiation of therapy. Thus, there is a pressing need for improved induction regimens and for strategies to control disease with the long-term goal of cure. Of note, sequential approaches consisting of induction followed by consolidation and maintenance with novel agents have been recently tested with the attempt of improving the clinical benefit of current treatments.[13] Consolidation improves responses after induction therapy (and transplantation when applicable), and maintenance further delays relapse/progression with the ultimate goal of improving OS. Consolidation consists of 2 to 4 cycles of combination therapies and maintenance of continuous therapy, usually with single agents, until disease progression.[14] Maintenance therapy is suggested for both transplant-ineligible patients (usually elderly patients 65 years of age and over) and transplant-eligible ones (patients younger than 65 years of age). However, no specific guidelines are available, and the optimal duration of maintenance remains to be established.[15]

Optimal MM maintenance therapy should maintain or increase response after induction and, when possible, AHSCT. Maintenance therapy should be easily given (preferably orally) and, if administered intravenously, convenient for the patient. Because of the lack of long-term efficacy and tolerability, agents such as melphalan, interferon-α, and glucocorticoids have not become widely used for maintenance.[16–19] Newer agents are more attractive as maintenance therapies because of improved efficacy and better tolerability. Most maintenance studies have used thalidomide and, more recently, bortezomib and lenalidomide. Different studies have assessed the benefits associated with maintenance treatment incorporating thalidomide, lenalidomide, and bortezomib, yet no clinical study has directly compared the advantages of one approach over the other. Despite the benefits associated with continuous novel-agent–based therapy, prolonged exposure to new drugs may increase toxicities and cause treatment discontinuation. Therefore, the optimal maintenance therapy must be effective with minimal toxicity and should be easily administered.[20]

MAINTENANCE APPROACHES FOR PATIENTS INELIGIBLE FOR TRANSPLANTATION

Patients 65 years of age and older do not tolerate intensive therapy and are usually ineligible for high-dose melphalan (MEL200; melphalan 200 mg/m^2) and AHSCT. For these patients, gentler strategies should be used. Combinations with novel agents, such as thalidomide, lenalidomide, and bortezomib, are widely adopted, for both newly diagnosed and relapsed patients with MM. In the 1970s, maintenance treatment of this subset of patients consisted of prolonging chemotherapy after successful induction treatment with melphalan-prednisone (MP).[17,21,22] Other attempts of maintenance therapies consisted of using single-agent interferon.[19,23]

Thalidomide

Thalidomide can be a suitable option for prolonged use because of the oral administration. Nevertheless, the neurologic toxicity associated with this drug is a major concern and should be carefully considered. To date, continuous thalidomide after melphalan-prednisone-thalidomide (MPT) induction has been evaluated in 4 trials (**Table 1**).[5,24–27] In one study, 100 mg/d thalidomide was given continuously. The median PFS was 25 months for patients who received thalidomide and 15 months for those who did not (P<.001). The median OS was 48 months and 45 months for the 2 arms, respectively (P = .79).[5,24] The incidence of grade 3 to 4 neurologic toxicity was 10% in patients receiving thalidomide therapy and 1% in those receiving no maintenance. In another study, thalidomide was administered at 200 mg/d at induction and was reduced to 50 mg/d during maintenance. The median event-free survival (EFS) time was 13 months for patients who received thalidomide and 9 months for those who did not (P<.001). A marginally significant OS advantage favoring thalidomide maintenance was also detected, with a median of 40 months versus 31 months (P = .05).[25] The incidence of grade 3 to 4 neurologic toxicities was particularly higher with thalidomide (23%) than no thalidomide (4%). In another study, thalidomide at a dose of 200 mg/d was administered continuously until relapse.[26] The median PFS (15 months vs 14 months, P = .84) and OS (29 months vs 32 months, P = .16) was similar between patients who received thalidomide and those who did not. The incidence of grade 3 to 4 peripheral neuropathy was quite low in both arms, 6% versus 1%, respectively. These findings support the concept that thalidomide maintenance should be administered at the minimal effective dose associated with the lowest toxicity (50–100 mg/d) to avoid early discontinuation.

Another randomized trial assessed the role of thalidomide-interferon or interferon alone as maintenance therapy after induction with either thalidomide-dexamethasone (TD) or MP.[28] The median PFS was 28 months for patients who received thalidomide maintenance and 13 months for those who received interferon alone (P = .007). The median OS was similar in the 2 groups (53 months vs 51 months, P = .81). The rate of grade 3 to 4 neuropathy was 7% versus 0%, respectively (P = .002). Finally, in another study, a total of 820 patients, both eligible and ineligible for AHSCT, were randomized to thalidomide maintenance or no maintenance. Patients ineligible for AHSCT had received MP or cyclophosphamide-TD induction.[29] In these patients, thalidomide maintenance improved PFS (23 vs 15 months, P<.001), and the advantage was more evident in patients who had received thalidomide also at induction. The median OS was not significantly different between the 2 arms (P = .40). In patients with adverse interphase Fluorescence In Situ Hybridization (iFISH), thalidomide maintenance had a negative impact on OS (P = .009).

All the studies including thalidomide maintenance reported an improvement in terms of PFS, although longer follow-up is needed to detect an OS benefit. The risk of peripheral neuropathy after long-term thalidomide exposure is a major limitation to its routine use. To avoid excessive neurologic toxicity and consequently treatment discontinuation, the preferred dose of thalidomide maintenance should range between 50 and 100 mg/d.[30] In case of occurrence of grade 3 to 4 neurotoxicity, it is highly recommended to temporarily interrupt treatment until resolution to at least grade 1; otherwise treatment should be stopped.

Lenalidomide

Lenalidomide, similarly to thalidomide, is administered orally and has the additional advantage of lower neurologic toxicity.

A phase 3 study evaluated the role of lenalidomide at 10 mg on days 1–21 of each 28-day cycle after melphalan-prednisone-lenalidomide (MPR-R) versus MPR versus MP.[31] The median PFS was 31 months with MPR-R, 14 months with MPR, and 13 months with MP. In a landmark analysis from start of lenalidomide maintenance,

Table 1
Main maintenance approaches for patients ineligible for MEL200 and transplantation

Drug	Study	Schedule	Response	Median PFS/TTP/EFS	Median OS	Previous Induction
Thalidomide	Palumbo et al,[5,24] 2006, 2008	T: 100 mg/d until relapse	16% CR	22 mo	45 mo	MPT
	Wijermans et al,[25] 2010	T: 50 mg/d until relapse	23% ≥VGPR	13 mo	40 mo	MPT
	Waage et al,[26] 2010	T: 200 mg/d until progression	13% CR	15 mo	29 mo	MPT
	Beksac et al,[27] 2011	T: 100 mg/d until relapse	9% CR	21 mo	26 mo	MPT
	Ludwig et al,[28] 2010	T: 200 mg/d until progression or intolerance; I: 3 Mega units 3 times a wk	—	28 mo	53 mo	MP or TD
	Morgan et al,[29] 2012	T: 50 mg/d increased to 100 mg/d after 4 cycles (if tolerated) until progression	—	23 mo	—	MP or CTDa
Lenalidomide	Palumbo et al,[31] 2012	R: 10 mg day 1–21 until disease progression	33% ≥VGPR	31 mo	70% @ 36 mo	MPR
	Gay et al,[35] 2013	R: 25 mg d 1–21; P: 50 mg qod for four 28-d cycles followed by R: 25 mg days 1–21 until disease progression	48% CR 53% CR	48 mo	63% @ 60 mo	PAD-MEL100[a]
Bortezomib	Mateos et al,[36] 2010	V: 1.3 mg/m² twice weekly, on days 1, 4, 8, 11, every 3 mo; P: 50 mg qod for up to 3 y	39% CR	32 mo	—	VMP or VTP
	Mateos et al,[36] 2010	V: 1.3 mg/m² twice weekly, on days 1, 4, 8, 11, every 3 mo; T: 50 mg/d for up to 3 y	44% CR	24 mo	—	VMP or VTP
	Palumbo et al,[37] 2014	V: 1.3 mg/m² every 14 d; T: 50 mg/d for 2 y	42% CR[b]	56% @ 36 mo	61% @ 60 mo	VMPT

Abbreviations: CTDa, cyclophosphamide-thalidomide-dexamethasone attenuated; I, interferon α-2b; MEL100, melphalan 100 mg/m²; MEL200, melphalan 200 mg/m²; P, prednisone; qod, every other day; R, lenalidomide; T, thalidomide; V, bortezomib; VGPR, very good partial response; VMP, bortezomib-melphalan-prednisone; VTP, bortezomib-thalidomide-prednisone.

[a] Treatment approach incorporating transplantation before consolidation and maintenance, enrolling patients 65–75 years.

[b] By exploratory analysis performed on the 82 patients treated with VMPT induction who received at least 6 months of maintenance with VT.

lenalidomide after MPR significantly prolonged the median PFS from 7 to 26 months (P<.001). No particular advantage was seen in terms of OS, and the 4-year OS was approximately 58% in the 3 treatment groups. One of the major toxicities associated with lenalidomide is neutropenia, which was reported in 7% of patients in the MPR-R arm. Some concerns about the increased risk of second primary malignancies (SPM) with prolonged exposure to lenalidomide were raised. In this study, the rate of SPM was 7% for both MPR-R and MPR, and 3% for MP. Nevertheless, the benefits associated with lenalidomide treatment outweigh the increased risk of SPM. A recent meta-analysis on 3218 patients found that patients treated with lenalidomide had an increased risk of developing hematologic SPM (hazard ratio [HR] 1.55; P = .037). Of note, the risk was increased when lenalidomide was given with melphalan compared with melphalan alone (HR 4.86; P<.0001), whereas exposure to lenalidomide plus cyclophosphamide (HR 1.26; P = .75) or lenalidomide plus dexamethasone (HR 0.86; P = .76) did not increase hematologic SPM risk versus melphalan alone. Thus, the use of alternative alkylating agents can be a possible option.[32]

A phase 2 study evaluated a sequential approach consisting of lenalidomide-prednisone (RP) induction followed by MPR consolidation and subsequent RP maintenance (lenalidomide 10 mg/d on days 1–21 of each 28-day cycle; prednisone 25 mg 3 times/wk).[33] Median age was 75 years; 59% of patients had at least one comorbidity and 35% at least 2 comorbidities. Median PFS was 18.4 months and 2-year OS was 80%. Grade 4 neutropenia occurred in 12% of patients. Therefore, this study demonstrated that the addition of prednisone increases the efficacy of lenalidomide alone in unfit elderly MM patients, with the advantage of a low toxicity and consequently improved quality of life.

A recent large phase 3 study compared lenalidomide plus low-dose dexamethasone (Rd) until relapse versus Rd for 18 cycles (72 weeks) versus MPT for 12 cycles (72 weeks).[34] Median age was 73 years. After a median follow-up of 37 months, Rd significantly improved PFS compared with MPT (HR 0.72; P = .00006) and marginally OS (HR 0.78, P = .01685). Relevant grade 3 to 4 adverse events with Rd until relapse versus MPT were neutropenia (28% vs 45%), thrombocytopenia (8% vs 11%), febrile neutropenia (1% vs 3%), infection (29% vs 17%), neuropathy (5% vs 15%), and deep vein thrombosis (5% vs 3%). The respective incidence of hematologic SPM was 0.4% versus 2.2%; the overall incidence of solid tumors was identical (2.8%). These results suggest the need for prolonging therapy until progression, because outcome after 18 cycles of therapy was similar between Rd and MPT. Continuous Rd is therefore a valid option in transplant-ineligible patients and may be preferred to the standard MPT with no maintenance.

Although elderly patients are usually not able to tolerate MEL200 and AHSCT, reduced intensity transplantation with melphalan 100 mg/m^2 (MEL100) can be safely adopted for fit elderly patients. A phase 2 study assessed bortezomib-adriamycin-dexamethasone (PAD) induction followed by tandem MEL100, AHSCT, RP consolidation, and lenalidomide maintenance in patients aged 65 to 75 years.[35] This approach induced a median PFS of 48 months and a 5-year OS of 63%. Consolidation and maintenance with lenalidomide considerably increased responses, mostly in subjects who had achieved a very good partial response after transplantation. During consolidation and maintenance, the main toxicities were hematologic; in particular, neutropenia (19% after consolidation and 23% after maintenance) and thrombocytopenia (15% after consolidation and 3% after maintenance).

Based on the data available, lenalidomide seems to be the most suitable choice for maintenance and can be preferred to thalidomide because of the higher efficacy and the lack of neurologic toxicity.

Bortezomib

Bortezomib is another possible option as maintenance therapy. Peripheral neuropathy associated with this drug may be a limitation, yet its incidence is lower than that reported with thalidomide.

In one study, bortezomib plus either thalidomide (VT) or prednisone (VP) was given after induction with either VMP or bortezomib-thalidomide-prednisone.[36] The median PFS was longer with VT (32 months) than VP (24 months), yet this difference was not statistically significant ($P = .1$). No OS advantage favoring one of the 2 options was detected, and the incidence of peripheral neuropathy was slightly higher with VT (7%) than VP (2%).

In another study, bortezomib-melphalan-prednisone-thalidomide (VMPT) induction followed by VT maintenance (VMPT-VT) was compared with VMP followed by no maintenance.[37] VT consisted of bortezomib at 1.3 mg/m^2 every 15 days and thalidomide at 50 mg per day for 2 years or until progression or relapse. The median PFS was significantly longer with VMPT-VT (35.3 months) than with VMP (24.8 months; HR 0.58; $P<.001$). The 5-year OS was greater with VMPT-VT (61%) than with VMP (51%; HR 0.70; $P = .01$). Of note, the use of once-weekly bortezomib instead of twice-weekly administration seemed to be an appropriate strategy to improve tolerability and decrease discontinuation.[38] During the maintenance phase with VT, the incidence of new or worsened grade 3 to 4 toxicities was low (less than 5%). Grade 3 to 4 neutropenia was reported in 4 patients (3%), peripheral neuropathy in 6 patients (4%), and cardiologic adverse events in 2 patients (1%).

Another study assessed the role of bortezomib alone as maintenance therapy (1.6 mg/m^2, days 1, 8, 15, 22 for five 35-day cycles) after induction with bortezomib-dexamethasone (VD), bortezomib-thalidomide-dexamethasone (VTD), or VMP.[39] The median PFS was 14.7 months with VD, 15.4 months with VTD, and 17.3 months with VMP. The respective median OS was 49.8, 51.5, and 53.1 months. Grade 3 to 4 adverse events were lower with VD (78%) than VTD (87%) and VMP (83%). Bortezomib maintenance was associated with limited additional toxicity compared with induction.

A recent study evaluated the role of a sequential strategy with VMP followed by Rd versus the same regimens in an alternating approach. A total of 18 cycles was planned for both approaches.[40] After a median follow-up of 12 months, the 18-month time to progression was 83% with the sequential strategy and 89% with the alternating approach. A trend in favor of the alternating approach was seen in patients with a high-risk cytogenetics profile (84% vs 94%). The respective 18-month OS was 83% and 93%. Nevertheless, the difference between the 2 options was not statistically significant. Hematologic toxicities were lower in the sequential strategy (neutropenia: 16% vs 23%; thrombocytopenia: 16% vs 20%). Nonhematologic toxicities were low, with infections being the most common (5% vs 4%, respectively). Both the sequential and the alternating approaches proved to be feasible and well tolerated.

In conclusion, bortezomib induces a lower rate of peripheral neuropathy than thalidomide, and maintenance with VT is effective and safe in patients ineligible for MEL200 and AHSCT. The lack of SPM and the possibility of the subcutaneous administration make bortezomib an advantageous strategy for maintenance. Although combining 2 agents associated with a potential risk of neurotoxicity can be a concern, the use of reduced dose intensities makes VT a valid maintenance option. Alternating VMP and Rd is an appealing option, particularly in high-risk patients, but further investigation is needed.

MAINTENANCE APPROACHES FOR PATIENTS ELIGIBLE FOR TRANSPLANTATION

The paradigm in 2014 for transplant-eligible patients consists of induction, stem-cell mobilization, AHSCT, followed by consolidation, and/or maintenance.[41,42] Recent studies have demonstrated improved outcomes in transplant-eligible patients receiving maintenance therapy, and new approaches to consolidation and maintenance are currently being investigated for transplant-eligible patients. This portion of the review focuses on maintenance therapy following AHSCT for transplant-eligible MM patients.

Thalidomide

The maintenance thalidomide studies resulted in improved EFS or PFS with OS that were improved, no different from maintenance, or worse for selected high-risk patients (**Table 2**). Four phase 3 studies looked at thalidomide maintenance until progression (see **Table 2**).[29,30,43-45] The Intergroupe Francophone du Myelome (IFM) randomized 400 patients after AHSCT to thalidomide versus no maintenance and demonstrated an improved 3-year EFS (52% vs 37%, $P<.009$) and an improved 4-year OS (87% vs 75%, $P<.04$).[30] A US single-institution study from the Arkansas group demonstrated a significant benefit for thalidomide versus no thalidomide maintenance. The 5-year EFS was 64% for thalidomide and 43% for no maintenance ($P<.001$), and the 8-year OS was 57% for thalidomide versus 44% for no maintenance ($P = .09$).[43] A Stichting Hemato-Oncologie voor Volwassensen Nederland (Dutch-Belgian Cooperative Trial Group for Hematology Oncology; HOVON) compared thalidomide and interferon-α maintenance and demonstrated that thalidomide improved the median EFS

Table 2
Thalidomide with and without glucocorticoid maintenance following AHSCT

Study	Number of Patients	Initial Dose, mg	Maintenance vs No Maintenance	
			EFS or PFS	OS
Attal et al,[30] 2006	597	400	3-y EFS 52 vs 37% ($P<.009$)	4-y OS 87 vs 75% ($P<.04$)
Barlogie et al,[43] 2008	668	400	5-y EFS 64 vs 43% ($P<.001$)	8-y OS 57 vs 44% ($P = .09$)
Lokhorst et al.[44]	556	50	Median EFS 43 vs 22 mo ($P<.001$)	Median OS 73 vs 60 mo ($P = .77$)
Morgan et al.[29,45] 2012, 2013	820[a]	50	Median PFS (HSCT) 30 vs 23 mo ($P = .003$)	3 y OS 75 vs 80% ($P = .26$)
Spencer et al,[46] 2009	243	200 and prednisolone	3-y PFS 42 vs 23% ($P<.001$)	3-y OS 86 vs 75% ($P = .004$)
Krishnan et al,[47] 2011	436[b]	200 and dexamethasone	3 y PFS 49 vs 43% ($P = .08$)	3 y OS 80 vs 81% ($P = .817$)
Maiolino et al,[48] 2012	108	200 and dexamethasone	2 y PFS 64 vs 30% ($P = .002$)	2 y OS 85 vs 70% ($P = .27$)
Stewart et al,[49] 2013	332	200 and prednisone	4 y PFS 32 vs 14% ($P<.0001$)	4 y OS 68 vs 60 ($P = .18$)

[a] This cohort was part of a larger 1910-patient study examining other nontransplant therapies.
[b] This cohort was part of a larger 710-patient study examining allogeneic and autologous HSCT.
Adapted from McCarthy PL. Part I: the role of maintenance therapy in patients with multiple myeloma undergoing autologous hematopoietic stem cell transplantation. J Natl Compr Canc Netw 2013;11(1):36.

(34 vs 22 months, $P<.001$) and resulted in a nonsignificant increase in median OS (73 vs 60 months, $P = .77$).[44] The Medical Research Council of the United Kingdom (MRC UK) Myeloma IX study examined intensive (transplant) and nonintensive (nontransplant) approaches for the treatment of newly diagnosed MM patients. For the transplant arm, thalidomide maintenance resulted in a median PFS of 22 months versus 15 months for the no-maintenance arm ($P<.0001$). The median OS was 60 months in both groups ($P = .70$).[29,45] The median PFS benefit due to thalidomide maintenance was seen only in the patients with low-risk cytogenetics analyses at diagnosis (29 vs 18 months, $P = .01$) but without OS benefit. For patients with high-risk cytogenetic analyses, the OS was inferior for patients receiving thalidomide maintenance when compared with no maintenance (35 vs 47 months, $P = .01$).

There have been 4 studies that have examined thalidomide plus glucocorticoids as maintenance after AHSCT.[46–49] An Australian study compared 243 patients receiving 1 year of thalidomide with prednisolone until progression to patients receiving prednisolone alone until progression.[46] The 3-year PFS for the thalidomide/prednisolone arm is 42%, and 23% for the prednisolone-only arm ($P<.001$). The 3-year OS for the thalidomide/prednisolone arm was 86%, and 75% for the prednisolone-only arm ($P = .004$). A US trial, BMT-CTN 0102, compared AHSCT followed by reduced-intensity allogeneic HSCT with tandem AHSCT as the primary objective.[47] Patients were assessed as low or high risk based on clinical and cytogenetic features. The tandem AHSCT patients received thalidomide and dexamethasone maintenance or observation alone. Following the first AHSCT, the 3-year PFS for low- (standard) risk MM patients randomized to thalidomide and dexamethasone was 49% and 43% in the observation arm ($P = .08$). There was no difference in the 3-year OS: 80% for the thalidomide and dexamethasone arm and 81% for the observation group ($P = .82$). A Brazilian study looked at 108 MM patients receiving single AHSCT by randomizing them to 12 months of either thalidomide and dexamethasone or dexamethasone-alone maintenance.[48] The 2-year PFS was 64% for the thalidomide and dexamethasone arm and 30% for the dexamethasone-only arm ($P = .002$). There was no difference in the 2-year OS: 85% for the thalidomide and dexamethasone arm and 70% for the dexamethasone-alone arm ($P = .27$). The National Cancer Institute of Canada Clinical Trials Group and the Eastern Cooperative Oncology Group maintenance study randomized 332 MM patients receiving a single AHSCT to thalidomide and prednisone versus observation after AHSCT.[49] The PFS for thalidomide-prednisone was superior to observation (4-year estimates: 32% vs 14%; HR 0.56; $P<.0001$). At 4 years median follow-up, the OS was 68% for thalidomide and prednisone and 60% for observation ($P = .18$). Lower-risk or standard-risk MM patients benefited the most from maintenance therapy. Prolonged maintenance was not tolerated by a significant proportion of patients in all of the thalidomide studies.

Zoledronate

Zoledronate was compared with clodronate as supportive care during induction and maintenance therapy for the MM patient receiving intensive (including AHSCT) and nonintensive (non-AHSCT) therapy for the initial treatment.[45,50] The primary maintenance question was the use of thalidomide therapy until progression with a secondary objective asking if every 3- to 4-week zoledronate therapy until progression would result in less skeletal-related events than daily oral clodronate. In the early report, for AHSCT patients, the median OS was not reached for the zoledronate arm and was 62 months for the clodronate arm (HR 0.84, 95% CI, 0.68–1.03; $P = .0854$). When combining both intensively and nonintensively treated patients, the median PFS was significantly longer in patients randomized to zoledronate when compared with patients randomized to clodronate (19 vs 18 months; HR 0.89; 95% CI, 0.80–0.98; $P = .02$). The median OS was significantly longer for patients receiving zoledronate (52 vs 46 months; HR, 0.86; 95% CI, 0.77–0.97; $P = .01$). There were more incidences of osteonecrosis of the jaw (ONJ) with zoledronate versus clodronate (3.7% vs 0.5%; $P<.0001$), and most ONJ events were considered low grade. These results imply that zoledronate may have an anti-MM effect as has been previously described.[51] Recent recommendations for bisphosphonate therapy were monthly for a year, then change to every 3 months in year 2, and then stop.[52] The early recognition and management of ONJ, the superiority of long-term use of zoledronate over pamidronate for decreasing skeletal-related events,[53] and the MRC IX trial results give consideration for zoledronate therapy until progression or at a minimum the continuation of zoledronate with active disease and resumption at disease progression.[45]

Lenalidomide

There are 2 phase 3 studies that have examined lenalidomide maintenance therapy after AHSCT.[54,55] A third study has reported preliminary results examining lenalidomide maintenance after chemotherapy or AHSCT.[56] A fourth study has examined lenalidomide alone versus lenalidomide plus prednisone after chemotherapy or AHSCT.[57] The studies are compared in **Table 3**.

The CALGB 100104 study randomized 462 newly diagnosed MM patients who had received various induction regimens to lenalidomide 10 mg daily (dose range 5–15 mg) versus placebo until progression after single AHSCT.[54] Of the induction regimens, 74% contained either thalidomide or lenalidomide in combination with other agents. There was no pre-AHSCT or post-AHSCT consolidation. The median time to progression (TTP) was 46 months for the lenalidomide arm and 27 months for the placebo arm ($P<.001$). The 3-year PFS was 66% for the lenalidomide arm and 39% for the placebo arm ($P<.001$). With a median follow-up of 34 months, the 3-year OS rate for the lenalidomide arm was 88% and 80% for the placebo arm ($P = .028$). The primary endpoint of TTP was met early and the study was unblinded 22 months before this analysis when 86 of 128 eligible (nonprogressing) placebo-arm patients crossed over and began lenalidomide. Despite the crossover, there has been a persistent TTP and OS benefit for the lenalidomide arm. An updated analysis was performed in 2013 at a median follow-up of 48 months: the OS was 80% for the lenalidomide group and 70% for the placebo group ($P = .008$).[58] A PFS advantage persisted for the lenalidomide arm. Patients receiving lenalidomide had an increased incidence of hematologic toxicities (neutropenia and thrombocytopenia) as well as an increase in SPM. There were 8 of 231 (3.5%) hematologic malignancies, primarily myeloid malignancies (acute myeloid leukemia/myelodysplastic syndrome [AML/MDS], n = 6) on the lenalidomide arm and 1 of 229 (0.4%), non-Hodgkin lymphoma (n = 1) on the placebo arm. There were 10 of 231 (4.3%) versus 5 (2.1%) solid tumors on the lenalidomide and 4 of 231 (1.7%) on the placebo arm. The SPM cumulative incidence risk was greater for the lenalidomide arm ($P<.008$). The cumulative incidence risks of progressive disease ($P<.001$) or death ($P<.002$) were greater for the placebo arm. When counting events as progressions, deaths, and SPMs, the median EFS was 43 months for the lenalidomide arm and 27 months for the placebo arm ($P<.001$).

The IFM 05-02 study examined 605 patients randomized to lenalidomide at the same dose range as CALGB 100104 versus placebo until progression after single (79%) or 2 AHSCT (21%). After the first or second AHSCT, all patients received a 2-cycle consolidation treatment of 25 mg lenalidomide for 3 weeks of 4 at approximately day 60 to day 120 post-AHSCT. Induction regimens consisted of vincristine, doxorubicin, and dexamethasone (VAD) or VD. Twenty-five percent of patients received

Table 3
Lenalidomide alone or with glucocorticoid maintenance after AHSCT

Study	Number of Patients	Initial Dose, mg	Maintenance vs No Maintenance	
			EFS or PFS	OS
McCarthy et al,[54] 2012	460	10	TTP 46 vs 27 mo (P<.001)	Median follow-up 34 mo 85 vs 77% (P = .028)
			3-y PFS rate 66% (95% CI, 59–73) vs 39% (95% CI, 33–48) EFS 43 vs 27 mo (P<.001)	3-y OS rate 88% (95% CI, 84–93) vs 80% (95% CI, 74–86)
McCarthy et al,[58] 2013				Median follow-up 48 mo 80 vs 70% (P = .008)
Attal et al,[55] 2012	614	10	PFS 41 vs 23 mo (P<.001)	Median follow-up 45 mo 74 vs 76% (P = .7)
			4 y PFS 43 vs 22% (P<.001) EFS 40 vs 23 mo (P<.001)	4-y OS 73 vs 75% (NS)
Attal et al,[59] 2013			5-y PFS 42% vs 18% (P<.001)	Median follow-up 70 mo 5-y OS 68 vs 67% (NS)
Gay et al,[56] 2013	202 (NIT) 200 (IT)	10 (3 of 4 wk monthly)	Landmark Analysis Median PFS (combining NIT and IT groups) 42 vs 18 mo (P<.001)	4-y OS (combining NIT and IT groups) 80 vs 62% (P = .01)
Palumbo et al,[57] 2013	194 (NIT) 195 (IT)	10: days 1–21 of 28 d +/− P 50: every other day	3-y PFS (combining NIT and IT groups) RP: 60% vs 38% for R alone (P = .003)	31-mo median follow-up (combining NIT and IT groups) 3-y OS (NIT and IT) ND

Abbreviations: EFS, event-free survival includes deaths, progressions, and second cancers; IT, intensive therapy; ND, no difference; NIT, nonintensive therapy; NS, not significant; P, prednisone; R, lenalidomide.

Adapted from McCarthy PL. Part I: the role of maintenance therapy in patients with multiple myeloma undergoing autologous hematopoietic stem cell transplantation. J Natl Compr Canc Netw 2013;11(1):37.

pre-AHSCT consolidation with dexamethasone, cyclophosphamide, etoposide, and cisplatin. The median PFS was 41 months for the lenalidomide-arm patients and 23 months for the placebo-arm patients (P<.001). At 4 years, the PFS was 43% for the lenalidomide-arm patients and 22% for the placebo-arm patients (P<.001). At a 45-month median follow-up, the OS was 74% for the lenalidomide arm and 76% for the placebo arm. The 4-year OS rates were 73% for the lenalidomide arm and 75% for the placebo arm (P = .7). The study was also unblinded 22 months before analysis. All maintenance was stopped at a median time of 2 years (range 1–3 years). There was no crossover for the placebo-arm patients. This study was updated recently.[59] Now, with a median follow-up of 60 months from randomization, the lenalidomide arm had an improved PFS (42%) compared with the placebo arm (18%) (P<.0001). At 5 years, the OS for the lenalidomide arm is 68% and 67% for the placebo arm (HR 1). After the first progression, the median survival is 29 months for the lenalidomide arm and 48 months for the placebo arm (P<.0001). There was an increased incidence of hematologic toxicities (primarily neutropenia and thrombocytopenia) and increased incidence of SPMs in the lenalidomide arm. There were 13 of 306 (4.2%) hematologic malignancies, primarily lymphoid malignancies (acute lymphocytic leukemia and Hodgkin lymphoma, n = 7) for lenalidomide-arm patients and 5 of 302 (1.6%) primarily AML/MDS (n = 4), for the placebo-arm patients. For solid tumors, there were 10 of 306 (3.3%) in lenalidomide-arm patients and 4 of 302 (1.3%) in placebo-arm patients. The median EFS (including progressions, deaths, and SPMs) was 40 months for the lenalidomide arm and 23 months for the placebo arm (P<.001).

The third lenalidomide maintenance study following chemotherapy (melphalan, prednisone, lenalidomide) versus tandem AHSCT with high-dose melphalan (MPR vs MEL200) was reported.[56] Both chemotherapy and tandem AHSCT maintenance patients were combined and compared with those chemotherapy and tandem AHSCT patients who did not receive lenalidomide maintenance. At 49 months median follow-up, from chemotherapy or tandem AHSCT and at 35 months median follow-up from randomization to lenalidomide maintenance or no maintenance, the 3-year PFS for the lenalidomide maintenance patients was 37 months and 26 months for patients not receiving maintenance (P<.0001). Five-year OS estimates were 75% for the lenalidomide arm and 58% for the no-maintenance arm (P = .02). The rate of SPMs was 4.5% in both maintenance arms (chemotherapy and tandem AHSCT). Another GIMEMA study examined maintenance therapy with lenalidomide plus prednisone versus lenalidomide alone following chemotherapy (cyclophosphamide, lenalidomide, prednisone) versus tandem AHSCT (CRD vs MEL200) in 389 newly diagnosed MM patients.[57] The chemotherapy and tandem AHSCT patients randomized to receive lenalidomide/prednisone maintenance were combined and compared with the chemotherapy and tandem AHSCT patients who were randomized to receive lenalidomide alone. At 31 months median follow-up from chemotherapy or tandem AHSCT, the 3-year PFS for the lenalidomide/prednisone arm was 60% and 38% for lenalidomide alone (P = .003). There was no difference in 3-year OS.

A meta-analysis of IFM 05 02, CALGB 100104, MPR versus Mel200, and MM 015[31] (a nontransplant trial) found that lenalidomide maintenance when compared with placebo improves PFS with a trend to an OS benefit.[60] **Table 4** compares the differences between CALGB 100104 and IFM 05-02, which may help to explain the differences in OS, and types of SPM. In particular, there are differences in induction regimens, number of transplants, use of consolidation pre-AHSCT and post-AHSCT, and length of maintenance therapy.

The SPM etiologic risk factors are not fully defined. MM and monoclonal gammopathy of unknown significance (MGUS) have been associated with the development of AML/MDS.[61] In this registry study, MGUS patients would have not received therapy, implying that there is an undefined stem cell defect in MGUS patients and by inference MM patients (who have the addition risk of chemotherapy exposure) predisposing to the development of myeloid malignancies. A recent meta-analysis of 7 randomized controlled trials of more than 3000 newly diagnosed MM patients found that those who received lenalidomide had an increased risk of developing hematologic SPMs, driven mainly by treatment strategies that included a combination of lenalidomide and oral melphalan.[32] Lenalidomide treatment with intravenous melphalan and other

Table 4
Differences between CALGB 100104 and IFM 05 02

Comparisons	CALGB 100104[54]	IFM 2005-02[55]
Induction	Thal- or Len-based (74%)	VAD (52%) and VD (44%)
Pre-AHSCT consolidation	None	DCEP (25%)
Number of AHSCT	One	1 (79%), 2 (21%)
Post-AHSCT consolidation before randomization	None	Len: 25 mg daily, 3 of 4 wk for 2 cycles before day 100
Median follow-up at unblinding	18 mo	33 mo
Median follow-up from randomization	65 mo	62 mo
Cytogenetic stratification	Not available	More high risk in Len arm
Dosing schedule	10 mg (5–15 mg)	10 mg (5–15 mg)
Time from first patient enrolled	90 mo	74 mo
Placebo patients crossed over to Len at unblinding	Yes (86 of 128 nonprogressing patients)	No cross-over
Second primary malignancies	3-fold increase	2.6-fold increase
Increase in AML/MDS	Yes	No
Increase in ALL/HL	No	Yes
Maintenance stopped	No	Yes at a median of 2 y (range 1–3)
OS after progression[a]	No difference between arms	Worse for Len than for placebo

Abbreviations: AHSCT, autologous hematopoietic stem cell transplant; ALL/HL, acute lymphocytic leukemia/Hodgkin lymphoma; DCEP, dexamethasone/cyclophosphamide/etoposide/cisplatin; Len, lenalidomide; Thal, thalidomide; VAD, vincristine/doxorubicin/dexamethasone; VD, bortezomib/dexamethasone.
[a] Preliminary analysis.
Adapted from McCarthy PL. Part I: the role of maintenance therapy in patients with multiple myeloma undergoing autologous hematopoietic stem cell transplantation. J Natl Compr Canc Netw 2013;11(1):38.

agents did not carry as high a risk as oral melphalan for the development of SPMs. Furthermore, with lenalidomide therapy, the risk of dying from MM or treatment-related adverse events remained higher than the risk of death due to SPMs. The HOVON-65/German-speaking-Myeloma Multicenter Group (GMMG)-HD4 2-year bortezomib maintenance was not associated with an increase in SPM.[62] The risk of SPM needs to be factored and balanced against the beneficial effects on PFS and OS when patients and clinicians decide on the use of maintenance treatment. So far, there is no OS benefit seen with the recent IFM 05-02 analysis. Future and ongoing studies should facilitate the understanding of the optimal maintenance strategies for long-term control of MM.

The IFM 05-02, MRC UK IX, Programa para el Estudio de la Terapéutica en Hemopatías Malignas (PETHEMA), and HOVON 65 GMMG HD4 studies used induction regimens that are being superseded by novel agent combinations. The CALGB 100104 study contained patients who received older thalidomide-based induction regimens in addition to lenalidomide-containing regimens. Thus, these studies need to be evaluated relative to the induction regimens in use today. New studies incorporating newer agents, in particular bortezomib and lenalidomide, are underway and are described later in this review. Unlike induction regimens, the standard AHSCT conditioning regimens remain high-dose melphalan alone or in combination with agents such as bortezomib.

MM patients receiving induction therapy followed by consolidation with high-dose melphalan and AHSCT often will have disease progression and relapse. Therefore, maintaining disease response is an important goal for MM management after AHSCT. Depth of response as manifested by the presence or absence of minimal residual disease correlates with long-term disease control.[63,64] However, factors such as disease staging, cytogenetics, and gene expression profiling predict long-term outcome.[65] Thus, there have been attempts to incorporate cytogenetic risk factors and minimal residual disease detection.[66] Determining the most effective combination of induction, transplant dose intensive therapy, consolidation, and maintenance will be accomplished with a goal of improved survival endpoints, patient tolerance, and patient quality of life.

AHSCT is a standard approach to the management of transplant-eligible MM patients after induction therapy. The superiority of AHSCT over prolonged lower-dose therapy has been demonstrated before use of bortezomib and lenalidomide in induction therapy.[67,68] A recent phase 3 study has shown a superior PFS and OS for early tandem transplant versus continued lower-dose therapy. There are recently completed and ongoing phase 3 studies that examine the utility of up-front versus delayed AHSCT, the role of consolidation and single versus tandem AHSCT, and the use of maintenance therapy.[69–72] The recently completed STAMINA trial (Stem cell transplant with lenalidomide maintenance in patients with multiple myeloma), BMT-CTN 0702, compared single, tandem AHSCT and single AHSCT, followed by lenalidomide, bortezomib, and dexamethasone consolidation.[69] Induction regimens were at the discretion of the enrolling centers. Originally, all 3 arms were to be followed by lenalidomide maintenance for 3 years. The protocol has been amended to extend maintenance until progression. The European Myeloma Network (EMN) trial, Study to Compare VMP With HDM Followed by VRD Consolidation, and Lenalidomide Maintenance in Patients With Newly Diagnosed Multiple Myeloma EMN 2 (HO95) will treat all NDMM patients with an induction regimen of bortezomib, cyclophosphamide, and dexamethasone. Patients are randomized to 3 arms: bortezomib, melphalan, prednisone therapy, single or tandem AHSCT. After completion of this segment of the protocol, patients will either receive no consolidation or consolidation with lenalidomide, bortezomib, and dexamethasone before all patients receive lenalidomide maintenance until progression.[70] The Dana Farber Cancer Institute (DFCI 10–106) (IFM DFCI 2009) randomized trial compares 8 cycles of lenalidomide, bortezomib, and dexamethasone, cyclophosphamide mobilization of hematopoietic stem cells, and AHSCT at relapse with 3 cycles of lenalidomide, bortezomib, and dexamethasone, cyclophosphamide mobilization of hematopoietic stem cells, and up-front AHSCT followed by 2 cycles of lenalidomide, bortezomib, and dexamethasone consolidation.[71] The IFM will treat patients with 1 year of lenalidomide maintenance. The study in the United States has been changed to maintenance lenalidomide until progression. The MRC myeloma XI trial, a randomized comparison of thalidomide and lenalidomide combinations in myeloma patients of all ages, will enroll patients on either an intensive (transplant) pathway or a nonintensive (nontransplant) pathway.[72] The intensive pathway compares 2 induction regimens and examines consolidation or no consolidation pre-AHSCT for patients with less than a very good partial response. After single AHSCT, patients will be randomized to no maintenance or lenalidomide maintenance until disease progression.

Bortezomib

Bortezomib, the first proteasome inhibitor approved for the treatment of MM, has been studied as part of both induction and maintenance therapy. The HOVON-65/GMMG-HD4 randomized 827 symptomatic and newly diagnosed MM patients to either of 2 induction regimens: VAD or PAD.[62] After induction, all patients underwent stem cell mobilization with cyclophosphamide, doxorubicin, and dexamethasone with granulocyte colony-stimulating factor followed by stem cell collection. Some high-risk patients eligible for allogeneic HSCT received VAD 5% and PAD 7%. German patients underwent tandem AHSCT due to clinical practice. Most VAD (84%) and PAD patients

Table 5
Bortezomib and zoledronate maintenance after AHSCT

Study	Number of Patients	Initial Dose	Maintenance vs No Maintenance	
			PFS	OS
Morgan et al,[50] 2010	1111 (IT) 851 (NIT)	Zoledronate: 4 mg IV every 3–4 wk or Clodronate 1600 mg orally daily	IT Median PFS 25 vs 25 mo	Median OS for IT patients Not reached vs 62.5 mo HR, 0.84 (95% CI, 0.68–1.03) $P = .0854$ Median OS for all patients 50 vs 45.5 mo HR 0.87 (95% CI 0.77–0.99) $P = .04$
Sonneveld et al,[62] 2012	827	Bortezomib: 1.3 mg/m² IV every 2 wk for 2 y or Thalidomide 50 mg daily	Median PFS 35 vs 28 mo $P = .002$	Median follow-up 41 mo OS (MV analysis) HR, 0.77 (95% CI, 0.60–1.00) $P = .049$
			Landmark analysis for those without progression at 1 y 45 vs 38% progression-free $P = .05$	5-y OS 61 vs 55% $P = .07$
Rosiñol et al,[73] 2012	386	Bortezomib 1.3 mg/m² IV on days 1, 4, 8, and 11 every 3 mo with thalidomide100 mg per day orally or thalidomide 100 mg per day orally alone or Interferon-α (3 million units SC 3 times weekly)	2 y PFS at a median follow-up of 24 mo 78 vs 63 vs 49% $P = .01$	OS not significantly different

Abbreviations: IT, intensive therapy; IV, intravenous; MV, multivariate; NIT, nonintensive therapy; OS, overall survival; PFS, progression-free survival; SC, subcutaneous.

Adapted from McCarthy PL. Part I: the role of maintenance therapy in patients with multiple myeloma undergoing autologous hematopoietic stem cell transplantation. J Natl Compr Canc Netw 2013;11(1):39.

(85%) underwent single or tandem AHSCT followed by 2 years of maintenance. The VAD arm received thalidomide and the PAD arm received bortezomib. The study was first reported at a median follow-up of 41 months. The median PFS for the PAD-P arm was 35 months and for the VAD-T arm was 28 months ($P = .002$) (**Table 5**). The multivariate analysis established an HR for PAD-P of 0.77 (95% CI, 0.60 to 1.00, $P = .049$). Patients with the poor-risk cytogenetic feature of del 17p13 receiving PAD-P had an improved median PFS (22 vs 12 months, $P = .01$) and improved OS (not reached at 54 months vs 24 months, $P = .003$) when compared with VAD-T. Patients in renal failure at diagnosis also had an improved PFS and OS when PAD-P was compared with VAD-T. There was no difference in PFS and OS for other cytogenetic risk groups. The Spanish Myeloma group (Grupo Espanol de Mieloma PETHEMA) conducted a 386-patient trial that randomized newly diagnosed MM patients to 3 different induction treatments: VTD versus TD versus alternating chemotherapy: vincristine, carmustine, melphalan, cyclophosphamide, prednisone/ vincristine, carmustine, doxorubicin, dexamethasone.[73] Following induction, all eligible patients received a single AHSCT. All 3 induction groups were randomized to maintenance therapy for 3 years with interferon-α versus T or VT. At a median follow-up of 2 years from maintenance initiation, the PFS for the VT maintenance treatment was significantly longer than T or interferon-α (78% vs 63% vs 49%; $P = .01$). For the 3 arms, there was no difference in OS (see **Table 2**).

SUMMARY

The introduction of novel agent-based maintenance therapy has considerably prolonged remission duration for MM patients. In transplant-ineligible patients, standard induction therapies consist of novel-agent–based 3-drug regimens. Two-drug regimens and gentler approaches with reduced doses are suggested in frail patients. The route of administration is fundamental while choosing maintenance therapy: thalidomide and lenalidomide have the advantage of oral administration in comparison with intravenous bortezomib. Of note, in patients ineligible for transplantation, an OS benefit was reported with bortezomib maintenance, while it was inconsistently detected with strategies including thalidomide and lenalidomide. The optimal maintenance approach should also be associated with a low toxicity to preserve quality of life. Peripheral neuropathy is a major concern with continuous thalidomide, less frequent with bortezomib, while it is not reported with lenalidomide. Nevertheless, lenalidomide is associated with an increased risk of SPM. Future trials are needed to establish which option is the most suitable as maintenance therapy for transplant-ineligible subjects, and head-to-head comparisons are therefore necessary. The optimal duration of treatment is another crucial point that needs further investigation. In conclusion, the data available show that a sequential approach including induction therapy followed by consolidation and maintenance therapy is an appropriate and effective strategy in MM.

The current treatment standard for the transplant-eligible patient is induction therapy, preferably with 3 agents, including novel agents (proteasome inhibitor and/or immunomodulatory drugs [IMiD]). Induction treatment is given to the best response with the goal of attainment of CR. Trials in the United States and Europe will help define the optimal induction regimen, the role of single or tandem AHSCT, or delayed AHSCT after salvage therapy at relapse. Consolidation therapy following AHSCT is discussed in another article in this issue. Following AHSCT with or without consolidation, maintenance therapy is becoming a standard approach to maintain response and control disease long term. The optimal maintenance strategy will be defined with future studies.

Understanding risk should allow for developing strategies for long-term disease control based on diagnostic disease characteristics. In addition to cytogenetic risk stratification, gene expression profiling has been developed for defining high-risk patients.[74,75] However, the optimal treatment approach for these high-risk patients has yet to be defined, and these high-risk patients should be evaluated for new approaches. Novel drugs with novel mechanisms of action may offer strategies that could convert high-risk disease into lower disease.[76] Ongoing studies will answer questions regarding the incorporation of new agents into induction treatment, the role of early versus delayed AHSCT, the role of consolidation, and standard approaches to maintenance therapy to prolong and control disease and improve outcome.

ACKNOWLEDGMENTS

The authors wish to thank the editorial assistant Giorgio Schirripa.

REFERENCES

1. Altekruse SF, Kosary CL, Krapcho M, et al, editors. SEER Cancer Statistics review, 1975-2007, National Cancer Institute. Bethesda (MD): Based on November 2009 SEER data submission, posted to the SEER website 2010. Available at: http://seer.cancer.gov/csr/1975_2007/. Accessed January 3, 2014.
2. Munshi NC, Anderson KC. New strategies in the treatment of multiple myeloma. Clin Cancer Res 2013;19(13):3337–44.
3. Kumar SK, Dispenzieri A, Lacy MQ, et al. Continued improvement in survival in multiple myeloma: changes in early mortality and outcomes in older patients. Leukemia 2014;28(5):1122–8.
4. Singhal S, Mehta J, Desikan R, et al. Antitumor activity of thalidomide in refractory multiple myeloma. N Engl J Med 1999;341:1565–71.
5. Palumbo A, Bringhen S, Musto P, et al. Oral melphalan, and prednisone chemotherapy plus thalidomide compared with melphalan and prednisone alone in elderly patients with multiple myeloma: randomized controlled trial. Lancet 2006;367:825–31.
6. Richardson PG, Schlossman RL, Weller E, et al. Immunomodulatory drug CC-5013 overcomes drug resistance and is well tolerated in patients with relapsed multiple myeloma. Blood 2002;100:3063–7.
7. Rajkumar SV, Hayman SR, Lacy MQ, et al. Combination therapy with lenalidomide plus dexamethasone (Rev/Dex) for newly diagnosed myeloma. Blood 2005;106:4050–3.
8. Richardson PG, Barlogie B, Berenson J, et al. A phase 2 study of bortezomib in relapsed, refractory myeloma. N Engl J Med 2003;348:2609–17.
9. Harousseau JL, Attal M, Leleu X, et al. Bortezomib plus dexamethasone as induction treatment prior to autologous stem cell transplantation in patients with newly diagnosed multiple myeloma: results of an IFM phase II study. Haematologica 2006;91:1498–505.
10. San Miguel JF, Schlag R, Khuageva NK, et al. Bortezomib plus melphalan and prednisone for initial treatment of multiple myeloma. N Engl J Med 2008;359: 906–17.
11. Cavo M, Tacchetti P, Patriarca F, et al. Bortezomib with thalidomide plus dexamethasone compared with thalidomide plus dexamethasone as induction therapy before, and consolidation therapy after, double autologous stem-cell

transplantation in newly diagnosed multiple myeloma: a randomized phase 3 study. Lancet 2010;376:2075–85.

12. Kumar S, Flinn I, Richardson PG, et al. Randomized, multicenter, phase 2 study (EVOLUTION) of combinations of bortezomib, dexamethasone, cyclophospha-mide, and lenalidomide in previously untreated multiple myeloma. Blood 2012;10(119):4375–82.

13. Kumar SK, Rajkumar SV, Dispenzieri A, et al. Improved survival in multiple myeloma and the impact of novel therapies. Blood 2008;111(5):2516–20.

14. Palumbo A, Rajkumar SV, San Miguel JF, et al. International Myeloma Working Group consensus statement for the management, treatment, and supportive care of patients with myeloma not eligible for standard autologous stem-cell transplantation. J Clin Oncol 2014;32(6):587–600.

15. Palumbo A, Anderson K. Multiple myeloma. N Engl J Med 2011;364(11): 1046–60.

16. Remission maintenance therapy for multiple myeloma. Arch Intern Med 1975; 135(1):147–52.

17. Belch A, Shelley W, Bergsagel D, et al. A randomized trial of maintenance versus no maintenance melphalan and prednisone in responding multiple myeloma patients. Br J Cancer 1988;57(1):94–9.

18. Fritz E, Ludwig H. Interferon-alpha treatment in multiple myeloma: meta-analysis of 30 randomised trials among 3948 patients. Ann Oncol 2000; 11(11):1427–36.

19. Berenson JR, Crowley JJ, Grogan TM, et al. Maintenance therapy with alternate-day prednisone improves survival in multiple myeloma patients. Blood 2002; 99(9):3163–8.

20. Ludwig H, Durie BG, McCarthy P, et al. IMWG consensus on maintenance ther-apy in multiple myeloma. Blood 2012;119(13):3003–15.

21. Alexanian R, Balcerzak S, Haut A, et al. Remission maintenance therapy for mul-tiple myeloma. Arch Intern Med 1975;135(1):147–52.

22. Alexanian R, Gehan E, Haut A, et al. Unmaintained remissions in multiple myeloma. Blood 1978;51(6):1005–11.

23. Myeloma Trialists' Collaborative Group. Interferon as therapy for multiple myeloma: an individual patient data overview of 24 randomized trials and 4012 patients. Br J Haematol 2001;113(4):1020–34.

24. Palumbo A, Bringhen S, Liberati AM, et al. Oral melphalan, prednisone, and thalidomide in elderly patients with multiple myeloma: updated results of a ran-domized controlled trial. Blood 2008;112(8):3107–14.

25. Wijermans P, Schaafsma M, Termorshuizen F, et al. Phase III study of the value of thalidomide added to melphalan plus prednisone in elderly patients with newly diagnosed multiple myeloma: the HOVON 49 Study. J Clin Oncol 2010; 28(19):3160–6.

26. Waage A, Gimsing P, Fayers P, et al. Melphalan and prednisone plus thalido-mide or placebo in elderly patients with multiple myeloma. Blood 2010;116(9): 1405–12.

27. Beksac M, Haznedar R, Firatli-Tuglular T, et al. Addition of thalidomide to oral melphalan/prednisone in patients with multiple myeloma not eligible for trans-plantation: results of a randomized trial from the Turkish Myeloma Study Group. Eur J Haematol 2011;86(1):16–22.

28. Ludwig H, Adam Z, Tóthová E, et al. Thalidomide maintenance treatment in-creases progression-free but not overall survival in elderly patients with myeloma. Haematologica 2010;95(9):1548–54.

29. Morgan GJ, Gregory WM, Davies FE, et al. The role of maintenance thalidomide therapy in multiple myeloma: MRC Myeloma IX results and meta-analysis. Blood 2012;119(1):7–15.

30. Attal M, Harousseau JL, Leyvraz S, et al. Maintenance therapy with thalidomide improves survival in patients with multiple myeloma. Blood 2006;108(10): 3289–94.

31. Palumbo A, Hajek R, Delforge M, et al. Continuous lenalidomide treatment for newly diagnosed multiple myeloma. N Engl J Med 2012;366(19): 1759–69.

32. Palumbo A, Bringhen S, Kumar SK, et al. Second primary malignancies with lenalidomide therapy for newly diagnosed myeloma: a meta-analysis of individual patient data. Lancet Oncol 2014;15(3):333–42.

33. Falco P, Cavallo F, Larocca A, et al. Lenalidomide-prednisone induction followed by lenalidomide-melphalan-prednisone consolidation and lenalidomide-prednisone maintenance in newly diagnosed elderly unfit myeloma patients. Leukemia 2013;27(3):695–701.

34. Facon T, Dimopoulos MA, Dispenzieri A, et al. Initial phase 3 results of the first (frontline investigation of lenalidomide + dexamethasone versus standard thalidomide) Trial (MM-020/IFM 07 01) in newly diagnosed multiple myeloma (NDMM) patients (Pts) ineligible for stem cell transplantation (SCT). Blood 2013;122(Suppl):21 [abstract 2].

35. Gay F, Magarotto V, Crippa C, et al. Bortezomib induction, reduced-intensity transplantation, and lenalidomide consolidation-maintenance for myeloma: updated results. Blood 2013;122(8):1376–83.

36. Mateos MV, Oriol A, Martínez-López J, et al. Bortezomib, melphalan, and prednisone versus bortezomib, thalidomide, and prednisone as induction therapy followed by maintenance treatment with bortezomib and thalidomide versus bortezomib and prednisone in elderly patients with untreated multiple myeloma: a randomised trial. Lancet Oncol 2010;11(10):934–41.

37. Palumbo A, Bringhen S, Larocca A, et al. Bortezomib-melphalan-prednisone-thalidomide followed by maintenance with bortezomib-thalidomide compared with bortezomib-melphalan-prednisone for initial treatment of multiple myeloma: updated follow-up and improved survival. J Clin Oncol 2014;32(7):634–40.

38. Bringhen S, Larocca A, Rossi D, et al. Efficacy and safety of once-weekly bortezomib in multiple myeloma patients. Blood 2010;116(23):4745–53.

39. Niesvizky R, Flinn I, Rifkin RM, et al. Efficacy and safety of three bortezomib-based induction and maintenance regimens in previously untreated, transplant-ineligible multiple myeloma (MM) patients (Pts): final results from the randomized, phase 3b, US community-based upfront study (NCT00507416). Blood 2013; 122(Suppl):21 [abstract 1966].

40. Mateos MV, Martínez-López J, Hernandez MT, et al. Comparison of sequential vs alternating administration of bortezomib, melphalan and prednisone (VMP) and lenalidomide plus dexamethasone (Rd) in elderly patients with newly diagnosed multiple myeloma (MM) patients: GEM2010MAS65 trial. Blood 2013; 122(Suppl):21 [abstract 403].

41. Reece D. Update on the initial therapy of multiple myeloma. Am Soc Clin Oncol Educ Book 2013;307–12.

42. McCarthy PL, Hahn T. strategies for induction, autologous hematopoietic stem cell transplantation, consolidation, and maintenance for transplantation-eligible multiple myeloma patients. Hematology Am Soc Hematol Educ Program 2013;2013:496–503.

43. Barlogie B, Pineda-Roman M, van Rhee F, et al. Thalidomide arm of total therapy 2 improves complete remission duration and survival in myeloma patients with metaphase cytogenetic abnormalities. Blood 2008;112(8):3115–21.
44. Lokhorst HM, van der Holt B, Zweegman S, et al. A randomized phase 3 study on the effect of thalidomide combined with adriamycin, dexamethasone, and high-dose melphalan, followed by thalidomide maintenance in patients with multiple myeloma. Blood 2010;115(6):1113–20.
45. Morgan GJ, Davies FE, Gregory WM, et al. Long-term follow-up of MRC myeloma IX trial: survival outcomes with bisphosphonate and thalidomide treatment. Clin Cancer Res 2013;19(21):6030–8.
46. Spencer A, Prince HM, Roberts AW, et al. Consolidation therapy with low-dose thalidomide and prednisolone prolongs the survival of multiple myeloma patients undergoing a single autologous stem-cell transplantation procedure. J Clin Oncol 2009;27(11):1788–93.
47. Krishnan A, Pasquini MC, Logan B, et al. Autologous haemopoietic stem-cell transplantation followed by allogeneic or autologous haemopoietic stem-cell transplantation in patients with multiple myeloma (BMT CTN 0102): a phase 3 biological assignment trial. Lancet Oncol 2011;12(13):1195–203.
48. Maiolino A, Hungria VT, Garnica M, et al. Thalidomide plus dexamethasone as a maintenance therapy after autologous hematopoietic stem cell transplantation improves progression-free survival in multiple myeloma. Am J Hematol 2012; 87(10):948–52.
49. Stewart AK, Trudel S, Bahlis NJ, et al. A randomized phase 3 trial of thalidomide and prednisone as maintenance therapy after ASCT in patients with MM with a quality-of-life assessment: the National Cancer Institute of Canada Clinicals Trials Group myeloma 10 trial. Blood 2013;121(9):1517–23.
50. Morgan GJ, Davies FE, Gregory WM, et al. First-line treatment with zoledronic acid as compared with clodronic acid in multiple myeloma (MRC Myeloma IX): a randomised controlled trial. Lancet 2010;376(9757):1989–99.
51. Corso A, Ferretti E, Lazzarino M. Zoledronic acid exerts its antitumor effect in multiple myeloma interfering with the bone marrow microenvironment. Hematology 2005;10(3):215–24.
52. Terpos E, Morgan G, Dimopoulos MA, et al. International Myeloma Working Group recommendations for the treatment of multiple myeloma-related bone disease. J Clin Oncol 2013;31(18):2347–57.
53. Rosen LS, Gordon D, Kaminski M, et al. Long-term efficacy and safety of zoledronic acid compared with pamidronate disodium in the treatment of skeletal complications in patients with advanced multiple myeloma or breast carcinoma: a randomized, double-blind, multicenter, comparative trial. Cancer 2003;98: 1735–44.
54. McCarthy PL, Owzar K, Hofmeister CC, et al. Lenalidomide after stem-cell transplantation for multiple myeloma. N Engl J Med 2012;366(19):1770–81.
55. Attal M, Lauwers-Cances V, Marit G, et al. Lenalidomide maintenance after stem-cell transplantation for multiple myeloma. N Engl J Med 2012;366(19):1782–91.
56. Gay F, Cavallo F, Caravita T, et al. Maintenance therapy with lenalidomide significantly improved survival of yong newly diagnosed multiple myeloma patients. Blood 2013;122:2089.
57. Palumbo A, Gay F, Spencer A, et al. A phase III study of ASCT vs cyclophosphamide-lenalidomide-dexamethasone and lenalidomide-prednisone maintenance vs lenalidomide alone in newly diagnosed myeloma patients. Blood 2013;122:763.

58. McCarthy P, Owzar K, Hofmeister CC, et al. Analysis of overall survival (OS) in the context of cross-over from placebo to lenalidomide and the incidence of second primary malignancies (SPM) in the phase III study of lenalidomide versus placebo maintenance therapy following autologous stem cell transplant (ASCT) for multiple myeloma (MM) CALGB (Alliance) ECOG BMTCTN. Clin Lymphoma Myeloma Leuk 2013;13(Suppl 1):S28 [abstract S15–5].

59. Attal M, Lauwers-Cances V, Marit G, et al. Lenalidomide maintenance after stem-cell transplantation for multiple myeloma: follow-up analysis of The IFM 2005-02 trial. Blood 2013;122:406a.

60. Singh PP, Kumar S, LaPlant BR, et al. Lenalidomide maintenance therapy in multiple myeloma: a meta-analysis of randomized trials. Blood 2013;122:407a.

61. Mailankody S, Pfeiffer RM, Kristinsson SY, et al. Risk of acute myeloid leukemia and myelodysplastic syndromes after multiple myeloma and its precursor disease (MGUS). Blood 2011;118:4086–92.

62. Sonneveld P, Schmidt-Wolf IG, van der Holt B, et al. Bortezomib induction and maintenance treatment in patients with newly diagnosed multiple myeloma: results of the randomized phase III HOVON-65/GMMG-HD4 trial. J Clin Oncol 2012;30(24):2946–55.

63. Paiva B, Vidriales MB, Cerveró J, et al. GEM (Grupo Español de MM)/PETHEMA (Programa para el Estudio de la Terapéutica en Hemopatías Malignas) Cooperative Study Groups. Multiparameter flow cytometric remission is the most relevant prognostic factor for multiple myeloma patients who undergo autologous stem cell transplantation. Blood 2008;112:4017–23.

64. Rawstron AC, Child JA, de Tute RM, et al. Minimal residual disease assessed by multiparameter flow cytometry in multiple myeloma: impact on outcome in the Medical Research Council Myeloma IX Study [Erratum appears in J Clin Oncol 2013;31(34):4383]. J Clin Oncol 2013;31(20):2540–7. http://dx.doi.org/10.1200/JCO.2012.46.2119.

65. Chng WJ, Dispenzieri A, Chim CS, et al. IMWG consensus on risk stratification in multiple myeloma. International Myeloma Working Group. Leukemia 2014;28(2):269–77.

66. Paiva B, Gutierrez NC, Rosinol L, et al. High-risk cytogenetics and persistent minimal residual disease by multiparameter flow cytometry predict unsustained complete response after autologous stem cell transplantation in multiple myeloma. Blood 2012;119(3):687–91.

67. Attal M, Harousseau JL, Stoppa AM, et al. A prospective, randomized trial of autologous bone marrow transplantation and chemotherapy in multiple myeloma. Intergroupe Francais du Myelome. N Engl J Med 1996;335(2):91–7.

68. Child JA, Morgan GJ, Davies FE, et al. High-dose chemotherapy with hematopoietic stem-cell rescue for multiple myeloma. N Engl J Med 2003;348(19):1875–83.

69. Stem cell transplant with lenalidomide maintenance in patients with multiple myeloma. Availabe at: http://clinicaltrials.gov/ct2/show/NCT01109004. Accessed July 17, 2014.

70. Study to compare VMP with HDM followed by VRD consolidation and lenalidomide maintenance in patients with newly diagnosed multiple myeloma EMN 2 (HO95). Available at: http://clinicaltrials.gov/ct2/show/NCT01208766. Accessed July 17, 2014.

71. Randomized trial of lenalidomide, bortezomib, dexamethasone vs high-dose treatment with SCT in MM patients up to age 65 (DFCI 10-106) (IFM DFCI 2009). Available at: http://clinicaltrials.gov/ct2/show/NCT01208662. Accessed July 17, 2014.

72. Thalidomide and lenalidomide combinations in newly diagnosed patients with symptomatic myeloma: a randomised, phase III, multi-centre, open-label trial. Available at: http://www.controlled-trials.com/ISRCTN49407852/myeloma+XI. Accessed July 17, 2014.

73. Rosiñol L, Oriol A, Teruel AI, et al. Superiority of bortezomib, thalidomide, and dexamethasone (VTD) as induction pretransplantation therapy in multiple myeloma: a randomized phase 3 PETHEMA/GEM study. Blood 2012;120: 1589–96.

74. Shaughnessy JD Jr, Haessler J, van Rhee F, et al. Testing standard and genetic parameters in 220 patients with multiple myeloma with complete data sets: superiority of molecular genetics. Br J Haematol 2007;137:530–6.

75. Kuiper R, Broyl A, de Knegt Y, et al. A gene expression signature for high-risk multiple myeloma. Leukemia 2012;26:2406–13.

76. Ocio EM, Richardson PG, Rajkumar SV, et al. New drugs and novel mechanisms of action in multiple myeloma in 2013: a report from the international myeloma working group (IMWG). Leukemia 2014;28:525–42.

Relapsed and Refractory Multiple Myeloma
New Therapeutic Strategies

Silvia Gentili, MD[a], Sagar Lonial, MD[b],*

KEYWORDS

- Multiple myeloma • Relapsed/refractory • Complete remission • Prognostic factors
- Immunomodulatory drugs • Proteasome inhibitors • Emerging agents

KEY POINTS

- Complete remission is becoming a crucial end point for longer survival in relapsed/refractory patients, especially for those not heavily pretreated.
- Disease-related and patient-related conditions should be considered in the management of relapsed and refractory multiple myeloma (RRMM), but the therapeutic choices presented by cytogenetic abnormalities are still untimely.
- Response to previous therapy may also contribute in deciding the treatment approach at the time of relapse, but no conclusive data outlining the most appropriate sequence of treatment of patients with RRMM exist.
- Carfilzomib and pomalidomide seem more effective and safer than their predecessors, and they may soon become the new standard in the treatment of multiple myeloma.
- Emerging agents with innovative mechanisms of action, like histone deacetylase inhibitors, monoclonal antibodies, and kinesin spindle protein inhibitors, are already proving to be effective in the relapsed setting.

INTRODUCTION

Improvements in treatment options over the last decade have contributed to a doubling in the median overall survival (OS) for patients with myeloma. Despite this progress, in large part because of the use of high-dose therapy (HDT) and autologous transplant as well as new drugs such as immunomodulatory drugs (IMiDs) and proteasome inhibitors (PI), multiple myeloma (MM) remains a disease of which few patients are cured, and most patients relapse and require additional therapy.[1]

In 2006, the International Myeloma Working Group (IMWG) modified the definition of relapse/refractory disease within the context of new response criteria for MM.[2,3] The

[a] Department of Hematology, Azienda Ospedaliero-Universitaria Ospedali Riuniti di Ancona, Via Conca 71, Ancona 60126, Italy; [b] Department of Hematology and Medical Oncology, Winship Cancer Institute of Emory University, 1365 Clifton Road, Building C, Room 4004, Atlanta, GA 30322, USA
* Corresponding author.
E-mail address: sloni01@emory.edu

Hematol Oncol Clin N Am 28 (2014) 861–890
http://dx.doi.org/10.1016/j.hoc.2014.06.008
0889-8588/14/$ – see front matter © 2014 Elsevier Inc. All rights reserved.

hemonc.theclinics.com

definition of relapsed myeloma is now based on laboratory or imaging criteria (25% increase from nadir in the serum or urine monoclonal protein, or difference between involved and uninvolved serum-free light chain levels), whereas the need to initiate therapy for a relapsed patient requires the development of symptomatic relapse such as the appearance of at least 1 clinical manifestation of organ damage summarized by the CRAB (increased calcium, renal failure, anemia, and bone disease) symptoms. For patients with nonsecretory myeloma, an increase in marrow plasma cells or bone disease is used to define progression, whereas symptomatic relapse is defined the same way as for patients with secretory myeloma. Refractory disease is defined as progression on therapy, or within 60 days from the last treatment. Patients who never achieve at least a minimal response (MR) to initial antimyeloma therapy and progress on therapy are defined as primary refractory patients with MM.[4]

Important advances have been made recently in understanding the biology and pathogenesis of the disease. The genomic instability of the myeloma cell predisposes patients to acquire new mutations or genetic events resulting in numerical and structural chromosomal abnormalities. The clinical heterogeneity of MM is caused by numerous different types of myeloma guided by different underlying genetic changes. Although on pathology plasma cells may look similar, using gene expression profiling or routine fluorescent in situ hybridization and cytogenetics, there are differences in disease biology between patients with hyperdiploid myeloma and with patients who harbor the t (4:14) or deletion of 17p. In addition to interpatient differences in disease biology, within a single patient there may be different clones of cells that harbor different mutational profiles resulting in disease evolution over time. The clinical significance of these different clones identified by whole-genome sequencing is currently under intense study; however, the sequence in which therapies are delivered may create new selective pressures and induce different biological responses in the different clones. If the disease is to be cured, aggressive therapy with the goal of eradication of all clones of disease to prevent emergence of more resistance subclones should remain a high priority.[5–7]

THE ACHIEVEMENT OF COMPLETE REMISSION

Although there is growing evidence that a deeper quality of response is associated with prolonged OS in newly diagnosed MM (NDMM), in the relapsed setting the impact of complete response (CR) on survival is still under debate.[8]

Emerging data in the early relapse setting (1–3 prior lines) suggests that a depth of response seen with 3 agents rather than 2 may predict longer OS, but additional studies are needed to confirm this benefit. Niesvizky and colleagues[9] analyzed the impact of quality of response on clinical benefit for patients who received bortezomib within the context of the phase III Assessment of Proteasome Inhibition for Extending Remissions (APEX) trial. Although median OS was not reached in the various response cohorts, it was observed that patients achieving CR had a substantially longer median treatment-free interval (24.1 months) compared with patients attaining very good partial remission (VGPR) (13.6 months) or partial remission (PR) (6.4 months). Furthermore, in this study the best outcomes were noted in the patients who experienced a MR to bortezomib compared with nonresponders in terms of time to progression (TTP) (4.9 vs 2.8 months) and OS (24.9 vs 18.7 months). Another study reported that a bortezomib-based regimen led to a trend toward an OS benefit in patients attaining at least a VGPR compared with those who reached only a PR, and event-free survival (EFS) was significantly longer in the first group (1-year EFS, 83% vs 16% respectively; $P = .02$).[10] The beneficial impact of CR was observed with 4-drug combination thalidomide-doxil-dexamethasone-bortezomib (ThaDD-V), which led to a longer TTP in patients obtaining CR (3-year TTP, 67%) compared with those achieving lower response (3-year TTP, 10%; P<.001).[11] A pooled analysis from 2 randomized phase III trials (MM-009 and MM-010) showed that response to lenalidomide plus dexamethasone improved over time, with better quality of response associated with improved clinical outcomes. With a follow-up of 48 months, median TTP and OS were longer in patients who achieved CR/VGPR compared with patients who obtained a PR (TTP, 27.7 vs 12.0 months; P<.001; OS, not yet reached vs 44.2 months; P<.021), regardless of when high-quality response was achieved.[12]

In the context of refractory or late relapse, the opposite situation is the case, because patients with MR seem to have a similar progression-free survival (PFS) and OS when treated with either carfilzomib or pomalidomide in the refractory setting.[13–15] Whether this discordance is a consequence of poor performance status and tolerance of therapy at the end stages of treatment or disease biology is unknown. Nonetheless, the impact of CR on outcomes in the late relapse setting seems to be less important.

PROGNOSTIC FACTORS

Among relapsed patients, the challenge is to select the best approach for each patient while balancing efficacy and toxicity. At present there are limited biomarker-driven approaches by which clinicians can optimally select the choice of salvage therapy. In practice, the decision of what to use in the relapsed setting is likely influenced by patient-related features (ie, preexisting toxicities, quality of life, age, performance status, and comorbidities), disease-related factors such as cytogenetic abnormalities, and treatment-related features such as the impact of previous therapies.

Impact of Cytogenetic Abnormalities

The prognostic value of chromosomal abnormalities such as del (13q), t (4;14), del (17p), or gain of 1q21 have not been well assessed in relapsed and refractory multiple myeloma (RRMM) in a prospective fashion because these data are often collected at individual sites, rather than through central review allowing standardization of methodology. Retrospective analysis of phase II-III trials including patients receiving single agents or new drug combinations often show benefit for new drugs to overcome poor-risk genetics; however, patients with poor-risk genetics who are enrolled in clinical trials of new drugs often have a different natural history because they are able to make it onto these trials. As such, these data should be viewed as retrospective and potentially limited in terms of broad applicability.

A Canadian group reported that amplification of 1q21 in patients with RRMM who received bortezomib-based therapy was associated with a significantly worse outcome (median PFS, 2.3 months vs 7.3 months for patients with 1q21 gains vs those who lacked this; P = .003; median OS, 5.3 months vs 24.6 months for patients with +1q21 and without +1q21; P = .0006), whereas no statistically significant difference in OS was observed for patients with other genetic risk factors like del (13q), t (4;14), del (17p), or del (1p21).[16] In a post-hoc subanalysis of an expanded access program, treatment with lenalidomide-dexamethasone (RD) overcame the poor prognosis conferred by deletions of chromosome 13q or t (4;14) with similar median TTP and OS to patients without these cytogenetic abnormalities.[17] However, Avet-Loiseau and colleagues[18] found that the patients with t (4;14) had a shorter survival compared with those without this translocation (median PFS, 5.5 months vs 10.6 months; P<.01; median OS, 9.4 months vs 15.4 months; P = .005). With another lenalidomide-based combination, the overall response rate (ORR) was similar for patients with or without del (13q) or t (4;14), but the presence of del (17p) was associated with a significantly poorer response (20% vs 87%; $P = .001$) and a significantly shorter median TTP (20 vs 45.5 weeks; $P = .025$) than in patients without this cytogenetic abnormality.[19] In the MM-016 study, the association RD similarly had poor activity in patients with RRMM and del (17p13), with significantly shorter median TTP (2.2 months; $P<.001$) and OS (4.7 months; $P<.001$) relative to patients without this cytogenetic abnormality.[20]

In a prospective study, Dimopoulos and colleagues[21] showed that the negative impact on outcome of +1(q21) was evident in the RD group ($P = .032$) but not in the VRD group ($P = .121$); the patients carrying del13q had shorter survivals in both arms, although it was more pronounced in the RD group, and the presence of t (4;14) was not associated with poor OS regardless of the use of bortezomib. However, despite the addition of bortezomib to lenalidomide-dexamethasone, the investigators found that del (17p) remained one of the most important negative prognostic factor for achieving a deeper response and longer survival.

In a recent study evaluating the impact of genetics on responses with carfilzomib, Jakubowiak and colleagues[22] found that carfilzomib as single agent was not able to overcome the poor prognosis associated with high-risk cytogenetics, with a significantly shorter OS in patients with del (17p), t (4;14), or t (14;16) compared with those with normal karyotypes (median OS, 9.3 months vs 19 months respectively; $P = .0003$). A phase III trial evaluated the combination of pomalidomide and low-dose dexamethasone versus high-dose dexamethasone revealed a substantially greater benefit in terms of response for patients with t (4;14) and del (17p) in the pomalidomide arm relative to those in steroid group (ORR, 23% vs 6% respectively; $P = .032$) and outcome (median PFS, 3.8 months vs 1.1 mo; hazard ratio [HR], 0.46; $P<.001$).[23]

In conclusion, at the moment there are conflicting data for overcoming poor-risk cytogenetics in the relapsed setting. It is likely that combination therapy is needed, in addition to long-term therapy. In a prospective study pomalidomide had activity among 17p-deleted patients, and perhaps combinations of pomalidomide and PI represent the current best approach for high-risk myeloma in the relapsed setting. Additional information is needed to use genetics more accurately to guide the choice of salvage therapy.

Impact of Previous Therapy, Retreatment, and Sequence of Drugs

Most NDMM are currently treated with combinations containing at least 1 new drug. There is concern that use of novel agents as part of induction may limit postrelapse survival because most data series suggest that, with each successive relapse, duration of response shortens progressively.[24] However, the duration of therapy with 1 or more novel agents does not limit practical options for management in the relapsed setting because most younger patients receive 4 cycles of induction followed by HDT consolidation. Krejci and colleagues[25] retrospectively compared outcomes following the use of thalidomide or bortezomib following induction, and at the time of first relapse they did not find significant differences between 2 treatment groups, suggesting that choice of induction, when used for a limited duration, does not affect the success of therapy in the early relapse setting.

In the refractory disease setting, In the MM-003 trial of pomalidomide and low-dose dexamethasone versus dexamethasone alone, pomalidomide/dexamethasone prolonged survival regardless of type or number of previous therapies, although the magnitude of OS benefit was greatest among patients who had received fewer than 3 prior regimens.[26]

When evaluating a similar question with second autologous transplant as the relapse therapy choice, Olin and colleagues[27] showed that the number of prior therapies ($\geq$5 vs <5 lines) was the strongest predictor of poor PFS and OS after salvage transplantation. This finding has recently been corroborated by a second group, with poorer outcomes among patients with more prior therapy (HR, 5.1; 95% confidence interval [CI], 1.1–22.1; $P = .04$).[28]

When evaluating the response rate and duration of response for the novel agents in the early relapsed setting, Vogl and colleagues[29] reported a poorer overall response among patients treated with bortezomib alone as salvage therapy after previous therapy with thalidomide relative to thalidomide-naive patients (ORR, 30% vs 46% respectively; $P<.005$) and this was associated with a shorter TTP ($P = .04$) and OS ($P<.001$), whereas this disparity was lost when the choice of salvage therapy was bortezomib plus pegylated liposomal doxorubicin.[30] Given the different mechanisms of action of IMiDs and PI, this difference is likely a line of therapy issue rather than the effect of induced drug resistance.

In a pooled analysis from the MM-009/MM-010 trials comparing lenalidomide and dexamethasone versus dexamethasone alone, the ORR was significantly higher among thalidomide-naive patients treated with lenalidomide and dexamethasone than among previously thalidomide-exposed patients (65% vs 54%; $P = .04$), as was the median TTP (13.9 months vs 8.4 months; $P = .004$) and PFS (13.2 months vs 8.4 months; $P = .02$). This difference did not translate into a difference in OS.[31] Patients receiving combination salvage therapy, such as the use of bortezomib, lenalidomide, and dexamethasone (VRD); bortezomib, thalidomide, and dexamethasone (VTD); or bortezomib, dexamethasone, and cyclophosphamide (VCD), showed improved responses if patients had not received prior treatment with or were resistant to thalidomide.[21,32,33]

Several studies have reported that prior bortezomib exposure is associated with a poorer outcome for patients receiving lenalidomide-dexamethasone at relapse.[18,20,34,35] However, results from the recent update analysis of the VISTA trial using bortezomib as part of induction showed no impact of bortezomib exposure as the response to either lenalidomide-thalidomide–based or bortezomib-based therapy in the relapsed setting.[36]

Although carfilzomib has shown significant clinical benefit among heavily pretreated patients, because of similar mechanism of action, better responses may be expected among bortezomib-naive or bortezomib-sensitive patients. A recent analysis suggests an improved response rate among patients who were bortezomib naive (ORR, 52%) relative to those who were bortezomib exposed (ORR, 17.1%).[37,38]

At present, no conclusive data outlining the most appropriate sequence of treatments for patients with RRMM exist. If the relapse occurs earlier (6–12 months) or while the patient is still undergoing treatment, the use of an alternative regimen should be considered, but, if the treatment-free period was greater than 6 months to 1 year, the National Comprehensive Cancer Network (NCCN) guidelines suggest that the agent can be used again. If relapse occurs following single-agent or doublet therapy, the addition of a novel agent can overcome the previous resistance, acting synergistically.

Studies have specifically addressed the issue of bortezomib retreatment in RRMM, confirming that it is feasible, without evidence of cumulative toxicity. In a retrospective multicenter survey of RRMM that responded to initial bortezomib treatment, toxicity with bortezomib retreatment was commonly identified, and efficacy data showed that 63% of patients responded to retreatment, with a median TTP of 9.3 months.[39] A recent prospective phase 2 trial showed an ORR of 40% in patients who received bortezomib as retreatment and a median duration of response (DOR) and TTP of 6.5 months and 8.4 months, respectively, after achieving at least a PR. The investigators noted a decrease in ORR with increasing number of prior therapies and also reported a trend for higher overall rates for bortezomib retreatment among patients who achieved a CR, rather than PR, following prior bortezomib therapy.[40]

CURRENT TREATMENT OPTIONS FOR RRMM
Thalidomide

Thalidomide was the first novel agent to be evaluated in RRMM, and since then many studies have shown its activity as a single agent or in combination. A systematic review of 42 clinical studies published by Glasmacher and colleagues[41] reported that thalidomide monotherapy produced at least a PR in 30% of RRMM, with a median OS of 14 months. The most frequent grade 3 or 4 toxicities were constipation (16%), sedation (11%), peripheral neuropathy (PN) (6%), and increased risk of venous thromboembolism (VTE) (3%). The neuropathy occurred more frequently if the daily dose exceeded 200 mg or particularly after prolonged exposure; 70% of patients treated for 12 months experienced at least mild PN.[42]

Many studies have shown that ORR can be significantly enhanced (to 50%) with the addition of concomitant dexamethasone.[43] Because thalidomide is not myelotoxic and potentiates the apoptotic activity of other agents, several conventional cytotoxic agents have been combined with thalidomide-dexamethasone (TD) in order to increase the depth and extent of response. One of the largest data sets of combination therapy has combined cyclophosphamide with TD, with high ORR; (57%–84%).[44–48] The use of thalidomide with continuous low-dose cyclophosphamide alone was also effective with 64% of patients reaching at least PR.[49] Other combinations containing thalidomide in RRMM include melphalan with or without prednisone or dexamethasone, liposomal doxorubicin (pegylated liposomal doxorubicin [PLD]), PLD-vincristine-dexamethasone, bendamustine-prednisolone, or dexamethasone-cisplatin-doxorubicin-cyclophosphamide-etoposide (DT-PACE) **(Table 1)**.[50–56]

The risk of VTE with thalidomide as a single agent is low but increases when it is used in combination with dexamethasone or anthracyclines. For this reason the IMWG has recommended low-molecular-weight heparins (LMWH), to patients receiving high-dose dexamethasone or doxorubicin regardless of the number of myeloma-related risk factors.[57]

The NCCN guidelines recommend thalidomide monotherapy for patients who are corticosteroid intolerant and consider TD and DT-PACE as category 2A options (uniform NCCN consensus that the intervention is appropriate based on low-level evidence) for RRMM.

Bortezomib

Bortezomib (BTZ) is a first-in-class proteasome inhibitor that blocks the 26S proteasome, with potent antimyeloma activity when used as a single agent and in combinations with other agents.

In the large randomized APEX trial, BTZ showed superiority compared with pulsed high-dose dexamethasone in 669 patients with myeloma who had received no more than 3 prior treatment regimens. Patients treated with bortezomib had higher ORRs (38% vs 18%; CR, 6% vs <1%; both P<.001), better TTP (6.2 months vs 3.5 months; P<.001), and longer 1-year OS (80% vs 66%; P = .003).[58] After an extended median follow-up period of 22 months, the ORR was 43% with BTZ and the data confirmed a survival benefit of 6 months for patients who received PI (29.8 months) compared with

Table 1
Selected thalidomide-based combination in the treatment of relapsed/refractory multiple myeloma

Study	Phase	N	Regimen	Schedule	Prior Treatment	ORR (%)	CR (%)	TTE	Key Toxicities (% of Patients)
Garcia-Sanz et al,[44] 2004	II	71	CTD	C: 50 mg continuously for 28-d cycle T: 200–800 mg (median dose 600 mg) continuously D: 40 mg days 1–4, 15–18	52% ≥2	55[a]	2[a]	2-y PFS: 57% 2-y OS: 66%	Grade ≥3 neutropenia: 10 Grade ≥3 infection: 7 Grade ≥2 PN: 6 Grade ≥3 venous thromboembolism: 7 Grade ≥2 constipation: 24
Kyriakou et al,[45] 2005	II	52	CTD	C: 300 mg/m² days 1, 8, 15, 22 of 28-d cycle T: 50–300 mg continuously D: 40 mg days 1–4	Median: 2	78.8	17.3	2-y EFS: 34% 2-y OS: 73%	All grade neutropenia: 38.5 Grade ≥3 infections: 19 Grade ≥3 PN: 0 Grade ≥3 venous thromboembolism: 7.5
Kropff et al,[46] 2003	II	60	CTD	C: 300 mg/m² days 1–8 of 28-d cycle T: 100–400 mg continuously D: 20 mg/m² days 1–4, 9–12, 17–20	Median: 2	72	4	Median EFS: 11 mo Median OS: 19 mo	Grade ≥3 neutropenia: 67 Grade ≥3 infection: 23 Grade ≥3 PN: 16
Palumbo et al,[51] 2006	I/II	24	MPT	M: 20 mg/m² days 1 every fourth month P: 12.5–50 mg every other day T: 100–400 mg continuously	Median: 3 T: 66%	41.7	0	Median PFS: 9 mo Median OS: 14 mo	Grade ≥3 neutropenia: 42 Grade ≥3 thrombocytopenia: 21 Grade ≥3 infection: 8 Grade ≥3 PN: 8
Offidani et al,[53] 2006	II	50	PLD-TD	PLD: 40 mg/m² day 1 of 28-day cycle T: 100 mg continuously D: 40 mg days 1–4, 9–12	54% >2	76	26	Median EFS: 17 mo Median PFS: 22 mo Median OS: NR	Grade ≥3 neutropenia: 16 Grade ≥3 infections: 16 Grade ≥3 PN: 2
Pönish et al,[55] 2008	I	28	BT-PNL	MTD: NR; highest dose level: B: 60 mg/m² days 1, 8, 15 of 28-d cycle T: 50–200 mg continuously PNL: 100 mg days 1, 8, 15, 22	Median: 2 T: 14% V: 28%	85.7	14.3	Median PFS: 11 mo Median OS: 19 mo	Grade ≥3 neutropenia: 43 Grade ≥3 thrombocytopenia: 7 Grade ≥3 infections: 21.5 Grade ≥3 PN: 0

Abbreviations: B, bendamustine; BT-PNL, bendamustine, thalidomide, thalidomide–prednisolone; C, cyclophosphamide; CR, complete response; CTD, cyclophosphamide, thalidomide, dexamethasone; D, dexamethasone; M, melphalan; MPT, melphalan, prednisone, thalidomide; NA, not applicable; NR, not reached; P, prednisone; PLD-TD, pegylated liposomal doxorubicin–thalidomide–dexamethasone; PNL, prednisolone; T, thalidomide; TTE, time to event.

[a] Responses available in 66 patients after 3 months of therapy.

steroid (23.7 months), despite a 62% crossover of patients from the dexamethasone to the bortezomib arm.[59] The addition of dexamethasone for patients with a suboptimal response or progression disease (PD) to BTZ alone, led to an improvement in the degree of response in 18% to 39% of patients, whereas this association from the onset of therapy produces ORRs ranging from 54% to 74% and did not seem to alter the safety profile of BTZ.[60–62]

Based on the results of a phase 1 study, a large randomized trial comparing single-agent bortezomib with bortezomib plus PLD showed an improvement with this combination in terms of longer median TTP (6.5 months vs 9.3 months) and 15-month OS (65% vs 76%).[63,64] A study has also reported an improved response rate (ORR, 67%) with the addition of low-dose dexamethasone to bortezomib plus doxorubicin.[10]

Based on the manageable toxicity profile of bortezomib and its synergistic activity with the other drugs characterized by different modes of action, multiple combinations have been evaluated in phase I to II trials, including bortezomib in combination with melphalan, dexamethasone-melphalan, low-dose cyclophosphamide-dexamethasone (VCD), or prednisone (VCP) and bendamustine-dexamethasone, showing high ORRs (60.9% to 82%) with promising DOR and OS (**Table 2**).[65–70]

Toxicities associated with bortezomib include cyclic transient thrombocytopenia, PN, herpes zoster infection, fatigue, nausea, and diarrhea. The PN occurs in about one-third of patients but it can be effectively managed with dose modifications, especially if associated with pain, and it is generally reversible in more than 50% of cases.[71] The use of bortezomib with weekly dosing or with subcutaneous administration, recently approved by US Food and Drug Administration (FDA), is able to reduce the risk of onset of this side effect.[72,73] Because of the high rate of varicella zoster virus reactivation, the routine use of antiviral prophylaxis is recommended.[74]

MLN9708 (Ixazomib) is a boronate PI similar to bortezomib and is the first orally available PI to advance into phase III trials. Because of its encouraging results in phase I study in RRMM, a phase III randomized trial in this setting is ongoing comparing lenalidomide and low-dose dexamethasone with or without the addition of ixazomib (TOURMALINE-MM1).[75]

Lenalidomide

Lenalidomide is a more potent derivate of thalidomide that has been found to be less toxic and more active than its older analogue. Single-agent lenalidomide was effective and well tolerated in both phase I and phase II studies with response rates ranging from 29% to 39% in patients with RRMM who had received a median of 3 prior therapeutic regimens. The maximum tolerated dose was 25 mg daily and, unlike thalidomide, no significant neuropathy, somnolence, or constipation were noted.[76–78]

Two randomized phase III trials (MM-009 and MM-010) compared RD with placebo plus dexamethasone in patients with RRMM who had received a median of 2 previous therapies. Patients receiving lenalidomide-dexamethasone obtained a better quality of response (ORRs, 60% and 61% for RD, compared with 24% and 20% for dexamethasone-monotherapy; CR rate, 16% and 14% for RD, compared with 3.4% and 0.6% for steroid as a single agent) and experienced a significantly longer median TTP (11.3 and 11.1 months in RD group vs 4.7 months in both dexamethasone groups) and prolonged survival (median OS, not reached and 29.6 months for RD, compared with 20.6 and 20.2 for dexamethasone single agent).[79,80] A pooled analysis of trials with a prolonged median follow-up of 48 months confirmed the significant improvements in ORRs (60.6 vs 21.9; $P<.001$) and a significantly longer DOR (15.8 vs 7 months; $P<.001$), which translated into longer TTP (median TTP, 13.4 vs 4.6; $P<.001$) and improved OS (median OS, 38 vs 31.6; $P = .045$) in the RD-treated patients, despite a crossover of 41.9% of the patients from the dexamethasone to lenalidomide-based treatment, as happened in the APEX trial.[81]

From these two pivotal phase III studies, RD was approved by the FDA and European Medicines Evaluation Agency for the treatment of patients with MM who had received at least 1 prior therapy, and it is listed in US and European treatment guidelines as a recommended treatment option.

Lenalidomide in combination with chemotherapeutics may be able to further improve the outcome of RRMM. The regimens tested in RRMM include lenalidomide in combination with adriamycin-dexamethasone (ORR, 73%), PLD-vincristine-dexamethasone (ORR, 75%), low-dose cyclophosphamide-prednisone (≥MR, 64%–94%), cyclophosphamide-dexamethasone (ORR, 65%–81%), bendamustine-dexamethasone (ORR, 52%), and bendamustine-prednisolone (ORR, 76%) (**Table 3**).[19,82–88]

The toxicity profile of lenalidomide includes fatigue, skin rash, thrombocytopenia, and neutropenia that may require dose reduction or granulocyte colony-stimulating factor (G-CSF), which can be given while maintaining the full lenalidomide dose.

If no increased risk of VTE has been reported with single-agent lenalidomide, with the addition of steroid the frequency of thromboembolic events will be significantly higher. Based on recommendations from the IMWG, prophylactic treatment with aspirin in patients at standard risk for VTE and LMWH or adjusted-dose warfarin for high-risk patients is suggested.[57]

Carfilzomib

Carfilzomib (CFZ) is a second-generation PI and is able to irreversibly and selectively inhibit the chymotrypsinlike site of the proteasome.[89] Carfilzomib has shown activity against cell lines resistant to conventional and novel agents, including bortezomib, and primary plasma cells models.[90] Several promising results reported in the phase I trials have led to development of phase II studies.[91,92] In the PX-171-003-A1 trial, 266 heavily pretreated patients with MM (most patients had 5 previous lines of therapy and 80% were refractory to lenalidomide and bortezomib) received carfilzomib monotherapy in the twice-weekly regimen. The investigators reported an ORR of 23.7%, with a median DOR of 7.8 months and a median OS of 15.6 months.[13] Another study, PX-171-004, evaluated CFZ in patients with RRMM but who were bortezomib naive in 2 different cohorts. Patients treated with escalated dosing from 20 to 27 mg/m^2 after a second cycle compared with the 20 mg/m^2 group had a better response rate (52% vs 42%), longer response durability (median DOR not reached vs 13.1 months), and TTP (median TTP not reached vs 8.3 months).[37] The results among previously bortezomib-exposed patients showed an ORR of 17.1%, DOR of greater than 10.6 months, and TTP of 4.6 months.[38]

An integrated safety analysis of 526 patients with RRMM enrolled in 4 phase II trials showed that CFZ was generally well tolerated and toxicities were manageable. The most common grades greater than or equal to 3 adverse events (AEs) were thrombocytopenia (23.4%), anemia (22.4%), lymphopenia (18.1%), pneumonia (10.5%), and neutropenia (10.3%). PN occurred in 13.9% of patients but 71.9% of these had active PN at study entry. However, only 1 patient discontinued treatment because of neuropathic pain, confirming the favorable toxicity profile of CFZ with regard to PN.[93]

From these studies, in 2012 the FDA approved carfilzomib for the treatment of patients with MM who have received at least 2 prior therapies, including bortezomib and IMiDs, and who have shown disease progression on or within 60 days of the completion of the last treatment.

Moreover, additional information will be obtained from the phase III trials currently ongoing in patients with RRMM involving CFZ. The FOCUS trial is evaluating CFZ

Table 2
Selected bortezomib-based combinations in the treatment of relapsed/refractory MM

Study	Phase	N	Regimen	Schedule	Prior Treatment	ORR (%)	CR (%)	TTE	Key Toxicities (% of Patients)
Orlowski et al,[64] 2007	III	324	PLD-V	PLD: 30 mg/m² day 4 of 21-d cycle V: 1.3 mg/m² days 1, 4, 8, 11	66% ≥2 T and L: 40% V: 0%	44	4	Median TTP: 9.3 mo 15-mo OS: 76%	Grade ≥3 neutropenia: 29 Grade ≥3 thrombocytopenia: 23 Grade ≥3 febrile neutropenia: 3 Grade ≥3 PN: 4
Palumbo et al,[10] 2008	II	64	V-DOX-D	V: 1.3 mg/m² days 1, 4, 8, 11 of 28-d cycle DOX: 20 mg/m² days 1, 4, or PLD 30 mg/m² day 1 D: 40 mg days 1–4	Median: 2 T: 75% V: 27%	67	9	1-y EFS: 34% 1-y OS: 66%	Grade ≥3 neutropenia: 36 Grade ≥3 thrombocytopenia: 48 Grade ≥3 infection: 15 Grade ≥3 PN: 10
Popat et al,[66] 2009	I/II	53	VMD	MTD: V: 1.3 mg/m² days 1, 4, 8, 11 of 28-day cycle M: 7.5 mg/m² day 2 D: 20 mg days 1–2, 4–5, 8–9, 11–12 in case of PD or SD after 2 or 4 cycles, respectively	Median: 3 T: 64% V: 9%	68	19	Median PFS: 10 mo Median OS: 28 mo	Grade ≥3 neutropenia: 57 Grade ≥3 thrombocytopenia: 62 Grade ≥3 infection: 21 Grade ≥3 PN: 15
Kropff et al,[67] 2007	II	54	VCD	V: 1.3 mg/m² days 1, 4, 8, 11 of 21-d cycle for the first 8 cycles, then same dose days 1, 8, 15, 22 of 35-d cycle for 3 cycles C: 50 mg/m² continuously D: 20 mg days 1–2, 4–5, 8–9, 11–12 for the first 8 cycles, then same dose days 1–2, 8–8, 15–16, 22–23	Median: 2 T: 30% V: 0%	82	16	Median EFS: 12 mo Median OS: 22 mo	Grade ≥3 leukopenia: 57 Grade ≥3 thrombocytopenia: 53 Grade ≥3 infection: 38 Grade ≥3 PN: 21 Grade ≥3 fatigue: 15

Reece et al,[68] 2008	I/II	37	VCP	MTD: NR; highest dose level: V: 1.5 mg/m² days 1, 8, 15 of 28-d cycle; C: 300 mg/m² days 1, 8, 15, 22; P: 100 mg every 2 d	Median: 2; T: 38%; V: 3%; L: 3%	68	32[a]	Median PFS: 15 mo; Median OS: 24 mo	Grade ≥3 neutropenia: 13; Grade ≥3 thrombocytopenia: 70; Grade ≥3 infection: 13; Grade ≥3 PN: 8
Ludwig et al,[69] 2014	II	79	BVD	B: 70 mg/m² days 1, 4 of 28-d cycle; V: 1.3 mg/m² days 1, 4, 8, 11; D: 20 mg days 1, 4, 8, 11	Median: 2; V: 63.3%; L: 53.2%	60.9	15	Median PFS: 9.7 mo; Median OS: 25.6 mo	Grade ≥3 leukopenia: 17; Grade ≥3 thrombocytopenia: 38; Grade ≥3 infections: 23; Grade ≥3 PN: 6
Offidani et al,[70] 2013	II	75	BVD	B: 70 mg/m² days 1, 8 of 28-d cycle; V: 1.3 mg/m² days 1, 4, 8, 11 for the first 2 cycles, then same dose days 1, 8, 15, 22; D: 20 mg days 1–2, 4–5, 8–9, 11–12 for the first 2 cycles, then same dose days 1, 8, 15, 22	Median: 1; T: 57%; V: 46.5%; L: 54.5%	77	20	Median PFS: 15.5 mo; 1-y OS: 78%	Grade ≥3 neutropenia: 18.5; Grade ≥3 thrombocytopenia: 30.5; Grade ≥3 infections: 12; Grade ≥3 PN: 8

Abbreviations: DOX, doxorubicin; L, lenalidomide; MTD, maximal tolerated dose; NR, not reached; PD, progressive disease; PLD, pegylated liposomal doxorubicin; SD, stable disease; TTP, time to progression; V, bortezomib.

[a] CR plus near CR.

Table 3
Selected lenalidomide-based combinations in the treatment of relapsed/refractory MM

Study	Phase	N	Regimen	Schedule	Prior Treatment	ORR (%)	CR (%)	TTE	Key Toxicities (% of Patients)
Dimopoulos et al,[79] 2007	III	176	RD	R: 25 mg days 1–21 of 28-d cycle D: 40 mg on days 1–4, 9–12, 17–20 for the first 4 cycles, then 40 mg days 1–4	Median: 2 T: 30.1% V: 4.5%	60.2	15.9	Median TTP: 11.3 mo Median OS: NR	Grade ≥3 neutropenia: 29.5 Grade ≥3 infection: 11.3 Grade ≥3 febrile neutropenia: 3.4 Grade ≥3 venous thromboembolism: 11.4
Weber et al,[80] 2007	III	177	RD	R: 25 mg days 1–21 of 28-d cycle D: 40 mg on days 1–4, 9–12, 17–20 for the first 4 cycles, then 40 mg days 1–4	Median: 2 T: 41.8% V: 10.7%	61	14.1	Median TTP: 11.1 mo Median OS: 29.6 mo	Grade ≥3 neutropenia: 41.2 Grade ≥3 thrombocytopenia: 14.7 Grade ≥3 infection: 21.4 Grade ≥3 venous thromboembolism: 14.7
Knop et al,[19] 2009	I/II	69	RAD	MTD: NR; highest dose level: R: 25 mg days 1–21 of 28-d cycle A: 9 mg/m² days 1–4 D: 40 mg on days 1–4, 17–20	Median: 2 T: 20% V: 57% L: 0%	73	15	Median TTP: 45 wk Median PFS: 40 wk 1-y OS: 88%	Grade ≥3 neutropenia: 48 Grade ≥3 thrombocytopenia: 38 Grade ≥3 infection: 10.5 Grade ≥3 venous thromboembolism: 1.5

Study	Phase	N	Regimen	Regimen details	Prior therapy			Outcomes	Toxicity
Reece et al,[84] 2010	I/II	32	CPR	MTD: NR; highest dose level: C: 300 mg/m² days 1, 8, 15 of 28-d cycle; R: 25 mg days 1–21; P: 100 mg every other day	Median: 2; T: 29%; V: 48%; L: 0%	94	19	1-y PFS: 78%; 1-y OS: 93%	Grade ≥3 neutropenia: 29; Grade ≥3 thrombocytopenia: 22; Grade ≥3 venous thromboembolism: 6
Schey et al,[86] 2010	I/II	31	RCD	MTD: C: 600 mg days 1, 8 of 28-d cycle; R: 25 mg days 1–21; D: 20 mg on days 1–4, 8–11	Median: 3; T: 90%; V: 26%; L: 0%	81	29	2-y PFS: 56%; OS at 30 mo: 80%	Grade ≥3 neutropenia: 19; Grade ≥3 infection: 3; Grade ≥3 venous thromboembolism: 6
Lentzsch et al,[87] 2012	I/II	29	BRD	MTD: B: 75 mg/m² days 1, 2 of 28-d cycle; R: 25 mg days 1–21; D: 40 mg on days 1, 8, 15, 22	Median: 3; T: 14%; V: 66%; L: 45%; T and L: 38%	52	0	Median PFS: 6.1 mo; 1-y OS: 93%; 2-y OS: 62%	Grade ≥3 anemia: 17; Grade ≥3 neutropenia: 62; Grade ≥3 thrombocytopenia: 38; Grade ≥3 febrile neutropenia: 3; Grade ≥3 infection: 3
Pönisch et al,[88] 2013	I	21	BR-PNL	B: 60–75 mg/m² days 1, 2 of 28-day cycle; R: 10–25 mg days 1–21; PNL: 100 mg days 1–4	Median: 2; T: 14%; V: 67%; L: 5%	76	5	18-mo PFS: 48%; 18-mo OS: 64%	Grade ≥3 anemia: 19; Grade ≥3 neutropenia: 52; Grade ≥3 thrombocytopenia: 19; Grade ≥3 fever: 14; Grade ≥3 infection: 14

Abbreviations: A, doxorubicin; R, lenalidomide.

versus best supportive care in heavily pretreated patients and the ENDEAVOR study is comparing BTZ and dexamethasone as a salvage regimen to CFZ and dexamethasone. The dosing of CFZ in the last study was 20 mg/m^2 on days 1 to 2 of cycle 1 and then 56 mg/m^2 for all the other doses. It was recently found that this dosage is well tolerated as a single agent or in combination with dexamethasone, with an ORR of 55% to 60% for patients with RRMM.[94]

Beyond the second-generation inhibitors, oprozomib is a truncated derivative of carfilzomib in clinical development and preliminary data highlight that oprozomib monotherapy has promising activity and also produces good responses in heavily pretreated patients.[95]

Pomalidomide

The third available IMiD, pomalidomide, has shown more potency and a more favorable toxicity profile than its predecessors, thalidomide and lenalidomide. Pomalidomide recently received FDA approval for the treatment of patients with RRMM in combination with low-dose dexamethasone.

The initial phase I studies showed immediately the effectiveness of this drug with or without dexamethasone in relapsed setting and established the maximum tolerated dose (MTD) initially at 2 mg and then 4 mg.[96–98] In the first reported phase II trial pomalidomide was given at 2 mg continuously in 28-day cycles along with low-dose dexamethasone and also confirmed its activity in patients previously treated with novel agents. The ORR was 63% and objective responses were also achieved in 37% of thalidomide-refractory patients, 40% of lenalidomide-refractory patients, and 60% of bortezomib-refractory patients.[99] This combination was tested in patients who were refractory to lenalidomide, and, as expected, the responses were lower in this group (ORR, 47%) but durable (median PFS, 9.1 months), with a median OS of 13.9 months.[100] Two studies explored the activity of pomalidomide in patients who were refractory to both bortezomib and lenalidomide. In the first trial, pomalidomide was given at either 2 mg or 4 mg daily with low-dose dexamethasone and the authors noted that there was no advantage with the higher dose. In this study, 49% of patients achieved at least an MR in the 2-mg cohort, whereas with the 4 mg dosing this figure was only 43% and the 6-month OS rates for these two groups were 78% and 67% respectively.[101] In the second trial, a French group randomized 84 patients to either 4 mg of pomalidomide for 21 days of each 28-day cycle or 28 days continuously. Both arms included dexamethasone 40 mg once a week. The response rates of the two cohorts were comparable (ORR, 35% in the 21-day groups and 34% in the other arm) as was the outcome (median OS, 14.9 months and 14.8 months respectively).[102] In a different study performed in the United States, pomalidomide and low-dose dexamethasone showed an improved response (ORR, 33% vs 18%; $P =$ .013) and superior outcome in terms of PFS (median PFS, 4.2 months vs 2.7 months; $P = $ .003), compared with pomalidomide alone. Most patients in the trial were double refractory (62% refractory to both lenalidomide and bortezomib).[14] In the first randomized phase III trial involving this IMiD, in 445 patients enrolled, pomalidomide plus low-dose dexamethasone significantly increased PFS and OS compared with high-dose dexamethasone (median PFS, 4 months vs 1.9 months; $P<$.001; median OS, 12.7 months vs 8.1 months; $P = $ .028), regardless of type or number of previous therapies, suggesting a lack of cross-resistance between pomalidomide and older IMiDs (**Table 4**).[15] From these promising findings, new combinations including pomalidomide are being developed. A phase I/II study recently combined pomalidomide with cyclophosphamide and prednisone and 51% of patients achieved at least a PR, whereas the association pomalidomide-clarithromycin and dexamethasone

Table 4
Selected combinations of novel agents in the treatment of relapsed/refractory MM

Study	Phase	N	Regimen	Schedule	Prior Treatment	ORR (%)	CR (%)	TTE	Key Toxicities (% of Patients)
Pineda-Roman et al,[32] 2008	I/II	85	VTD	V: 1.3 mg/m² days 1, 4, 8, 11 of 21-d cycle T: 150 mg continuously D: 20 mg days 1–2, 4–5, 8–9, 11–12 in case of no PR after 4 cycles	Median: ≥2 T: 74% V: 0%	63	6	Median EFS: 6 mo Median OS: 22 mo	Dose-limiting toxicity: grade 4 thrombocytopenia and grade 4 neutropenia
Garderet et al,[106] 2012	III	135	VTD	V: 1.3 mg/m² days 1, 4, 8, 11 of 21-d cycle for the first 8 cycles, then days 1, 8, 15, 22 of 42-d cycle for other 4 cycles T: 200 mg continuously D: 40 mg days 1–4	T: 10% V: 20%	86	25	Median TTP: 19.5 mo Median PFS: 18.3 mo 2-y OS: 71%	Grade ≥3 neutropenia: 11 Grade ≥3 thrombocytopenia: 17 Grade ≥3 PN: 31 Grade ≥3 infection: 14 Grade ≥3 venous thromboembolism: 6
Offidani et al,[11] 2011	II	46	PLD-VTD	PLD: 30 mg/m² day 4 of 28-d cycle V: 1.3 mg/m² days 1, 4, 8, 11 T: 100 mg continuously D: 20 mg days 1–2, 4–5, 8–9, 11–12	Median: 1 T: 59% V: 17.3%	76	37	Median TTP: 18.5 mo Median PFS: 17.5 mo Median OS: 40 mo	Grade ≥3 neutropenia: 8.5 Grade ≥3 thrombocytopenia: 16 Grade ≥3 PN: 11 Grade ≥3 infection: 15 Grade ≥3 venous thromboembolism: 4.5
Terpos et al,[108] 2008	II	62	VMTD	V: 1 mg/m² days 1, 4, 8, 11 of 28-d cycle M: 0.15 mg/kg days 1–5 T: 100 mg days 1–4, 17–20 D: 12 mg/m² days 1–4, 17–20	Median: 2 T: 55% V: 10%	66	13	Median TTP: 9.3 mo 2-y OS: 63%	Grade ≥3 neutropenia: 10 Grade ≥3 thrombocytopenia: 23 Grade ≥3 PN: 10 Grade ≥3 infection: 15
Palumbo et al,[109] 2007	I/II	30	VMPT	MTD: V: 1.3 mg/m² days 1, 4, 15, 22 of 35-d cycle M: 6 mg/m² days 1–5 P: 60 mg/m² days 1–5 T: 50 mg continuously	Median: 2 T: 30%	67	17	1-y PFS: 61% 1-y OS: 84%	Grade ≥3 neutropenia: 43 Grade ≥3 thrombocytopenia: 33 Grade ≥3 PN: 6 Grade ≥3 infection: 16

(continued on next page)

Table 4
(continued)

Study	Phase	N	Regimen	Schedule	Prior Treatment	ORR (%)	CR (%)	TTE	Key Toxicities (% of Patients)
Kim et al,[107] 2010	II	70	VCTD	V: 1.3 mg/m² days 1, 4, 8, 11 of 21-d cycle C: 150 mg/m² days 1–4 T: 50 mg continuously D: 20 mg/m² days 1, 4, 8, 11	Median: 2 TD: 49% CTD: 57% V: 0%	88	46	Median PFS: 14.6 mo Median OS: 31.6 mo	Grade ≥3 neutropenia: 4 Grade ≥3 thrombocytopenia: 12 Grade ≥3 PN: 3 Grade ≥3 pneumonia: 14
Palumbo et al,[110] 2010	II	44	RMPT	R: 10 mg days 1–21 of 28-d cycle M: 0.18 mg/kg days 1–4 P: 2 mg/kg days 1–4 T: 50 mg or 100 mg continuously	Median: 1 T: 23% V: 20%	75	2	1-y PFS: 51% 1-y OS: 72%	Grade ≥3 neutropenia: 63 Grade ≥3 thrombocytopenia: 34 Grade ≥3 PN: 0 Grade ≥3 infection: 21
Richardson et al,[111] 2014	II	64	RVD	R: 15 mg days 1–14 of 21-d cycle V: 1 mg/m² days 1, 4, 8, 11 D: 20 or 40 mg days 1–2, 4–5, 8–9, 11–12 for the first 4 cycles, then 10 or 20 mg same days, cycles 5–8	Median: 2 T: 75% V: 53% R: 6%	64	11	Median PFS: 9.5 mo Median OS: 30 mo	Grade ≥3 neutropenia: 30 Grade ≥3 thrombocytopenia: 22 Grade ≥3 PN: 3 Grade ≥3 infection: 9
Wang et al,[112] 2013	II	52	CFZ-RD	CFZ: 20 mg/m² for days 1–2 first cycle, then 27 mg/m² mg days 1–2, 8–9, 15–16 of 28-d cycle R: 25 mg days 1–21 D: 40 mg days 1, 8, 15, 22	Median: 3 T: 46% V: 80% R: 73%	77	6[a]	Median PFS: 15 mo	Grade ≥3 neutropenia: 33 Grade ≥3 thrombocytopenia: 19 Grade ≥3 anemia: 19 Grade ≥3 fatigue: 11 Grade ≥3 pneumonia: 10
Shah et al,[114] 2013	I/II	72	CFZ-POM-D	CFZ: 20 mg/m² for days 1–2 first cycle, then 27 mg/m² mg days 1–2, 8–9, 15–16 of 28-d cycle P: 4 mg days 1–21 D: 40 mg days 1, 8, 15, 22	Median: 6 V: 87% R: 100%	64	1.5	Median PFS: 12 mo Median OS: 16.3 mo	Grade ≥3 neutropenia: 40 Grade ≥3 thrombocytopenia: 34 Grade ≥3 anemia: 34 Grade ≥3 fatigue: 48 Grade ≥3 diarrhea: 20

Study	Phase	N	Regimen	Dose/Schedule				
San Miguel et al,[15] 2013	III	302	POM-D	POM: 4 mg days 1–21 of 28-d cycle D: 40 mg on days 1, 8, 15, 22 of 28-d cycle	Median: 5 T: 57% V: 100% R: 100%	31	1	Median PFS: 4 mo Median OS: 12.7 mo	Grade ≥3 anemia: 33 Grade ≥3 neutropenia: 48 Grade ≥3 thrombocytopenia: 22 Grade ≥3 infections/infestations: 34 Grade ≥3 pneumonia: 14 Grade ≥3 febrile neutropenia: 10
Richardson et al,[113] 2013	I	20	POM-VD	MTD: POM: 4 mg days 1–14 of 21-d cycle V: 1.3 mg/m² days 1, 4, 8, 11 for the first 8 cycles, then days 1, 8 for subsequent cycles D: 10 or 20 mg days 1–2, 4–5, 8–9, 11–12 for the first 8 cycles, then days 1–2, 8–9 for subsequent cycles	Median: 2 V: 100% R: 100%	75	30[b]	NA	Grade ≥3 neutropenia: 29 Grade ≥3 thrombocytopenia: 19
La Rocca et al,[103] 2013	I/II	69	POM-CP	MTD: POM: 2.5 mg continuously of 28-d cycle C: 50 mg every other day P: 50 mg every other day	Median: 3 T: 19% V: 84% R: 100%	51[c]	5[c]	Median PFS: 10.4 mo 1-y OS: 69%	Grade ≥3 neutropenia: 42 Grade ≥3 thrombocytopenia: 11 Grade ≥3 infection: 9 Grade ≥3 neurologic events: 7 Grade ≥3 dermatologic events: 7

Abbreviations: CFZ, carfilzomib; NA, not applicable; POM, pomalidomide; R, lenalidomide.

[a] Stringent CR plus CR.
[b] Stringent CR plus CR plus very good partial response.
[c] Evaluable patients: 55.

yielded an ORR of 61.4% in 114 patients enrolled and of 56.4% in patients with double-refractory MM.[103,104]

Adverse events frequently associated with pomalidomide are myelosuppression and fatigue. PN and thromboembolic events are rare, but, as with the other IMiDs, patients require deep vein thrombosis prophylaxis.

Combinations of Novel Agents

New combinations including PI and IMiDs have been studied to further improve the outcome of RRMM. The use of agents with complementary mechanisms of action is becoming an attractive means of increasing efficacy and overcoming resistance to standard treatment regimens. This approach could reinforce the quality of response, with an additive positive effect, without excessive toxicity.[105]

The thalidomide-bortezomib combination has been tested with dexamethasone (VTD; ORR, 63%–86%), PLD-dexamethasone (ORR, 76%), cyclophosphamide-dexamethasone (VCTD; ORR, 88%) melphalan-dexamethasone (VMDT; ORR, 66%), and melphalan-prednisone (ORR, 67%) with encouraging results, but several studies reported a significant rate of high-grade PN (see **Table 4**).[11,32,106–109]

The 4-drug combination of lenalidomide, melphalan, prednisone, and thalidomide (RMPT) led to a high response rate ($\geq$PR, 75%; $\geq$VGPR, 32%), but the investigators noted increased hematologic toxicities relative to regimens including lenalidomide alone.[110] Based on the synergistic activity of lenalidomide with PI and its good toxicity profile compared with thalidomide, the addition of lenalidomide to bortezomib and dexamethasone yielded a promising response rate (RVD; ORR, 64%) and was well tolerated.[111]

Several studies have evaluated combinations with the most recent generation of agents between PI and IMiDs. A phase II dose-expansion study showed that carfilzomib combined with lenalidomide and dexamethasone (CRD) is effective in the relapsed setting (ORR, 77%).[112] A phase III trial, the ASPIRE study, is currently comparing lenalidomide and low-dose dexamethasone with or without CFZ for RRMM. Combining pomalidomide with bortezomib and dexamethasone (PVD) also results in an effective and promising regimen with at least PR in 75% of lenalidomide-refractory patients.[113] This finding led to efforts to identify the optimal dose of these drugs in a phase III trial, which is presently evaluating the impact of the addition of pomalidomide to bortezomib and dexamethasone in patients with relapsed myeloma (OPTIMISMM). A phase I/II study is investigating carfilzomib plus pomalidomide and dexamethasone in heavily pretreated lenalidomide-refractory patients (median of 6 previous lines of therapy). Preliminary results show an impressive overall response rate ($\geq$MR) of 81%, including 64% greater than or equal to PR and 28% greater than or equal to VGPR.[114]

THE FUTURE OF THERAPY: EMERGING AGENTS AND NOVEL TREATMENT STRATEGIES

Patients with advanced refractory or relapsed and refractory myeloma who do not benefit from newly developed PI or IMiDs have a median OS of only 9 months.[115]

For this reason, in addition to development of more next-generation PI and IMiDs, several other drug classes that target other novel pathogenic mechanisms of the MM cells are actively being explored. The challenge in the relapsed setting is to identify novel agents able to overcome resistance to previous treatment in order to prolong the survival of patients with MM but also with better toxicity profiles compared with their predecessors, to preserve a good quality of life in this frail population.

Among these novel agents, this article focuses on the most promising groups of agents used in RRMM, most of which have already reached phase III and are close to approval in the relapsed setting.

Histone Deacetylase Inhibitors

Panobinostat (LBH589) and vorinostat are histone and protein-deacetylase inhibitors that regulate proteins involved in multiple oncogenic pathways, including the aggresome protein degradation pathway.

Although the activity of these deacetylase inhibitors (DACi) as single agents is limited, when they combine in RRMM with dexamethasone and/or bortezomib, these drugs seem to be able to overcome bortezomib resistance. Thus, the encouraging data reported in phase I studies led to phase II trials evaluating panobinostat plus bortezomib plus low-dose dexamethasone and vorinostat plus bortezomib plus dexamethasone in bortezomib-refractory patients.[116,117] Richardson and colleagues[118] recently described the results of the first study, PANORAMA-2, which showed an ORR of 34.5%, a clinical benefit response (CBR) rate of 52.7%, and a median PFS of 5.4 months. The updated analysis also showed a promising median OS of 17.5 months (**Table 5**).[119] In a similar refractory study combining vorinostat with bortezomib among heavily pretreated patients (median of 4 previous therapies, including 87% of IMiD-refractory patients), 17% of patients achieved at least a PR, whereas the CBR rate was 31%. The median OS was 11.2 months and the OS rate at 2 years was 32%.[120] A randomized, placebo-controlled, phase III trial of vorinostat plus bortezomib has been completed and disappointing results have been shown. Despite an improved response rate in the vorinostat arm compared with the placebo group (ORR, 56% vs 41% respectively; $P<.0001$), only a minimal advantage was found in PFS (median PFS, 7.6 months vs 6.8 months; HR, 0.77; 95% CI, 0.64–0.94; $P = .01$) and no differences in OS.[121] Better results are expected from a similar randomized, phase III trial with panobinostat instead of vorinostat (PANORAMA-1). Preliminary data reported a significant clinical benefit with this association.[122]

Because of their wide spectrum of action, several toxicities, including fatigue, gastrointestinal symptoms, and myelosuppression, have frequently been reported with DACi, which limits their use in combination regimens. Rocilinostat (ACY1215) is a histone deacetylase (HDAC)-6–specific inhibitor, developed to minimize the general toxicity associated with the other nonspecific DACi, maintaining the efficacy. Although similar to other agents in this class, the efficacy of rocilinostat as monotherapy is modest, and a phase I/II trial is investigating rocilinostat plus bortezomib and low-dose dexamethasone in heavily pretreated patients (range of previous therapies 2–11, including 69% of bortezomib-refractory patients). Preliminary results showed promise with 4 out of 16 evaluable patients achieving an MR or better and a good toxicity profile.[123]

Monoclonal Antibodies

Among the most promising classes of drugs currently in development in MM are the monoclonal antibodies.

Elotuzumab is a humanized monoclonal antibody that targets the cell surface adhesion molecule CS1, which is selectively expressed on more than 95% of plasma cells and has little to no expression on normal tissues.

Elotuzumab as a single agent was not very effective with stable disease in 27% of patients and showed no objective responses. Elotuzumab infusion-related side effects included cough, fever, chills, nausea, back pain, and headache.[124] However, in a phase I study, treatment with elotuzumab, lenalidomide, and low-dose dexamethasone

Table 5
Selected emerging agents: trials in the treatment of relapsed/refractory MM

Study	Phase	N	Regimen	Schedule	Prior Treatment	ORR (%)	CR (%)	TTE	Key Toxicities (% of Patients)
Dimopoulos et al,[121] 2013	III	317	VRN-V	VRN: 400 mg days 1–14 of 21-d cycles V: 1.3 mg/m² days 1, 4, 8, 11	Median: 2 T: 52% V: 25% R: 12%	56.2	7.9	Median TTP: 7.3 mo Median PFS: 7.6 mo Median OS: NA	Grade ≥3 anemia: 17 Grade ≥3 neutropenia: 28 Grade ≥3 thrombocytopenia: 45 Grade ≥3 diarrhea: 16 Grade ≥3 fatigue: 16
Richardson et al,[118,119] 2013	II	55	PNB-VD	PNB: 20 mg days 1, 3, 5, 8, 10, 12 of 21-d cycle for the first 8 cycles, then same dose days 1, 3, 5, 8, 10, 12, 22, 24, 26, 29, 31, 33 of 42-d cycle V: 1.3 mg/m² days 1, 4, 8, 11 for the first 8 cycles, then same dose days 1, 8, 22, 29 D: 20 mg days 1–2, 4–5, 8–9, 11–12 for the first 4 cycles, then same dose days 1–2, 8–9, 22–23, 29–30	Median: 4 T: 69.1% V: 100% R: 98.2%	34.5	0	Median PFS: 5.4 mo Median OS: 17.5 mo	Grade ≥3 neutropenia: 15 Grade ≥3 thrombocytopenia: 63.6 Grade ≥3 diarrhea: 20 Grade ≥3 fatigue: 20 Grade ≥3 infections: 29.1
Richardson et al,[126] 2012	II	77	ELO-RD	ELO: 10 or 20 mg/kg days 1, 8, 15, 22 of 28-d cycle for the first 2 cycles, then same dose days 1, 15 of 28-d cycle R: 25 mg days 1–21 D: 40 mg days 1, 8, 15, 22	55% ≥2 T: 62% V: 60% R: 0%	84 92[a] 76[b]	NA	Median PFS: 25 mo Median PFS: 26.9 mo[a] Median PFS: 18.6 mo[b]	Grade ≥3 neutropenia: 18 Grade ≥3 thrombocytopenia: 16 Grade ≥3 diarrhea: 7 Grade ≥3 fatigue: 7 Grade ≥3 pneumonia: 7

Abbreviations: ELO, elotuzumab; PBN, panobinostat; VRN, vorinostat.
[a] With ELO, 10/kg.
[b] With ELO, 20 mg/kg.

yielded an impressive ORR of 82%, with 94% of patients having received prior thalidomide and 83% being refractory to their last line of therapy. In addition, the investigators did not find dose-limiting toxicities up to a dose of 20 mg/kg.[125] These findings provided the rationale for phase II studies, in which the same combination led to an ORR of 92% for the patients in the 10 mg/kg cohort and 76% in the 20 mg/kg cohort, with a longer PFS using the 10 mg/kg dose (33 months and 19 months for the 10-mg/kg and 20-mg/kg cohorts, respectively).[126] Based on these encouraging results, the ongoing phase III trial (ELOQUENT 2) is comparing the efficacy and the safety of lenalidomide plus low-dose dexamethasone with or without 10-mg/kg elotuzumab in patients with RRMM.

Moreover, elotuzumab combined with bortezomib again was well tolerated in a phase I dose-escalation study, and no MTD was identified within the tested range. PR or better was seen in 48% of patients, including 2 of 3 patients who were refractory to bortezomib, and the median TTP was 9.46 months.[127]

Daratumumab, an anti-CD38 monoclonal antibody, induces plasma cell killing mainly via antibody-dependent cellular cytotoxicity and complement-dependent cytotoxicity. The results of a phase I/II study were recently reported and confirmed the antitumor activity of daratumumab as a single agent. Patients in this study (N = 22) had received a median of 5.5 prior regimens and 75% were double refractory. An ORR of 42% has been seen to date, and the CBR was 67%.[128] Preclinical in vivo study has recently reported that daratumumab induces high rates of tumor cell lysis in lenalidomide-refractory and bortezomib-refractory patients, but this activity increased in a synergistic way when the monoclonal antibody was used in combination with lenalidomide or bortezomib.[129] On this basis, a phase I dose-escalation trial is currently investigating daratumumab plus lenalidomide and dexamethasone and preliminary data revealed significant clinical benefit in the 6 patients enrolled to date.[130]

In addition, another anti-CD38 antibody, SAR650984 (SAR), has been developed and shows similar encouraging clinical activity. SAR is currently being evaluated in a phase I study and early data of 17 heavily pretreated patients, who received SAR in the active dose range (1–10 mg/kg), showed a manageable safety profile and encouraging responses.[131]

Kinesin Spindle Protein Inhibitors

ARRY-520 is a kinesin spindle protein (KSP) inhibitor that, by targeting this protein, induces mitotic catastrophe in tumor cells. A phase I/II study of ARRY-520 monotherapy yielded an ORR of 16% and, in combination with low-dose dexamethasone, this drug has also shown good activity (ORR, 16%; CBR, 22%) and tolerability in very heavily pretreated patients who are triple refractory to bortezomib, lenalidomide, and dexamethasone, indicating a lack of cross-resistance. The survival for patients with low α-1 acid glycoprotein (AAG) levels was 23 months versus only 4.5 months for those with high baseline AAG, suggesting the possibility of selecting the candidates who will most benefit from this treatment.[132] A phase I study is investigating the safety, tolerability, and activity of ARRY-520 with carfilzomib. The MTD for the KSP inhibitor in this combination was 1.5 mg/m^2 and the available data showed an MR or better in 58% of evaluable patients.[133]

Another trial with ARRY-520, bortezomib, and dexamethasone is currently ongoing but preliminary results indicate an excessive toxicity arising from this association, whereas the combination with only bortezomib seems well tolerated and effective. However, both trials highlighted the need to use a growth factor support with ARRY-520 to limit the hematologic toxicity.[134]

SUMMARY

New treatment options for patients with myeloma have helped to change the natural history of this disease even in the context of relapsed disease. At this time, there is no simple formula for defining a path for treatment of patients with early or late relapse. It seems that, for standard-risk patients, doublet-based therapy may offer benefit, whereas for patients with aggressive or genetically high-risk disease combinations of agents are needed for adequate disease control. Second-generation agents including carfilzomib and the newest IMiD, pomalidomide, offer significant activity for patients with refractory myeloma, and new categories of agents including mono-clonal antibodies and HDAC inhibitors provide even newer targets for future study and clinical use. Combinations of these agents in selected patient populations repre-sent the next stage in the quest to cure myeloma.

REFERENCES

1. Palumbo A, Anderson K. Multiple myeloma. N Engl J Med 2011;364(11): 1046–60.
2. Durie BG, Harousseau JL, Miguel JS, et al. International uniform response criteria for multiple myeloma. Leukemia 2006;20:1467–73.
3. Kyle RA, Rajkumar SV. Criteria for diagnosis, staging, risk stratification and response assessment of multiple myeloma. Leukemia 2009;23:3–9.
4. Anderson KC, Kyle RA, Rajkumar SV, et al. Clinically relevant end points and new drug approvals for myeloma. Leukemia 2008;22:231–9.
5. Keats JJ, Chesi M, Egan JB, et al. Clonal competition with alternating domi-nance in multiple myeloma. Blood 2012;120(5):1067–76.
6. Egan JB, Shi CX, Tembe W, et al. Whole-genome sequencing of multiple myeloma from diagnosis to plasma cell leukemia reveals genomic initiating events, evolution, and clonal tides. Blood 2012;120(5):1060–6.
7. Magrangeas F, Avet-Loiseau H, Gouraud W, et al. Minor clone provides a reser-voir for relapse in multiple myeloma. Leukemia 2013;27(2):473–81.
8. Lonial S, Anderson KC. Association of response endpoints with survival out-comes in multiple myeloma. J Clin Oncol 2014;28(2):258–68.
9. Niesvizky R, Richardson PG, Rajkumar SV, et al. The relationship between qual-ity of response and clinical benefit for patients treated on the bortezomib arm of the international, randomized, phase 3 APEX trial in relapsed multiple myeloma. Br J Haematol 2008;143:46–53.
10. Palumbo A, Gay F, Bringhen S, et al. Bortezomib, doxorubicin and dexametha-sone in advanced multiple myeloma. Ann Oncol 2008;19(6):1160–5.
11. Offidani M, Corvatta L, Polloni C, et al. Thalidomide, dexamethasone, Doxil and Velcade (ThaDD-V) followed by consolidation/maintenance therapy in patients with relapsed-refractory multiple myeloma. Ann Hematol 2011;90:1449–56.
12. Harousseau JL, Dimopoulos MA, Wang M, et al. The quality of response to lena-lidomide plus dexamethasone is associated with improved clinical outcomes in patients with relapsed or refractory multiple myeloma. Haematologica 2010; 95(10):1738–44.
13. Siegel DS, Martin T, Wang M, et al. A phase 2 study of single-agent carfilzomib (PX-171-003-A1) in patients with relapsed and refractory multiple myeloma. Blood 2012;120(14):2817–25.
14. Richardson PG, Siegel DS, Vij R, et al. Pomalidomide alone or in combination with low-dose dexamethasone in relapsed and refractory multiple myeloma: a randomized phase 2 study. Blood 2014;123:1826–32.

15. San Miguel J, Weisel K, Moreau P, et al. Pomalidomide plus low-dose dexamethasone versus high-dose dexamethasone alone for patients with relapsed and refractory multiple myeloma (MM-003): a randomised, open-label, phase 3 trial. Lancet 2013;14(11):1055–66.

16. Chang H, Trieu Y, Qi X, et al. Impact of cytogenetics in patients with relapsed or refractory multiple myeloma treated with bortezomib: adverse effect of 1q21 gains. Leuk Res 2011;35(1):95–8.

17. Chen C, Reece DE, Siegel D, et al. Expanded safety experience with lenalidomide plus dexamethasone in relapsed or refractory multiple myeloma. Br J Haematol 2009;146(2):164–70.

18. Avet-Loiseau H, Soulier J, Fermand JP, et al. Impact of high-risk cytogenetics and prior therapy on outcomes in patients with advanced relapsed or refractory multiple myeloma treated with lenalidomide plus dexamethasone. Leukemia 2010;24(3):623–8.

19. Knop S, Gerecke C, Liebisch P, et al. Lenalidomide, adriamycin, and dexamethasone (RAD) in patients with relapsed and refractory multiple myeloma: a report from the German Myeloma Study Group DSMM (Deutsche Studiengruppe Multiples Myelom). Blood 2009;113(18):4137–43.

20. Reece D, Song K, Fu T, et al. Influence of cytogenetics in patients with relapsed or refractory multiple myeloma treated with lenalidomide plus dexamethasone: adverse effect of deletion 17p13. Blood 2009;114(3):522–5.

21. Dimopoulos MA, Kastritis E, Christoulas D, et al. Treatment of patients with relapsed/refractory multiple myeloma with lenalidomide and dexamethasone with or without bortezomib: prospective evaluation of the impact of cytogenetic abnormalities and of previous therapies. Leukemia 2010;24(10):1769–78.

22. Jakubowiak AJ, Siegel DS, Martin T, et al. Treatment outcomes in patients with relapsed and refractory multiple myeloma and high-risk cytogenetics receiving single-agent carfilzomib in the PX-171-003-A1 study. Leukemia 2013;27(12):2351–6.

23. Dimopoulos MA, Weisel K, Song KW, et al. Final analysis, cytogenetics, long-term treatment, and long-term survival in MM-003, a phase 3 study comparing pomalidomide + low-dose dexamethasone (POM + LoDEX) vs high-dose dexamethasone (HiDEX) in relapsed/refractory multiple myeloma (RRMM). ASH Annual Meeting Abstract 2013;122(21):408.

24. Kumar SV, Therneau TM, Gertz MA, et al. Clinical course of patients with relapsed multiple myeloma. Mayo Clin Proc 2004;79(7):867–74.

25. Krejci M, Gregora E, Straub J, et al. Similar efficacy of thalidomide- and bortezomib-based regimens for first relapse of multiple myeloma. Ann Hematol 2011;90(12):1441–7.

26. San Miguel JF, Weisel K, Song KW, et al. Patient outcomes by prior therapies and depth of response: analysis of MM-003, a phase 3 study comparing pomalidomide + low-dose dexamethasone (POM + LoDEX) vs high-dose dexamethasone (HiDEX) in relapsed/refractory multiple myeloma (RRMM). ASH Annual Meeting Abstract 2013;122(21):686.

27. Olin RL, Vogl DT, Porter DL, et al. Second auto-SCT is safe and effective salvage therapy for relapsed multiple myeloma. Bone Marrow Transplant 2009;43(5):417–22.

28. Gonsalves WI, Gertz MA, Lacy MQ, et al. Second auto-SCT for treatment of relapsed multiple myeloma. Bone Marrow Transplant 2013;48(4):568–73.

29. Vogl DT, Stadtmauer EA, Richardson PG, et al. Impact of prior therapies on the relative efficacy of bortezomib compared with dexamethasone in patients with relapsed/refractory multiple myeloma. Br J Haematol 2009;147(4):531–4.

30. Sonneveld P, Hajek R, Nagler A, et al. Combined pegylated liposomal doxorubicin and bortezomib is highly effective in patients with recurrent or refractory multiple myeloma who received prior thalidomide/lenalidomide therapy. Cancer 2008;112(7):1529–37.

31. Wang M, Dimopoulos MA, Chen C, et al. Lenalidomide plus dexamethasone is more effective than dexamethasone alone in patients with relapsed or refractory multiple myeloma regardless of prior thalidomide exposure. Blood 2008; 112(12):4445–51.

32. Pineda-Roman M, Zangari M, van Rhee F, et al. VTD combination therapy with bortezomib-thalidomide-dexamethasone is highly effective in advanced and refractory multiple myeloma. Leukemia 2008;22:1419–27.

33. Kropff M, Bisping G, Schuck E, et al. Bortezomib in combination with intermediate-dose dexamethasone and continuous low-dose oral cyclophosphamide for relapsed multiple myeloma. Br J Haematol 2007;138(3):330–7.

34. Klein U, Neben K, Hielscher T, et al. Lenalidomide in combination with dexamethasone: effective regimen in patients with relapsed or refractory multiple myeloma complicated by renal impairment. Ann Hematol 2011;90(4):429–39.

35. Chang H, Jiang A, Connie Q, et al. Impact of genomic aberrations including chromosome 1 abnormalities on the outcome of patients with relapsed or refractory multiple myeloma treated with lenalidomide and dexamethasone. Leuk Lymphoma 2010;51(11):2084–91.

36. Mateos MV, Richardson PG, Schlag R, et al. Bortezomib plus melphalan and prednisone compared with melphalan and prednisone in previously untreated multiple myeloma: updated follow-up and impact of subsequent therapy in the phase III VISTA trial. J Clin Oncol 2010;28(13):2259–66.

37. Vij R, Wang M, Kaufman JL, et al. An open-label, single-arm, phase 2 (PX-171-004) study of single- agent carfilzomib in bortezomib-naive patients with relapsed and/or refractory multiple myeloma. Blood 2012;119(24):5661–70.

38. Vij R, Siegel DS, Jagannath S, et al. An open-label, single-arm, phase 2 study of single-agent carfilzomib in patients with relapsed and/or refractory multiple myeloma who have been previously treated with bortezomib. Br J Haematol 2012;158(6):739–48.

39. Hrusovsky I, Emmerich B, Von Rohr A, et al. Bortezomib retreatment in relapsed multiple myeloma - results from a retrospective multicenter survey in Germany and Switzerland. Oncology 2010;79(3–4):247–54.

40. Petrucci MT, Giraldo P, Corradini P, et al. A prospective, international phase 2 study of bortezomib retreatment in patients with relapsed multiple myeloma. Br J Haematol 2013;160:649–59.

41. Glasmacher A, Hahn C, Hoffmann F, et al. A systematic review of phase-II trials of thalidomide monotherapy in patients with relapsed or refractory multiple myeloma. Br J Haematol 2006;132(5):584–93.

42. Palumbo A, Facon T, Sonneveld P, et al. Thalidomide for treatment of multiple myeloma: 10 years later. Blood 2008;111(8):3968–77.

43. von Lilienfeld-Toal M, Hahn-Ast C, Furkert K, et al. A systematic review of phase II trials of thalidomide/dexamethasone combination therapy in patients with relapsed or refractory multiple myeloma. Eur J Haematol 2008;81(4):247–52.

44. Garcia-Sanz R, Gonzalez-Porras JR, Hernandez JM, et al. The oral combination of thalidomide, cyclophosphamide and dexamethasone (ThaCyDex) is effective in relapsed/refractory multiple myeloma. Leukemia 2004;18(4):856–63.

45. Kyriakou C, Thomson K, D'Sa S, et al. Low-dose thalidomide in combination with oral weekly cyclophosphamide and pulsed dexamethasone is a well tolerated

and effective regimen in patients with relapsed and refractory multiple myeloma. Br J Haematol 2005;129(6):763–70.

46. Kropff MH, Lang N, Bisping G, et al. Hyperfractionated cyclophosphamide in combination with pulsed dexamethasone and thalidomide (hyperCDT) in primary refractory or relapsed multiple myeloma. Br J Haematol 2003;122(4): 607–16.

47. Dimopoulos MA, Hamilos G, Zomas A, et al. Pulsed cyclophosphamide, thalidomide and dexamethasone: an oral regimen for previously treated patients with multiple myeloma. Hematol J 2004;5(2):112–7.

48. Sidra G, Williams CD, Russell NH, et al. Combination chemotherapy with cyclophosphamide, thalidomide and dexamethasone for patients with refractory, newly diagnosed or relapsed myeloma. Haematologica 2006;91(6):862–3.

49. Hovenga S, Daenen SM, de Wolf JT, et al. Combined thalidomide and cyclophosphamide treatment for refractory or relapsed multiple myeloma patients: a prospective phase II study. Ann Hematol 2005;84(5):311–6.

50. Offidani M, Marconi M, Corvatta L, et al. Thalidomide plus oral melphalan for advanced multiple myeloma: a phase II study. Haematologica 2003;88(12): 1432–3.

51. Palumbo A, Avonto I, Bruno B, et al. Intravenous melphalan, thalidomide and prednisone in refractory and relapsed multiple myeloma. Eur J Haematol 2006;76(4):273–7.

52. Srkalovic G, Elson P, Trebisky B, et al. Use of melphalan, thalidomide, and dexamethasone in treatment of refractory and relapsed multiple myeloma. Med Oncol 2002;19(4):219–26.

53. Offidani M, Corvatta L, Marconi M, et al. Low dose thalidomide with pegylated liposomal doxorubicin and high-dose dexamethasone for relapsed/refractory multiple myeloma: a prospective, multicenter, phase II study. Haematologica 2006;91(1):133–6.

54. Hussein MA, Baz R, Srkalovic G, et al. Phase 2 study of pegylated liposomal doxorubicin, vincristine, decreased-frequency dexamethasone, and thalidomide in newly diagnosed and relapsed-refractory multiple myeloma. Mayo Clin Proc 2006;81(7):889–95.

55. Pönisch W, Rozanski M, Goldschmidt H, et al. Combined bendamustine, prednisolone and thalidomide for refractory or relapsed multiple myeloma after autologous stem-cell transplantation or conventional chemotherapy: results of a phase I clinical trial. Br J Haematol 2008;143(2):191–200.

56. Lee CK, Barlogie B, Munshi N, et al. DTPACE: an effective, novel combination chemotherapy with thalidomide for previously treated patients with myeloma. J Clin Oncol 2003;21(14):2732–9.

57. Palumbo A, Rajkumar SV, Dimopoulos MA, et al. Prevention of thalidomide- and lenalidomide-associated thrombosis in myeloma. Leukemia 2008;22(2): 414–23.

58. Richardson PG, Sonneveld P, Schuster MW, et al, Assessment of Proteasome Inhibition for Extending Remissions (APEX) Investigators. Bortezomib or high-dose dexamethasone for relapsed multiple myeloma. N Engl J Med 2005; 352(24):2487–98.

59. Richardson PG, Sonneveld P, Schuster M, et al. Extended follow-up of a phase 3 trial in relapsed multiple myeloma: final time-to-event results of the APEX trial. Blood 2007;110(10):3557–60.

60. Jagannath S, Barlogie B, Berenson JR, et al. Updated survival analyses after prolonged follow-up of the phase 2, multicenter CREST study of bortezomib

in relapsed or refractory multiple myeloma. Br J Haematol 2008;143(4): 537–40.

61. Mikhael JR, Belch AR, Prince HM, et al. High response rate to bortezomib with or without dexamethasone in patients with relapsed or refractory multiple myeloma: results of a global phase 3b expanded access program. Br J Haematol 2009;144(2):169–75.

62. Kropff MH, Bisping G, Wenning D, et al. Bortezomib in combination with dexamethasone for relapsed multiple myeloma. Leuk Res 2005;29:587–90.

63. Orlowski RZ, Voorhees PM, Garcia RA, et al. Phase 1 trial of the proteasome inhibitor bortezomib and pegylated liposomal doxorubicin in patients with advanced hematologic malignancies. Blood 2005;105(8):3058–65.

64. Orlowski RZ, Nagler A, Sonneveld P, et al. Randomized phase III study of pegylated liposomal doxorubicin plus bortezomib compared with bortezomib alone in relapsed or refractory multiple myeloma: combination therapy improves time to progression. J Clin Oncol 2007;25(25):3892–901.

65. Berenson JR, Yang HH, Sadler K, et al. Phase I/II trial assessing bortezomib and melphalan combination therapy for the treatment of patients with relapsed or refractory multiple myeloma. J Clin Oncol 2006;24(6):937–44.

66. Popat R, Oakervee H, Williams C, et al. Bortezomib, low-dose intravenous melphalan, and dexamethasone for patients with relapsed multiple myeloma. Br J Haematol 2009;144(6):887–94.

67. Kropff M, Bisping G, Schuck E, et al. Bortezomib in combination with intermediate-dose dexamethasone and continuous low-dose oral cyclophosphamide for relapsed multiple myeloma. Br J Haematol 2007;138(3):330–7.

68. Reece DE, Rodriguez GP, Chen C, et al. Phase I-II trial of bortezomib plus oral cyclophosphamide and prednisone in relapsed and refractory multiple myeloma. J Clin Oncol 2008;26(29):4777–83.

69. Ludwig H, Kasparu H, Leitgeb C, et al. Bendamustine-bortezomib-dexamethasone is an active and well tolerated regimen in patients with relapsed or refractory multiple myeloma. Blood 2014;123:985–91.

70. Offidani M, Corvatta L, Maracci L, et al. Efficacy and tolerability of bendamustine, bortezomib and dexamethasone in patients with relapsed-refractory multiple myeloma: a phase II study. Blood Cancer J 2013;3(11):162.

71. Richardson PG, Briemberg H, Jagannath S, et al. Frequency, characteristics, and reversibility of peripheral neuropathy during treatment of advanced multiple myeloma with bortezomib. J Clin Oncol 2006;124(19):3113–20.

72. Bringhen S, Larocca A, Rossi D, et al. Efficacy and safety of once-weekly bortezomib in multiple myeloma patients. Blood 2010;116(23):4745–53.

73. Moreau P, Pylypenko H, Grosicki S, et al. Subcutaneous versus intravenous administration of bortezomib in patients with relapsed multiple myeloma: a randomised, phase 3, non-inferiority study. Lancet Oncol 2011;12(5):431–40.

74. Chanan-Khan A, Sonneveld P, Schuster MW, et al. Analysis of herpes zoster events among bortezomib-treated patients in the phase III APEX study. J Clin Oncol 2008;26:4784–90.

75. Kumar S, Bensinger W, Zimmerman TM, et al. Weekly MLN9708, an investigational oral proteasome inhibitor (PI), in relapsed/refractory multiple myeloma (MM): results from a phase I study after full enrollment. ASCO Meeting Abstracts 2013;31(15):8514.

76. Richardson PG, Schlossman RL, Weller E, et al. Immunomodulatory drug CC-5013 overcomes drug resistance and is well tolerated in patients with relapsed multiple myeloma. Blood 2002;100(9):3063–7.

77. Richardson PG, Blood E, Mitsiades CS, et al. A randomized phase 2 study of lenalidomide therapy for patients with relapsed or relapsed and refractory multiple myeloma. Blood 2006;108(10):3458–64.
78. Richardson P, Jagannath S, Hussein M, et al. Safety and efficacy of single-agent lenalidomide in patients with relapsed and refractory multiple myeloma. Blood 2009;114(4):772–8.
79. Dimopoulos M, Spencer A, Attal M, et al. Lenalidomide plus dexamethasone for relapsed or refractory multiple myeloma. N Engl J Med 2007;357(21):2123–32.
80. Weber DM, Chen C, Niesvizky R, et al. Lenalidomide plus dexamethasone for relapsed multiple myeloma in North America. N Engl J Med 2007;357(21): 2133–42.
81. Dimopoulos MA, Chen C, Spencer A, et al. Long-term follow-up on overall survival from the MM-009 and MM-010 phase III trials of lenalidomide plus dexamethasone in patients with relapsed or refractory multiple myeloma. Leukemia 2009;23(11):2147–52.
82. Baz R, Walker E, Karam MA, et al. Lenalidomide and pegylated liposomal doxorubicin-based chemotherapy for relapsed or refractory multiple myeloma: safety and efficacy. Ann Oncol 2006;17(12):1766–71.
83. van de Donk NW, Wittebol S, Minnema MC, et al. Lenalidomide (Revlimid) combined with continuous oral cyclophosphamide (endoxan) and prednisone (REP) is effective in lenalidomide/dexamethasone-refractory myeloma. Br J Haematol 2010;148(2):335–7.
84. Reece DE, Masih-Khan E, Khan A, et al. Phase I-II trial of oral cyclophosphamide, prednisone and lenalidomide (Revlimid) (CPR) for the treatment of patients with relapsed and refractory multiple myeloma. ASH Annual Meeting Abstract 2010;116(21):3055.
85. Morgan GJ, Schey SA, Wu P, et al. Lenalidomide (Revlimid), in combination with cyclophosphamide and dexamethasone (RCD), is an effective and tolerated regimen for myeloma patients. Br J Haematol 2007;137(3):268–9.
86. Schey S, Morgan GJ, Ramasamy K, et al. The addition of cyclophosphamide to lenalidomide and dexamethasone in multiply relapsed/refractory myeloma patients; a phase I/II study. Br J Haematol 2010;150(3):326–33.
87. Lentzsch S, O'Sullivan A, Kennedy RC, et al. Combination of bendamustine, lenalidomide, and dexamethasone (BLD) in patients with relapsed or refractory multiple myeloma is feasible and highly effective: results of phase 1/2 open-label, dose escalation study. Blood 2012;119(20):4608–13.
88. Pönisch W, Heyn S, Beck J, et al. Lenalidomide, bendamustine and prednisolone exhibits a favourable safety and efficacy profile in relapsed or refractory multiple myeloma: final results of a phase 1 clinical trial OSHO - #077. Br J Haematol 2013;162(2):202–9.
89. Wang Z, Yang J, Kirk C, et al. Clinical pharmacokinetics, metabolism, and drug-drug interaction of carfilzomib. Drug Metab Dispos 2013;41(1):230–7.
90. Kuhn DJ, Chen Q, Voorhees PM, et al. Potent activity of carfilzomib, a novel, irreversible inhibitor of the ubiquitin-proteasome pathway, against preclinical models of multiple myeloma. Blood 2007;110(9):3281–90.
91. O'Connor OA, Stewart AK, Vallone M, et al. A phase 1 dose escalation study of the safety and pharmaco-kinetics of the novel proteasome inhibitor carfilzomib (PR-171) in patients with hematologic malignancies. Clin Cancer Res 2009; 15(22):7085–91.
92. Alsina M, Trudel S, Furman RR, et al. A phase I single-agent study of twice-weekly consecutive-day dosing of the proteasome inhibitor carfilzomib in

patients with relapsed or refractory multiple myeloma or lymphoma. Clin Cancer Res 2012;18(17):4830–40.

93. Siegel D, Martin T, Nooka A, et al. Integrated safety profile of single-agent car-filzomib: experience from 526 patients enrolled in 4 phase II clinical studies. Haematologica 2013;98(11):1753–61.

94. Badros AZ, Papadopoulos KP, Zojwalla N, et al. A phase 1b study of 30-minute infusion carfilzomib 20/45 and 20/56 mg/m^2 plus 40 mg weekly dexamethasone in patients with relapsed and/or refractory (R/R) multiple myeloma. ASH Annual Meeting Abstract 2012;120(21):4036.

95. Kaufman JL, Siegel D, Ghobrial IM, et al. Clinical profile of once-daily, modified-release oprozomib tablets in patients with hematologic malignancies: results of a phase IB/2 trial. EHA Annual Meeting Abstracts 2013;P233.

96. Schey SA, Fields P, Bartlett JB, et al. Phase I study of an immunomodulatory thalidomide analog, CC-4047, in relapsed or refractory multiple myeloma. J Clin Oncol 2004;22(16):3269–76.

97. Streetly MJ, Gyertson K, Daniel Y, et al. Alternate day pomalidomide retains anti-myeloma effect with reduced adverse events and evidence of in vivo immuno-modulation. Br J Haematol 2008;141(1):41–51.

98. Richardson PG, Siegel D, Baz R, et al. Phase 1 study of pomalidomide MTD, safety, and efficacy in patients with refractory multiple myeloma who have received lenalidomide and bortezomib. Blood 2013;121(11):1961–7.

99. Lacy MQ, Hayman SR, Gertz MA, et al. Pomalidomide (CC4047) plus low-dose dexamethasone as therapy for relapsed multiple myeloma. J Clin Oncol 2009; 27(30):5008–14.

100. Lacy MQ, Hayman SR, Gertz MA, et al. Pomalidomide (CC4047) plus low dose dexamethasone (Pom/dex) is active and well tolerated in lenalidomide refractory multiple myeloma (MM). Leukemia 2010;24(11):1934–9.

101. Lacy MQ, Allred JB, Gertz MA, et al. Pomalidomide plus low-dose dexameth-asone in myeloma refractory to both bortezomib and lenalidomide: compari-son of 2 dosing strategies in dual-refractory disease. Blood 2011;118(11): 2970–5.

102. Leleu X, Attal M, Arnulf B, et al. Pomalidomide plus low-dose dexamethasone is active and well tolerated in bortezomib and lenalidomide-refractory multiple myeloma: intergroupe Francophone du Myelome 2009-02. Blood 2013; 121(11):1968–75.

103. Larocca A, Montefusco V, Bringhen S, et al. Pomalidomide, cyclophosphamide, and prednisone for relapsed/refractory multiple myeloma: a multicenter phase 1/2 open-label study. Blood 2013;122(16):2799–806.

104. Mark TM, Boyer A, Rossi AC, et al. ClaPD (clarithromycin, pomalidomide, dexa-methasone) therapy in relapsed or refractory multiple myeloma. ASH Annual Meeting Abstract 2013;122(21):1955.

105. Lonial S, Mitsiades C, Richardson PG. Treatment options for relapsed and re-fractory multiple myeloma. Clin Cancer Res 2011;17(6):1264–77.

106. Garderet L, Iacobelli S, Moreau P, et al. Superiority of the triple combination of bortezomib-thalidomide-dexamethasone over the dual combination of thalidomide-dexamethasone in patients with multiple myeloma progressing or relapsing after autologous transplantation: the MMVAR/IFM 2005-04 random-ized phase III Trial from the Chronic Leukemia Working Party of the European Group for blood and marrow transplantation. J Clin Oncol 2012;30(20):2475–82.

107. Kim YK, Sohn SK, Lee JH, et al. Clinical efficacy of a bortezomib, cyclophospha-mide, thalidomide, and dexamethasone (Vel-CTD) regimen in patients with

relapsed or refractory multiple myeloma: a phase II study. Ann Hematol 2010; 89:475–82.

108. Terpos E, Kastritis E, Roussou M, et al. The combination of bortezomib, melphalan, dexamethasone and intermittent thalidomide is an effective regimen for relapsed/refractory myeloma and is associated with improvement of abnormal bone metabolism and angiogenesis. Leukemia 2008;22(12):2247–56.

109. Palumbo A, Ambrosini MT, Benevolo G, et al. Bortezomib, melphalan, prednisone and thalidomide for relapsed multiple myeloma. Blood 2007;109(7): 2767–72.

110. Palumbo A, Larocca A, Falco P, et al. Lenalidomide, melphalan, prednisone and thalidomide (RMPT) for relapsed/refractory multiple myeloma. Leukemia 2010; 24(5):1037–42.

111. Richardson PG, Xie W, Jagannath S, et al. A phase II trial of lenalidomide, bortezomib and dexamethasone in patients with relapsed and relapsed/refractory myeloma. Blood 2014;123:1461–9.

112. Wang M, Martin T, Bensinger W, et al. Phase 2 dose-expansion study (PX-171-006) of carfilzomib, lenalidomide, and low-dose dexamethasone in relapsed or progressive multiple myeloma. Blood 2013;122(18):3122–8.

113. Richardson PG, Hofmeister CG, Siegel D, et al. MM-005: a phase 1 trial of pomalidomide, bortezomib, and low-dose dexamethasone (PVD) in relapsed and/ or refractory multiple myeloma (RRMM). ASH Annual Meeting Abstract 2013; 122(21):1969.

114. Shah JJ, Stadtmauer EA, Abonour R, et al. Phase I/II dose expansion of a multi-center trial of carfilzomib and pomalidomide with dexamethasone (Car-Pom-d) in patients with relapsed/refractory multiple myeloma. ASH Annual Meeting Abstract 2013;122(21):690.

115. Kumar SK, Lee JH, Lahuerta JJ, et al. Risk of progression and survival in multiple myeloma relapsing after therapy with IMiDs and bortezomib: a multicenter international myeloma working group study. Leukemia 2012;26:149–57.

116. San-Miguel JF, Richardson PG, Günther A, et al. Phase Ib study of panobinostat and bortezomib in relapsed or relapsed and refractory multiple myeloma. J Clin Oncol 2013;31(29):3696–703.

117. Badros A, Burger AM, Philip S, et al. Phase I study of vorinostat in combination with bortezomib for relapsed and refractory multiple myeloma. Clin Cancer Res 2009;15(16):5250–7.

118. Richardson PG, Schlossman RL, Alsina M, et al. PANORAMA 2: panobinostat in combination with bortezomib and dexamethasone in patients with relapsed and bortezomib-refractory myeloma. Blood 2013;122(14):2331–7.

119. Richardson PG, Schlossman RL, Alsina M, et al. Time to event analyses in PANORAMA 2: a phase 2 study of panobinostat, bortezomib, and dexamethasone in patients with relapsed and bortezomib-refractory multiple myeloma. ASH Annual Meeting Abstract 2013;122(21):1970.

120. Siegel DS, Dimopoulos MA, Yoon SS, et al. Vantage 095: vorinostat in combination with bortezomib in salvage multiple myeloma patients: final study results of a global phase 2b trial. ASH Annual Meeting Abstracts 2011;118(21):480.

121. Dimopoulos M, Siegel DS, Lonial S, et al. Vorinostat or placebo in combination with bortezomib in patients with multiple myeloma (VANTAGE 088): a multi-centre, randomised, double-blind study. Lancet Oncol 2013;14(11):1129–40.

122. San-Miguel JF, Moreau P, Yoon SS, et al. Phase III study of panobinostat with bortezomib and dexamethasone in patients with relapsed multiple myeloma (PANORAMA 1). ASCO Meeting Abstracts 2012;30(15 Suppl):18572.

123. Raje N, Vogl DT, Hari PN, et al. ACY-1215, a selective histone deacetylase (HDAC) 6 inhibitor: interim results of combination therapy with bortezomib in patients with multiple myeloma (MM). ASH Annual Meeting Abstracts 2011; 118(21):759.

124. Zonder JA, Mohrbacher AF, Singhal S, et al. A phase 1, multicenter, open-label, dose escalation study of elotuzumab in patients with advanced multiple myeloma. Blood 2012;120(3):552–9.

125. Lonial S, Vij R, Harousseau JL, et al. Elotuzumab in combination with lenalidomide and low-dose dexamethasone in relapsed or refractory multiple myeloma. J Clin Oncol 2012;30(16):1953–9.

126. Richardson PG, Jagannath S, Moreau P, et al. A phase 2 study of elotuzumab (Elo) in combination with lenalidomide and low-dose dexamethasone (Ld) in patients (pts) with relapsed/refractory multiple myeloma (R/R MM): updated results. ASH Annual Meeting Abstracts 2012;120(21):202.

127. Jakubowiak AJ, Benson DM, Bensinger W, et al. Phase I trial of anti-CS1 monoclonal antibody elotuzumab in combination with bortezomib in the treatment of relapsed/refractory multiple myeloma. J Clin Oncol 2012;30(16):1960–5.

128. Lokhorst HM, Plesner T, Gimsing P, et al. Phase I/II dose-escalation study of daratumumab in patients with relapsed or refractory multiple myeloma. ASCO Meeting Abstracts 2013;31(15 Suppl):8512.

129. Nijhof IS, Noort WA, van Bueren JL, et al. CD38-targeted immunochemotherapy of multiple myeloma: preclinical evidence for its combinatorial use in lenalidomide and bortezomib refractory/intolerant MM patients. ASH Annual Meeting Abstract 2013;122(21):277.

130. Plesner T, Arkenau T, Lokhorst H, et al. Preliminary safety and efficacy data of daratumumab in combination with lenalidomide and dexamethasone in relapsed or refractory multiple myeloma. ASH Annual Meeting Abstract 2013; 122(21):1986.

131. Martin TG III, Strickland SA, Glenn M, et al. SAR650984, a CD38 monoclonal antibody in patients with selected CD38+ hematological malignancies- data from a dose-escalation phase I study. ASH Annual Meeting Abstract 2013; 122(21):284.

132. Lonial S, Shah JJ, Zonder J, et al. Prolonged survival and improved response rates with ARRY-520 in relapsed/refractory multiple myeloma (RRMM) patients with low α-1 acid glycoprotein (AAG) levels: results from a phase 2 study. ASH Annual Meeting Abstract 2013;122(21):285.

133. Shah JJ, Feng L, Thomas SK, et al. Phase 1 study of the novel kinesin spindle protein inhibitor ARRY-520 + carfilzomib (Car) in patients with relapsed and/or refractory multiple myeloma (RRMM). ASH Annual Meeting Abstract 2013; 122(21):1982.

134. Chari A, Htut M, Zonder J, et al. A phase 1 study of ARRY-520 with bortezomib (BTZ) and dexamethasone (dex) in relapsed or refractory multiple myeloma (RRMM). ASH Annual Meeting Abstract 2013;122(21):1938.

Allogeneic Stem Cell Transplantation for Multiple Myeloma

William Bensinger, MD

KEYWORDS

- Multiple myeloma • Allogeneic stem cell transplant • Autologous stem cell transplant
- Peripheral blood stem cells • Myeloablative transplant • Nonmyeloablative transplant

KEY POINTS

- Allogeneic stem cell transplantation can result in durable remissions for some patients with multiple myeloma; however, transplant morbidity and mortality limit its wider application.
- Reduced intensity allografts improve the safety, but are still limited by graft-versus-host disease and high rates of relapse.
- Prospective trials comparing autologous with allogeneic transplants based on donor availability have shown conflicting outcomes with respect to survival and disease-free intervals.
- Allogeneic stem cell transplants will remain investigational until improvements in conditioning regimens, and control of graft-versus-host disease and relapse are achieved.

INTRODUCTION

Despite significant progress in the treatment of multiple myeloma, most patients will have recurrent disease and die. New drugs and autologous stem cell transplantation (ASCT) have increased rates of remission, improved remission durations, and prolonged overall survival rates by 3 to 5 years. Relapses, however, continue for most patients, emphasizing the need for new drugs and treatment strategies. Allogeneic stem cell transplantation (AlloSCT) offers the potential of harnessing an immunologic graft-versus-myeloma (GVM) effect capable of controlling residual disease and offering the potential for cure. Unfortunately, the complexity, complications, and relatively poor outcomes of AlloSCT for myeloma have limited its application and relegated this therapy to investigational studies. As survival of patients with myeloma has improved with new drugs and ASCT, the role of AlloSCT, if any, in the treatment of myeloma has been further questioned.[1] This article reviews the current knowledge about AlloSCT for myeloma and discusses current research activities.

Division of Oncology, University of Washington, Fred Hutchinson Cancer Research Center, 1100 Fairview Avenue North, D5-390, Seattle, WA 98109, USA
E-mail address: wbensing@fhcrc.org

Hematol Oncol Clin N Am 28 (2014) 891–902
http://dx.doi.org/10.1016/j.hoc.2014.06.001
0889-8588/14/$ – see front matter © 2014 Elsevier Inc. All rights reserved.

HISTORY

An initial attempt at treating refractory myeloma with total body irradiation (TBI) and bone marrow from an unmatched cadaver, reported in 1957, was unsuccessful.[2] Success with AlloSCT for the treatment of multiple myeloma was first reported in 1982[3] and again in 1984.[4] One patient with progressive myeloma received cyclophosphamide and 800 cGy TBI followed by HLA identical sibling marrow and achieved engraftment and a remission. Two patients with advanced myeloma received cyclophosphamide and TBI followed by sibling bone marrow. Both patients engrafted with subsequent resolution of their myeloma; however, one died of disseminated zoster at 6 months, while the other relapsed at 3 years. These reports were followed by small series from Seattle[5] and the European Bone Marrow Transplant Cooperative Group (EBMT)[6] showing the feasibility of this procedure in myeloma. As experience accumulated in the 1980s and 1990s, it became clear that AlloSCT using ablative techniques was associated with high morbidity and mortality, as a consequence, many transplant centers abandoned myeloablative allograft conditioning for myeloma.[7] A US trial of early versus late ASCT had an option of AlloSCT for patients with matched sibling donors.[8] Patients received myeloablative conditioning with melphalan plus TBI. After 36 patients were enrolled in the AlloSCT arm, this group was closed to further accrual because of transplant-related mortality (TRM) exceeding 50%. Interestingly, after more than 7 years of follow-up, the overall survival (OS) rate of the AlloSCT group was 40%, better than either arm of the ASCT groups. Because of the GVM effect of AlloSCT, deeper and more durable remissions were observed, resulting in a reduced rate of relapse in the AlloSCT group compared with either ASCT group. Studies using patient-specific primers to look for minimal residual disease in myeloma patients achieving a complete response (CR) reported higher rates of minimal residual disease negativity among recipients of AlloSCT compared with ASCT. Furthermore, patients with minimal residual disease–negative remissions have much longer disease-free intervals than patients whose marrow is minimal residual disease positive at any time after transplant.[9,10]

By the mid-1990s the EBMT reported a retrospective comparison of 189 patients with myeloma who received myeloablative AlloSCT and were matched for gender and prior courses of chemotherapy with 189 patients with myeloma who received ASCT.[11] The groups were comparable except the median age of the AlloSCT group was 6 years younger, with 16-month longer median follow-up. OS was superior for the ASCT group (median, 34 vs 18 months; $P = .001$) because of a much higher TRM in the AlloSCT group (41% vs 13%; $P = 0001$). This higher TRM was not offset by the lower rates of relapse seen in the AlloSCT group (at 4 years, 50% vs 70%; $P = .04$).

Thus, the perception of an increase in morbidity and mortality after AlloSCT for patients with myeloma draws directly from outcomes of patients reported in the literature. Recently, this idea has been challenged by pooled analyses of 56,000 transplants reported to EBMT.[12] Patients were given a risk score of 0 to 7 based on age, disease stage, time from diagnosis to transplant, donor type, and donor-recipient gender. Patients with myeloma had a greater mortality risk after AlloSCT but were also observed to have a higher risk score because of more advanced age, longer interval from diagnosis to transplant, and more advanced disease stage. When similar risk score patients with myeloma or acute leukemia underwent transplant, the mortality was similar. Although interesting, as a practical matter, these observations are of limited benefit, because the diagnosis of myeloma is frequent at advanced age, and most patients do not achieve complete remission before transplant. Furthermore, the EBMT observed a marked reduction in nonrelapse mortality after 2 years from 46% for patients undergoing transplant between 1983 and 1993 to 30% for patients undergoing transplant between 1994 and 1998, likely because of improvements in supportive care and more careful patient selection.[13] Nevertheless, with a mortality rate of even 30%, most transplant centers began to explore alternatives to myeloablative AlloSCT in patients with myeloma and other hematologic malignancies.

REDUCED-INTENSITY CONDITIONING REGIMENS

In the late 1990s, interest in exploiting the GVM effects of AlloSCT was adopted by several groups using a reduced-intensity conditioning designed to minimize early toxicity and mortality associated with high intensity, myeloablative treatments.[14,15] A reduced-intensity regimen delivers therapy that is immunosuppressive and designed mainly to facilitate donor engraftment. This reduced-intensity approach relies heavily on the immunologic effect of the graft for disease control, as prior demonstrations of the GVM effect in recipients of donor lymphocyte infusions showed.[16] Several conditioning regimens have been reported ranging from minimal conditioning using 2 Gy TBI to ablative yet reduced doses of melphalan or busulfan. A summary of the principal reduced intensity regimens evaluated in clinical trials of 40 or more patients is shown in **Table 1**. Almost all of these series used peripheral blood stem cells rather than bone marrow from matched related or unrelated donors because of higher rates of graft failure or rejection observed with marrow.[14] Trials using a single dose of 2 Gy TBI, mycophenolic acid, and cyclosporine for GVHD prophylaxis with matched related donors have reported 8% grades 3 to 4 GVHD, 11% to 22% nonrelapse mortality rate, and 50% to 60% CR rates.[17] The addition of fludarabine to 2 Gy TBI in a mix of related and unrelated donors was associated with more severe GVHD (24%) but similar nonrelapse mortality.[18,19] Fludarabine melphalan combinations with cyclosporine, methotrexate, and antithymocyte globulin (ATG, unrelated donors only) reported 21%, severe GVHD, less than 20% nonrelapse mortality, and CR rates of approximately 50%.[20] Intermediate dose (100 mg/m^2) melphalan, with or without 2.5 Gy TBI and cyclosporine and prednisone for GVHD prophylaxis, was associated with high rates of severe GVHD (42%) and nonrelapse mortality (38%).[21] A regimen of fludarabine and ablative but reduced doses of busulfan, 8 mg/kg, and ATG resulted in low (7%) severe GVHD, moderate (17%) nonrelapse mortality, and low (27%) rates of CR.[22] It is likely that the relatively high doses of ATG used in this trial interfered with the GVM effects of the allograft. A novel 3-drug regimen of thiotepa, 5 mg/kg, fludarabine, and melphalan reported low rates (5%) of severe GVHD, 13% nonrelapse mortality rate, and a relatively high (62%) CR rate.[23] None of the regimens in **Table 1** have been directly compared with one another, and differences in the mix of patient characteristics, donor types, and the GVHD prophylaxis may account for many of the outcome disparities.

GVHD AND RELAPSE

Multiple trials show a strong association between the development of acute or chronic GVHD and improved progression-free survival (PFS). An analysis of registry data after reduced-intensity AlloSCT for myeloma found that patients who had chronic extensive or chronic limited GVHD had superior OS and PFS compared with patients who had no chronic GVHD (84% and 46% vs 29% and 12%, respectively).[24] A subsequent multivariate analysis found a lower risk of relapse and better event free-survival with limited chronic GVHD, but this failed to translate to improved OS.[25]

Because of the increased morbidity and mortality associated with AlloSCT for myeloma, it is recommended by some experts that this treatment be deferred until

Table 1
Principal reduced intensity regimens used for AlloSCT for multiple myeloma

Reference	No. of Patients	Regimen	Donors (No. of Patients)	GVHD Proph	AGVHD 3 to 4 (%)	CGVHD (%)	TRM (%)	CR (%)
Bruno et al,[17] 2009	100	2 Gy TBI[a]	MRD	MMF/Csa	3 (4 only)	50	11	53
Rotta[18]	102	2 Gy TBI[a] ±fludarabine	MRD	MMf/Csa	8	74	19	62
Gerull[19]	52	2 Gy TBI Fludarabine 90	MRD 32 MUD 20	Mmf/Csa	24	70	17	NR
Kroger[20]	120	Fludarabine 150–180 Melphalan 70–140[a]	MRD 85 MUD 35	Csa Mtx, ATG	21	47	18	49
Lee[21]	45	Melphalan 100 ±2.5 Gy TBI	MRD 34 MUD 11	Csa Prednisone	42	58	38	64
Mohty[22]	41	Fludarabine 180 Busulfan 8	MRD	Csa, ATG ±Mtx	7	41	17	27
Majolino[23]	53	Thiotepa 5 Fludarabine 90 Melphalan 80	MRD	Csa Mtx	5	64	13	62

Abbreviations: ATG, anti-thymocyte globulin; Csa, cyclosporine; MMf, mycofenolic acid; MRD, matched related donors; Mtx, methotrexate; MUD, matched unrelated donors; NR, not reported.
[a] Some or all as tandem after ASCT.

ASCT fails. Relapse after ASCT, however, is an important negative risk factor for outcome after AlloSCT.[20,26] Several studies report that patients whose disease has progressed after ASCT and who are then offered AlloSCT, have increased rates of TRM and relapse. A retrospective study has compared outcomes in a multicenter analysis of patients with myeloma who progressed after ASCT.[27] The study compared 68 patients who had relapse after ASCT and were treated with AlloSCT from matched related or unrelated donors with 94 patients who had relapse after ASCT but did not have suitable donors and received salvage chemotherapy with novel agents. The groups were comparable, except for a 4-year median greater age in the no-donor group and slightly more patients with extramedullary disease in the donor group. Two-year TRM was 22% versus 1% in the donor versus no-donor groups ($P<.0001$), and PFS at 2 years was 43% versus 18% ($P<.001$), but 2-year OS was not different at 54%. Of the 68 patients, 19 (28%) were reported to be in CR at 29 months, indicating that a proportion of patients can achieve long-term control with AlloSCT, even after ASCT relapse. The above studies would indicate that waiting until failure of ASCT may not be the best strategy for considering AlloSCT.

HI-RISK MYELOMA

Another recommendation is that AlloSCT be reserved for patients with myeloma who have the highest risk of disease relapse with conventional therapy, with or without ASCT, based on the hypothesis that the GVM effect of the donor graft is independent of chemosensitivity. Indeed, high β-2 microglobulin, conventional cytogenetic abnormalities such as deletion of chromosome 13, and certain chromosomal abnormalities detected by fluorescence in situ hybridization (FISH) including translocation 4;14 or deletion 17p have been associated with PFS intervals as short as 9 to 20 months after ASCT. Data using newer drugs such as bortezomib for both induction before ASCT and maintenance or consolidation after ASCT have indicated improved PFS and OS of certain high-risk groups compared with patients not receiving bortezomib.[28] Unfortunately, outcomes with bortezomib were still not as good as in the group of patients without these high-risk features.

Retrospective analyses of AlloSCT suggest that this approach may overcome high-risk cytogenetics such as del17 or 4;14, and very small prospective trials have validated this theory.[10] The German myeloma study group reported the preliminary results of a prospective trial, DSMM V, for patients with high-risk myeloma based on del13 by FISH who received one ASCT followed by either a reduced-intensity AlloSCT or a second ASCT based on the availability of a related or unrelated donor.[29] Of 199 patients enrolled, 126 received AlloSCT using fludarabine and melphalan 140 mg/m^2, whereas 73 received ASCT after a second course of melphalan. At 1 year, the CR rate was significantly higher for ASCT-AlloSCT (59% vs 32%; $P = .003$). TRM for the ASCT-AlloSCT group was 12.6%. With short follow-up of 25 to 34 months, the OS was 72% for the tandem ASCT group versus 60% for the ASCT-AlloSCT group ($P = .22$). A longer follow-up and analysis of this trial is currently underway.

PROSPECTIVE COMPARISONS OF TANDEM ASCT VERSUS ASCT-AlloSCT

Six trials comparing 1 to 2 ASCTs with single ASCT followed by reduced-intensity AlloSCT have been published; major features are summarized in **Table 2**. In general, none of these trials were strictly randomized; the randomization to AlloSCT was based on the availability of an human leukocyte antigen (HLA)-matched family donor. All trials compared ASCT with tandem ASCT followed by AlloSCT as part of the initial therapy, immediately after initial induction therapy. All trials used reduced intensity, but not

Table 2
Prospective trials comparing single or double ASCT with ASCT followed by AlloSCT

Reference	Treatment	No Allo vs Auto	Response CR (%)	EFS/PFS	OS	Comments, Significance
Garban[30]	Auto-allo (RIC) vs auto-auto	65 vs 219 del13 FISH, B2>3	62 vs 51	Median EFS, 31.7 vs 35 mo	Median OS, 35 vs 47.2 mo	Short median follow-up 2 y, no difference in EFS, OS
Bruno[31] Giaccone[32]	Auto-allo (TBI) vs auto-auto	80 vs 82	55 vs 26	Median EFS, 2.8 vs 2.4 y	Median OS, NR vs 4.25 y	Median 7-y follow-up, $P = .005$ for EFS and $P = .001$ OS favoring auto-allo
Rosinol[33]	Allo vs 2nd auto	25 vs 85 <nCR after first ASCT	40 vs 11	Median PFS, not reached vs 31 mo	5-y OS, 62% vs 60%	$P = .001$ for CR; improved PFS trend for auto-allo ($P = .08$); OS ns
Krishnan[34]	Auto-allo vs auto-auto	156 vs 356, standard risk	13 vs 9	3-y PFS, 43% vs 46%	3-y OS; 77% vs 80%	Patients referred for study after HLA typing, short follow-up, PFS, OS ns
Bjorkstrand et al,[35] 2011 Gahrton et al,[36] 2013	Auto-allo vs auto-auto	108 vs 249	51 vs 41	22% vs 12%	49% vs 36%	Median 8-y follow-up, $P = .02$ for CR, $P = .027$ EFS, $P = .030$ for OS
Lokhorst et al,[37] 2012	Auto then allo vs auto #2	122 vs 138	43 vs 37	28% vs 22%	55% vs 55%	Median follow-up 6 y, EFS, OS ns

Abbreviations: MEL 200, melphalan 200 mg/m^2; NR, not reported; ns, not significant; RIC, reduced-intensity conditioning.

always nonmyeloablative, regimens for AlloSCT. The first reported study by a French consortium compared myeloma patients considered to have high risk features based on del13 by FISH or a β-2 microglobulin greater than 3.[30] This report included 2 parallel studies for patients with or without donors, rather than a randomization. All patients received a single ASCT after melphalan, 200 mg/m². The donor group received a reduced, but myeloablative, preparative regimen of busulfan, fludarabine, and antithymocyte globulin. The no-donor group received a second ASCT after melphalan 220 mg/m². There were no differences in response rates (RR), PFS, or OS. The second study was conducted by an Italian consortium comparing melphalan, 200 mg/m², and single ASCT in all patients, followed by an AlloSCT after 2 Gy TBI or a second ASCT with 100 to 140 mg melphalan.[31] CR rates were 55% versus 26% favoring the AlloSCT arm. With follow-up of 7 years in a recent update, continued improved PFS and OS rates for the AlloSCT group were observed.[32] The third trial, conducted by a Spanish consortium, looked only at patients who achieved less than a near CR after a single ASCT with melphalan, 200 mg/m².[33] A small number of patients with donors (N = 25) proceeded to AlloSCT after a reduced-intensity ablative regimen of fludarabine and melphalan. They were compared with 85 patients without donors who received a second ASCT after a regimen of cyclophosphamide, etoposide, and carmustine or melphalan, 200 mg/m². There was a statistically better CR rate and a nonsignificant trend for improved PFS in the AlloSCT arm, but no differences in OS. The fourth study was a US consortium comparing 156 patients with donors to 356 patients without donors. As in other studies, all patients received a single ASCT with melphalan, 200 mg/m², followed by genetically assigned second ASCT or nonablative AlloSCT with fludarabine and 2 Gy TBI.[34] An important difference of this trial is that patients could be enrolled after results of family HLA typing were completed. Thus, there was a potential referral bias created, as both the patient and referring physician already knew the treatment group assignment. In this trial, there were no observed differences in RR, PFS, or OS. Follow-up in this trial was relatively short at just over 3 years. In contrast, a European intergroup trial compared 108 patients assigned to a tandem ASCT-AlloSCT treatment with fludarabine and 2 Gy TBI to 249 patients who received 1 or 2 ASCTs with melphalan, 200 mg/m².[35] This trial observed a statistically better CR, PFS, and OS in both the initial report and extended follow-up at 8 years.[36] Because of the disparate outcomes of the last 2 trials, some suggest that longer follow-up for the clinical trials network (CTN) was needed. The sixth trial was a prospectively followed subset of patients from a large Dutch-German consortium who all received a single ASCT after melphalan 200 mg/m², followed by an AlloSCT with 2 Gy TBI for the 122 patients with donors or only maintenance after their single ASCT in the 138 patients with no donors.[37] There were no differences in RR, event-free survival (EFS), or OS, even though this trial had a median follow-up of 6 years.

Thus, among 6 prospective trials with differing designs, only 2 studies show significantly better PFS and OS for AlloSCT, whereas the other 4 studies show equivalence between ASCT and AlloSCT. In a recently published meta-analysis that examined 4 of 6 trials, there was a statistically better CR rate but no differences in PFS or OS.[38] The failure of most prospective trials to show superiority of AlloSCT has led to the recommendation that patients with myeloma only receive AlloSCT within the context of clinical trials, and some have called for the abandonment of any front-line AlloSCT.[39]

RECENT REPORTS

Several updates were presented at the recent American Society of Hematology meeting 2013 on allogeneic transplants in patients with myeloma. A group from

Hackensack, NJ reported on 56 patients receiving a nonablative fludarabine, low dose TBI regimen, or an ablative busulfan, melphalan regimen.[40] AlloSCT was performed either as consolidation after a partial response or better (N = 26) or as salvage therapy in resistant patients. The complete response rate was 57%, with 50% chronic GVHD and 23% nonrelapse mortality. Survival was significantly better for patients with responsive disease transplanted as consolation and for patients who had chronic GVHD because of lower rates of recurrence. The EBMT retrospectively examined the effect of a planned autologous SCT before reduced-intensity AlloSCT.[41] Both PFS and OS were significantly better at 5 years (34% vs 22% and 59% vs 43%, respectively) for patients who received a planned ASCT before a reduced-intensity AlloSCT (N = 444) when compared with patients who had a reduced-intensity AlloSCT without a prior ASCT (N = 172). This trial importantly suggests the value of cytoreduction with an ASCT before a reduced-intensity AlloSCT. The Hopkins group reported on their experience with 39 patients with myeloma who received posttransplant cyclophosphamide to reduce GVHD.[42] Patients received myeloablative (N = 9) or reduced-intensity (N = 30) conditioning and were then received transplants from matched related (N = 30), haploidentical related (N = 7) or matched unrelated (N = 2) donors. Marrow was used for 28 transplants, with peripheral blood stem cells for the remainder. High-risk cytogenetics were present in 15 patients, and 13 patients had International Staging System class III myeloma. Transplant mortality rate was only 2.5%, grade 3 acute GVHD occurred in only 3 patients, and there was no grade 4 GVHD. Chronic GVHD occurred in only 5 patients. Twenty patients are alive and 6 remain in sustained complete remission. As in other reports, the major cause of treatment failure was disease progression, suggesting once again that efforts to prevent GVHD are often associated with impaired GVM.

A recent report updated, with extended follow-up, the Hovon 50/54 trial comparing outcomes in patients who did not have a donor and received 1 or 2 autologous transplants versus patients with donors who received a reduced-intensity AlloSCT after 1 ASCT.[43] With a median follow-up of 7.5 years, no differences in PFS (median 29 months vs 30 months; P = .25) or OS (76 months vs 81 months; P = .61) were observed.

SUMMARY AND FUTURE STUDIES

Although AlloSCT can clearly result in long-term disease control for some patients with multiple myeloma, only some patients will benefit from this approach because of the relatively high transplant mortality rate, even with reduced-intensity conditioning, and significant rates of relapse. Several strategies may improve conditioning regimens. [153]Sammarium-EDTMP, a bone-seeking radioisotope, has been used to intensify the conditioning regimen of ASCT and may have utility after AlloSCT.[44] In Seattle, we are studying the utility of a ^{90}Y-CD45 isotope-antibody conjugate to deliver radiation to bone marrow, lymph nodes, and spleen in patients with myeloma, as has been done in acute leukemia.[45] Bortezomib has been added to conditioning regimens for AlloSCT in an effort to deliver greater myeloma-specific therapy.[46] After AlloSCT maintenance with lenalidomide, bortezomib or the newer oral proteasome inhibitor, ixazomib, could reduce rates of recurrence.[47,48] It was shown several years ago that idiotypic vaccines could be used to preimmunize donors and that donor specific immunity could be transferred to patients during AlloSCT.[49] Several myeloma-specific anti-CD38 antibodies have shown single-agent activity in relapsed myeloma and could be studied post-AlloSCT.[50] Finally, efforts to modulate GVHD by selective T cell depletion continue.[51] Until it is possible to improve the conditioning regimens, reduce transplant mortality by modulation of GVHD, and improve the GVM effect, AlloSCT will continue to be relegated to investigational status.

REFERENCES

1. Bensinger W. Stem-cell transplantation for multiple myeloma in the era of novel drugs. J Clin Oncol 2008;26:480–92.
2. Thomas ED, Lochte HL Jr, Lu WC, et al. Intravenous infusion of bone marrow in patients receiving radiation and chemotherapy. N Engl J Med 1957;257: 491–6.
3. Higby DJ, Brass C, Fitzpatick J, et al. Bone marrow transplantation in multiple myeloma: a case report with protein studies. ASCO Abstracts 1982;192:C-747.
4. Ozer H, Han T, Nussbaum-Blumenson A, et al. Allogeneic BMT and idiotypic monitoring in multiple myeloma. AACR Abstracts 1984;84:161.
5. Buckner CD, Fefer A, Bensinger WI, et al. Marrow transplantation for malignant plasma cell disorders: Summary of the Seattle Experience. Eur J Haematol 1989;43:186–90.
6. Gahrton G, Tura S, Flesch M, et al. Bone marrow transplantation in multiple myeloma: report from the European Cooperative Group for bone marrow transplantation. Blood 1987;69:1262–4.
7. Bensinger WI, Buckner CD, Anasetti C, et al. Allogeneic marrow transplantation for multiple myeloma: an analysis of risk factors on outcome. Blood 1996;88: 2787–93.
8. Barlogie B, Kyle RA, Anderson KC, et al. Standard chemotherapy compared with high-dose chemoradiotherapy for multiple myeloma: final results of phase III US Intergroup Trial S9321. J Clin Oncol 2006;24:929–36 [Erratum appears in J Clin Oncol 2006;24(17):2687].
9. Corradini P, Cavo M, Lokhorst H, et al. Molecular remission after myeloablative allogeneic stem cell transplantation predicts a better relapse-free survival in patients with multiple myeloma. Blood 2003;102:1927–9.
10. Kröger N, Badbaran A, Zabelina T, et al. Impact of high-risk cytogenetics and achievement of molecular remission on long-term freedom from disease after autologous-allogeneic tandem transplantation in patients with multiple myeloma. Biol Blood Marrow Transplant 2013;19(3):398–404.
11. Björkstrand B, Ljungman P, Svensson H, et al. Allogeneic bone marrow transplantation versus autologous stem cell transplantation in multiple myeloma - a retrospective case-matched study from the European Group for Blood and Marrow transplantation. Blood 1996;88:4711–8.
12. Gratwohl A, Stern M, Brand R, et al. Risk score for outcome after allogeneic hematopoietic stem cell transplantation: a retrospective analysis. Cancer 2009;115:4715–26.
13. Gahrton G, Svensson H, Cavo M, et al. Progress in allogeneic bone marrow and peripheral blood stem cell transplantation for multiple myeloma: a comparison between transplants performed 1983-93 and 1994-98 at European Group for Blood and Marrow Transplantation centres. Br J Haematol 2001;113:209–16.
14. McSweeney PA, Niederwieser D, Shizuru JA, et al. Hematopoietic cell transplantation in older patients with hematologic malignancies: replacing high-dose cytotoxic therapy with graft-versus-tumor effects. Blood 2001;97:3390–400.
15. Champlin R, Khouri I, Kornblau S, et al. Allogeneic hematopoietic transplantation as adoptive immunotherapy. Induction of graft-versus-malignancy as primary therapy [review]. Hematol Oncol Clin North Am 1999;13:1041–57.

16. Verdonck LF, Petersen EJ, Lokhorst HM, et al. Donor leukocyte infusions for recurrent hematologic malignancies after allogeneic bone marrow transplantation: impact of infused and residual donor T cells. Bone Marrow Transplant 1998;22:1057–63.

17. Bruno B, Rotta M, Patriarca F, et al. Non-myeloablative allografting for newly diagnosed multiple myeloma: the experience of the Gruppo Italiano Trapianti di Midollo. Blood 2009;113:3375–82.

18. Rotta M, Storer BE, Sahebi F, et al. Long-term outcome of patients with multiple myeloma after autologous hematopoietic cell transplantation and nonmyeloablative allografting. Blood 2009;113:3383–91.

19. Gerull S, Goerner M, Benner A, et al. Long-term outcome of nonmyeloablative allogeneic transplantation in patients with high-risk multiple myeloma. Bone Marrow Transplant 2005;36:963–9.

20. Kroger N, Perez-Simon JA, Myint H, et al. Relapse to prior autograft and chronic graft-versus-host disease are the strongest prognostic factors for outcome of melphalan/fludarabine-based dose-reduced allogeneic stem cell transplantation in patients with multiple myeloma. Biol Blood Marrow Transplant 2004;10: 698–708.

21. Lee CK, Badros A, Barlogie B, et al. Prognostic factors in allogeneic transplantation for patients with high-risk multiple myeloma after reduced intensity conditioning. Exp Hematol 2003;31:73–80.

22. Mohty M, Boiron JM, Damaj G, et al. Graft-versus-myeloma effect following antithymocyte globulin-based reduced intensity conditioning allogeneic stem cell transplantation. Bone Marrow Transplant 2004;34:77–84.

23. Majolino I, Davoli M, Carnevalli E, et al. Reduced intensity conditioning with thiotepa, fludarabine, and melphalan is effective in advanced multiple myeloma. Leuk Lymphoma 2007;48:759–66.

24. Crawley C, Lalancette M, Szydlo R, et al. Outcomes for reduced-intensity allogeneic transplantation for multiple myeloma: an analysis of prognostic factors from the Chronic Leukemia Working Party of the EBMT. Blood 2005;105: 4532–9.

25. Ringdén O, Shrestha S, da Silva GT, et al. Effect of acute and chronic GVHD on relapse and survival after reduced-intensity conditioning allogeneic transplantation for myeloma. Bone Marrow Transplant 2012;47:831–7.

26. Bensinger W, Rotta M, Storer B, et al. Allo-SCT for multiple myeloma: a review of outcomes at a single transplant center. Bone Marrow Transplant 2012;47: 1312–7.

27. Patriarca F, Einsele H, Spina F, et al. Allogeneic stem cell transplantation in multiple myeloma relapsed after autograft: a multicenter retrospective study based on donor availability. Biol Blood Marrow Transplant 2012;18(4):617–26.

28. Sonneveld P, Schmidt-Wolf IG, van der Holt B, et al. Bortezomib induction and maintenance treatment in patients with newly diagnosed multiple myeloma: results of the randomized phase III HOVON-65/GMMG-HD4 trial. J Clin Oncol 2012;30(24):2946–55.

29. Knop S, Liebisch P, Hebart H, et al. Allogeneic stem cell transplant versus tandem high-dose melphalan for front-line treatment of deletion 13q14 myeloma-an interim analysis of the German DSMM V Trial. Blood 2009;114:22.

30. Garban F, Attal M, Michallet M, et al. Prospective comparison of autologous stem cell transplantation followed by dose-reduced allograft (IFM99-03 trial) with tandem autologous stem cell transplantation (IFM99-04 trial) in high-risk de novo multiple myeloma. Blood 2006;107:3474–80.

31. Bruno B, Rotta M, Patriarca F, et al. A comparison of allografting with autografting for newly diagnosed myeloma. N Engl J Med 2007;356:1110–20.
32. Giaccone L, Storer B, Patriarca F, et al. Long-term follow-up of a comparison of nonmyeloablative allografting with autografting for newly diagnosed myeloma. Blood 2011;117:6721–7.
33. Rosinol L, Perez-Simon JA, Sureda A, et al. A prospective PETHEMA study of tandem autologous transplantation versus autograft followed by reduced-intensity conditioning allogeneic transplantation in newly diagnosed multiple myeloma. Blood 2008;112:3591–3.
34. Krishnan A, Pasquini MC, Logan B, et al. Autologous haemopoietic stem-cell transplantation followed by allogeneic or autologous haemopoietic stem-cell transplantation in patients with multiple myeloma (BMT CTN 0102): a phase 3 biological assignment trial. Lancet Oncol 2011;12:1195–203.
35. Bjorkstrand B, Iacobelli S, Hegenbart U, et al. Tandem autologous/reduced-intensity conditioning allogeneic stem-cell transplantation versus autologous transplantation in myeloma: long-term follow-up. J Clin Oncol 2011;29:3016–22.
36. Gahrton G, Iacobelli S, Bjorkstrand B, et al. Autologous/reduced-intensity allogeneic stem cell transplantation vs autologous transplantation in multiple myeloma: long-term results of the EBMT-NMAM2000 study. Blood 2013;121:5055–63.
37. Lokhorst HM, van der Holt B, Cornelissen JJ, et al. Donor versus no-donor comparison of newly diagnosed myeloma patients included in the HOVON-50 multiple myeloma study. Blood 2012;119:6219–25.
38. Kharfan-Dabaja MA, Hamadani M, Reljic T, et al. Comparative efficacy of tandem autologous versus autologous followed by allogeneic hematopoietic cell transplantation in patients with newly diagnosed multiple myeloma: a systematic review and meta-analysis of randomized controlled trials. J Hematol Oncol 2013;6:2.
39. Donato ML, Siegel DS, Vesole DH, et al. Long-term follow-up of patients with multiple myeloma who received allogeneic hemaotpoietic stem cell transplantation. Blood 2013;122:2154.
40. Sahebi F, Iacobelli S, Van Biezen A, et al. Reduced intensity allogeneic stem cell transplant in patients with multiple myeloma: a comparison of planned Autologous-Reduced Intensity Allogeneic Stem Cell Transplant (Auto-Allo) and Reduced Intensity Allogeneic Stem Cell Transplant (RIC) as upfront transplant in patients with multiple myeloma, an EBMT analysis. Blood 2013;122:920.
41. Ghosh N, Ye X, Bolaños-Meade J, et al. Outcomes Of Allogeneic Blood Or Marrow Transplantation (AlloBMT) in multiple myeloma with post-transplantation cyclophosphamide. Blood 2013;122:3407.
42. Lokhorst H, van der Holt B, Cornelissen J, et al. No improvement of overall survival after extended follow-up of donor versus no donor analysis of newly diagnosed myeloma patients included in the HOVON 50/54 study. Blood 2013;122: 2132.
43. Moreau P. Death of frontline allo-SCT in myeloma. Blood 2012;119(26):6178–9.
44. Dispenzieri A, Wiseman GA, Lacy MQ, et al. A Phase II study of (153)Sm-EDTMP and high-dose melphalan as a peripheral blood stem cell conditioning regimen in patients with multiple myeloma. Am J Hematol 2010;85:409–13.
45. Orozco JJ, Zeller J, Pagel JM. Radiolabeled antibodies directed at CD45 for conditioning prior to allogeneic transplantation in acute myeloid leukemia and myelodysplastic syndrome. Ther Adv Hematol 2012;3:5–16.
46. Caballero-Velázquez T, López-Corral L, Encinas C, et al. Phase II clinical trial for the evaluation of bortezomib within the reduced intensity conditioning regimen

(RIC) and post-allogeneic transplantation for high-risk myeloma patients. Br J Haematol 2013;162(4):474–82.

47. Bensinger WI, Green DJ, Burwick N, et al. A prospective study of lenalidomide monotherapy for relapse after Allo-SCT for multiple myeloma. Bone Marrow Transplant 2014;49(4):492–5. http://dx.doi.org/10.1038/bmt.2013.219.

48. El-Cheikh J, Crocchiolo R, Furst S, et al. Lenalidomide plus donor-lymphocytes infusion after allogeneic stem-cell transplantation with reduced-intensity conditioning in patients with high-risk multiple myeloma. Exp Hematol 2012;40:521–7.

49. Kwak LW, Taub DD, Duffey PL, et al. Transfer of myeloma idiotype-specific immunity from an actively immunised marrow donor. Lancet 1995;345:1016–20.

50. de Weers M, Tai YT, van der Veer MS, et al. Daratumumab, a novel therapeutic human CD38 monoclonal antibody, induces killing of multiple myeloma and other hematological tumors. J Immunol 2011;186(3):1840–8.

51. Mavroudis DA, Dermime S, Molldrem J, et al. Specific depletion of alloreactive T cells in HLA-identical siblings: a method for separating graft-versus-host and graft-versus-leukaemia reactions. Br J Haematol 1998;101(3):565–70.

Novel Targeted Agents in the Treatment of Multiple Myeloma

Cindy Varga, MD, Jacob Laubach, MD, Teru Hideshima, MD, PhD,
Dharminder Chauhan, PhD, Kenneth C. Anderson, MD,
Paul G. Richardson, MD*

KEYWORDS

- Multiple myeloma • Second-generation proteasome inhibitors
- Histone deacetylase inhibitors • Heat shock protein 90 inhibitors
- PIK3/Akt/mTOR inhibitors • BET bromodomain inhibitors
- Deubiquitinating enzyme inhibitors • Wnt

KEY POINTS

- New, next-generation targeted treatment strategies are urgently required to improve out-comes in patients with multiple myeloma (MM).
- Monoclonal antibodies, cell signaling inhibitors, and selective therapies targeting the bone marrow microenvironment have demonstrated encouraging results with generally manageable toxicity in therapeutic trials of patients with relapsed and refractory disease, each critically informed by preclinical studies.
- A combination approach of these newer agents with immunomodulators and/or protea-some inhibitors as part of a treatment platform seems to consistently improve the efficacy of anti-MM regimens, even in heavily pretreated patients.
- Future studies continue to be required to better understand the complex mechanisms of drug resistance in MM.
- Incorporating molecular correlates to further personalize treatment and to, thus, better integrate these agents into clinical practice is a clear priority.

INTRODUCTION

Multiple myeloma (MM) is the second most common hematologic malignancy after non-Hodgkin lymphoma and remains incurable despite major advances in therapy over the last decade, with the use of bortezomib, thalidomide, and lenalidomide as

Department of Hematology/Oncology, Jerome Lipper Multiple Myeloma Center, Dana-Farber Cancer Institute, Harvard Medical School, 450 Brookline Avenue, Boston, MA 02215, USA
* Corresponding author. Dana-Farber Cancer Institute, 450 Brookline Avenue, Mayer 228, Boston, MA 02215.
E-mail address: paul_richardson@dfci.harvard.edu

Hematol Oncol Clin N Am 28 (2014) 903–925
http://dx.doi.org/10.1016/j.hoc.2014.07.001
0889-8588/14/$ – see front matter © 2014 Elsevier Inc. All rights reserved.

first-generation novel therapies in particular impacting favorably on prognosis. MM remains challenging because of both tumor-specific factors, including adverse mutations that result in both inherent and acquired resistance to therapy, and enhanced tumor survival derived from the surrounding bone marrow microenvironment. Newer targeted treatment strategies are currently under development and show considerable promise in overcoming this resistance; these include second-generation proteasome inhibitors (PIs) (such as carfilzomib), third-generation immunomodulators (specifically pomalidomide), monoclonal antibodies in particular, and other cell signaling inhibitors, as well as specific therapies targeting the bone marrow microenvironment. Some of these agents already have proven highly efficacious in the relapsed and refractory (RR) setting, specifically carfilzomib and pomalidomide; this leads to their recent regulatory approval. This review focuses on novel targeted therapies currently under investigation and in various stages of clinical trials, with approvals pending and/or breakthrough designation assigned to several agents.

SECOND-GENERATION PROTEOSOME INHIBITORS
Ixazomib (MLN9708)

MLN9708 is a dipeptidilic boronic acid that immediately hydrolyzes to MLN2238, an active form, on exposure to aqueous solutions. MLN2238 reversibly and selectively inhibits the 20S proteasome. It has a 6-fold faster dissociation half-life and greater tissue penetration as compared with bortezomib (**Fig. 1**).[1] In a xenograft model, MLN2238 showed significantly longer survival in tumor-bearing mice treated with MLN2238 than mice receiving bortezomib. MLN2238 was found to be active even in bortezomib-resistant cells.[2] MLN2238 can synergize with lenalidomide, vorinostat, and/or dexamethasone in combination.[2] Importantly, MLN9708 did not demonstrate significant inhibition of neuronal cell survival, which may explain the lack of major peripheral neuropathy (PN) seen so far with this PI.[2]

MLN9708 was the first oral PI to be incorporated into clinical trials. Several phase I studies have evaluated the safety of MLN9708 using both oral and intravenous (IV) routes of administration. Data from these studies have demonstrated linear pharmacokinetics, regardless of administration route.[3]

Two phase I studies, one using weekly dosing[4] and the other using biweekly dosing,[5] have evaluated the oral administration of MLN9708 as a single agent in heavily pretreated patients with RR MM previously exposed to PIs. In the 41 evaluable patients receiving weekly dosing, responses included 1 very good partial response (VGPR), 5 partial responses (PR), 1 minimal response (MR), and 15 with stable disease (SD).[4] In the 46 evaluable patients receiving biweekly dosing, 6 patients achieved PR or more, including 1 stringent complete remission (sCR) and 5 PR.[5]

The most common all-grades adverse events (AEs) included fatigue (30%–40%), thrombocytopenia (30%–40%), nausea (30%), diarrhea (25%), vomiting (20%), as well as rash and neutropenia. Drug-related PN was minimal at 4% to 8%, and none were grade 3 or more. Toxicities proved generally manageable with dose reduction and supportive care, and tolerability overall was considered favorable.

Preliminary data from phase I/II studies of once-weekly and biweekly oral MLN9708 in combination with lenalidomide and dexamethasone in patients with newly diagnosed myeloma were recently reported. Drug-related AEs were similar to the phase I studies, although more frequent with twice-weekly administration. Among evaluable patients who received biweekly dosing, 95% achieved PR or better, with a 27% CR/sCR rate. The depth of response increased over the course of treatment. The median time to best response was 1.96 months.[6] MLN9708 in combination with lenalidomide

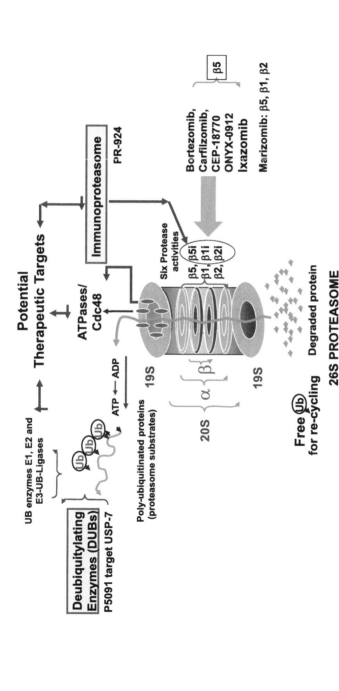

Fig. 1. Proteasome: present and future therapies. UB, ubiquitin. (*Adapted from* Lawasut P, Chauhan D, Laubach J, et al. New proteasome inhibitors in myeloma. Curr Hematol Malig Rep 2012;7:258–66, with permission; and *Data from* Refs.[9,13,60,127,128])

and dexamethasone is currently being investigated in a phase III trial in newly diagnosed patients as well as having been recently completed in patients with relapsed disease, with results expected next year. The benefit of maintenance therapy with this agent is also being evaluated both as a single agent and in combination with lenalidomide.

Oprozomib (ONX 0912)

Oprozomib (ONX 0192) is an epoxyketone PI and is an orally available analogue of carfilzomib. Both carfilzomib and ONX 0912 are irreversible PIs that selectively inhibit the chymotrypsin-like (CT-L) subunit (β5 and β5i) and, thus, have minimal off-target effects (see **Fig. 1**).[7–9] This PI has shown a significant anti-MM response in vitro and in vivo studies.[9,10] ONX 0912 is currently being evaluated in phase I and II dose-escalating studies.[11] Reported adverse effects are mainly gastrointestinal and similar to observations in preclinical animal models.[12] Although promising activity has been seen, serious gastrointestinal toxicity has been reported; concerted efforts to improve tolerability are underway.

NPI-0052 (Marizomib)

NPI-0052 (Marizomib) is part of a unique class of PIs, in that it is a natural β-lactone compound that can irreversibly inhibit CT-L, trypsin-like (T-L), and caspase-like (C-L) proteasomal activities in vitro and in vivo (see **Fig. 1**).[13] Through its covalent binding of all 3β subunits, NPI-0052 demonstrates comparable or even greater proteasome inhibition compared with bortezomib and carfilzomib in preclinical models.[13] NPI-0052 is also highly synergistic with either lenalidomide or pomalidomide in vitro and overcomes bortezomib resistance preclinically.[14,15]

Subsequent results from a dose-escalating study in patients with RR MM with twice-weekly IV NPI-0052 has been reported,[16] with 20% (3 of 15) of bortezomib-resistant patients achieving PR, and 73% of all evaluable patients (n = 22) achieving at least SD. Reported dose-limiting toxicities (DLTs) included predominantly mild to moderate hallucinations, cognitive changes, and loss of balance, which were transient and reversible with dose reduction. Importantly, there was no evidence of treatment-emergent PN or significant myelosuppression. A twice-weekly regimen is currently being investigated, and combination studies with pomalidomide and dexamethasone are underway.

CELL SIGNALING AGENTS
Histone Deacetylases Inhibitors

Epigenetic modification plays a diverse role in both physiologic and pathologic cellular processes. Acetylation, one of the most frequent alterations in epigenetics, serves as a key player in the regulation of gene expression by altering chromatin structure without modifying the underlying DNA.[17,18] Acetylation is tightly regulated by 2 opposing enzymes: histone deacetylases (HDACs) and histone acetyltransferases (HATs). Although hyperacetylation of the histone NH2 tail by HATs results in open chromatin and gene expression, HDACs have shown to have a repressive effect on transcription by mediating a closed chromatin conformation.[19,20] Transcriptional repression by HDACs is implicated in carcinogenesis,[21] making them a promising therapeutic target. HDACs also act on many other nonhistone substrate proteins involved in the modulation of transcription.[22,23]

HDAC inhibitors bind to the catalytic sites of HDACs, preventing accessibility of transcription factors to promoter regions[22,23] and also upregulate negative cell cycle modulators of the G1 phase, such as p21^{WAF1} and p27^{Kip1}.[24,25] HDAC inhibitors can be categorized as class–specific inhibitors or as pan-deacetylase (pan-DAC) inhibitors, the latter denoting activity against both class I and II recombinant HDACs.[26]

Panobinostat

Panobinostat is a potent pan-DAC inhibitor, which has potent inhibitory activity at low nanomolar concentrations against all class I, II, and IV HDACs (**Fig. 2**).[27] Panobinostat leads to the acetylation of lysine residues across intracellular targets.[28] In preclinical studies, panobinostat had an antimyeloma effect using in vitro and in vivo myeloma models.[28–30] Based on this data, a phase II study of oral panobinostat as monotherapy in heavily pretreated patients with RR MM was investigated.[31] Patients had at least 2 prior treatments, including bortezomib, thalidomide, and lenalidomide. Panobinostat was administered at a dosage of 20 mg 3 times weekly out of a 21-day treatment cycle. Overall, one PR and one MR were observed out of 38 evaluable patients; however, these responses were maintained for 19 and 28 months, respectively.[31] All grade AEs reported included gastrointestinal toxicity (80.0%) and hematologic effects, which included grade 3/4 neutropenia (31.6%), thrombocytopenia (26.3%), and anemia (18.4%).

Panobinostat was next evaluated in combination with bortezomib in patients with RR MM, based on preclinical studies, which demonstrated synergy.[29,30,32] Specifically, in a phase Ib study of panobinostat and bortezomib,[33] clinical responses were observed (including complete responses) in patients with bortezomib-refractory MM; toxicity proved manageable.

PANORAMA 2 was a multicenter phase II study examining the combination of oral panobinostat with bortezomib and dexamethasone in 55 heavily pretreated patients

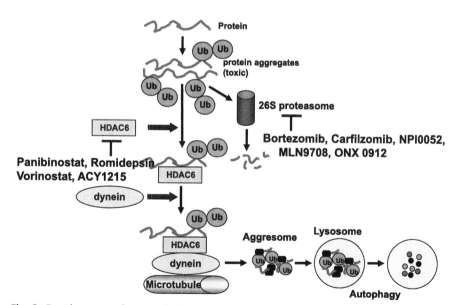

Fig. 2. Development of rationally based combination therapies (HDAC and PIs). (*Adapted from* Hideshima T, Bradner JE, Chauhan D, et al. Intracellular protein degradation and its therapeutic implications. Clin Cancer Res 2005;11:8530, with permission; and Catley L, Weisberg E, Kiziltepe T, et al. Aggresome induction by proteasome inhibitor bortezomib and alpha-tubulin hyperacetylation by tubulin deacetylase (TDAC) inhibitor LBH589 are synergistic in myeloma cells. Blood 2006;108(10):3441–9.)

with relapsed and bortezomib-refractory MM.[34] The overall response rate (ORR) was 34.5% (including 1 near PR and 18 PRs), with 10 patients achieving an MR, resulting in a clinical benefit rate (CBR) of 52.7%. Among patients with adverse cytogenetics (n = 14), the ORR was 43% and the CBR was 71%. The median progression-free survival (PFS) was 5.4 months. Common grade 3/4 AEs included thrombocytopenia (63.6%), fatigue (20.0%), and diarrhea (20.0%).[34]

Based on these encouraging data, a phase III clinical trial was performed. PANORAMA 1 was an international, randomized, double-blinded study of panobinostat (vs placebo) in combination with bortezomib and dexamethasone in patients with RR MM. A total of 768 patients were randomized. Preliminary results demonstrated an ORR of 61% in the panobinostat arm versus 55% in the placebo arm, with an near CR (nCR)/CR rate of 28% versus 16% ($P = .00006$), respectively. The median PFS was 12.0 months versus 8.1 months ($P<.0001$; hazard ratio 0.63, 95% confidence interval [0.52, 0.76]) in favor of the panobinostat arm. Common grade 3/4 AEs in the panobinostat versus placebo arms included thrombocytopenia (67% vs 31%), neutropenia (35% vs 11%), and diarrhea (26% vs 8%), which were generally manageable with dose reduction and/or supportive care.[35] Given the PFS benefit of 4 months in favor of panobinostat and its activity in high-risk groups in particular, as well as the encouraging quality of response differences seen, regulatory approval is anticipated this year.

Vorinostat

Similar to panobinostat, vorinostat is also a pan-DAC inhibitor in the hydroxamic class (see **Fig. 2**).[36] Mitsiades and colleagues demonstrated in vitro antimyeloma activity when MM cells were irreversibly committed to cell death after hours of incubation with vorinostat. Using microarray analyses, vorinostat-induced apoptosis was associated with suppression of genes mediating cytokine-driven proliferation and survival, drug-resistance, DNA synthesis/repair, and proteasome function.[37] In MM cell lines, vorinostat successfully induced apoptosis in all tumor cells with increased levels of proapoptotic protein levels of p21 and p53. Vorinostat also inhibited the secretion of interleukin 6 (IL-6) produced by bone marrow stromal cells (BMSCs), suggesting that HDAC inhibitors can overcome cell adhesion–mediated drug resistance (CAM-DR).[38] An ongoing phase I trial examined the combination of vorinostat with lenalidomide, bortezomib, and dexamethasone in patients with newly diagnosed MM. Vorinostat was administered orally at 100, 200, 300, or 400 mg daily on days 1 to 14 of each cycle. Thirty patients were enrolled with an ORR (PR or better) of 100%, with a VGPR or better of 52%, and a CR rate of 28%. At a median follow-up of 11.5 months (range 1–31 months), there has been only one patient with progressive disease.[39] Similarly encouraging results with vorinostat in combination with lenalidomide in RR MM were seen in a phase I combination study with an ORR of 47% and favorable tolerability.[40] In contrast, efforts with vorinostat combined with bortezomib proved challenging; ultimately, the prospective international randomized phase III trial of vorinostat combined with bortezomib versus bortezomib alone failed to demonstrate a meaningful clinical benefit. This finding was despite significantly higher rates of response in favor of the combination and largely because of the excessive toxicity seen with the particular dose and schedule of vorinostat used, as well as the absence of dexamethasone use, resulting in only a minimal PFS improvement of less than a month seen between the doublet and the monotherapy control.[41]

ACY-1215 (Rocilinostat)

HDAC6 plays an important role in the breakdown of ubiquitinated proteins and in the formation of perinuclear aggresomes. Blocking HDAC6 activity results in the accumulation of polyubiquitinated proteins, which, in turn, induces cell stress followed by apoptosis.[42] HDAC6 inhibition markedly enhances the action of PIs, making HDAC6 a promising novel target for this approach as well as with other combinations. Furthermore, the more selective inhibition of HDAC6 may reduce the off-target toxicity previously seen with pan-HDAC inhibitors.[42,43]

ACY-1215 is a novel, selective HDAC6 inhibitor that is orally available (see **Fig. 2**). Santo and colleagues[44] evaluated the action of ACY-1215 alone and in combination with bortezomib in the preclinical setting. In this study, the combination of both proteasome and HDAC6 inhibition lead to synergistic cytotoxicity, resulting in apoptosis of MM cells by activation of the caspase pathway. In vivo experiments using 2 xenograft severe combined immunodeficiency (SCID) mouse models, confirmed the anti-MM effects of ACY-1215 when combined with bortezomib. The mouse treated with both agents experienced a significantly prolonged overall survival and delayed tumor growth.[44] This study prompted the rationale to use ACY-1215 in clinical trials.

ACY-100 is a single arm, open-label, dose-escalation trial using ACY-1215 in patients with RR MM as monotherapy (phase Ia) and in combination with bortezomib (phase Ib) followed by a phase II extension. ACY-1215 was given orally on days 1 to 5 and 8 to 12 of a 21-day cycle. Most AEs were grade 1 to 2, whereas 2 patients had grade 3 AEs (anemia and neutropenia). No DLTs were observed. Six patients had SD as their best response.[45]

In the combination cohort, treatment-related AEs were mainly low grade, with the majority not considered related to ACY-1215. The first cohort was expanded because of a DLT of asymptomatic increase in amylase, but no other DLTs have been observed. Grade 3 to 4 AEs included asymptomatic elevated amylase, thrombocytopenia, anemia, stomach cramps, and an increase in creatinine. Of the 16 evaluable patients, 1 VGPR, 2 PR, 1 MR, and 5 SD were reported. Of the patients who were previously refractory to bortezomib, the best outcome at the time of presentation was 1 VGPR, 1 MR, and 4 SD,[45] with recent updates suggesting greater ORR with more time on therapy.

Based on synergy observed between ACY-1215 and lenalidomide in preclinical studies, a phase I trial investigating this combination treatment regimen in patients with RR MM is being carried out. In part A, patients were treated with escalating doses of oral ACY-1215 on days 1 to 5 and 8 to 12 of a 28-day cycle, with lenalidomide 25 mg on day 1 to 21 and dexamethasone 40 mg weekly.[46] Most treatment-related events were low grade and included fatigue (43%), upper respiratory infection (36%), anemia and peripheral edema (21% each), neutropenia (29%) and muscle spasms (21%). There were 9 grade 3 to 4 events in 6 patients, which were primarily hematologic. Nine patients (69%) achieved responses of PR or greater, including 1 CR, 4 VGPR, and 3 PR. Of the 6 patients who were previously refractory to lenalidomide, the best responses included 1 PR, 1 VGPR, 2 MR, and 2 SD.[46] Future studies are now evaluating the combination of ACY-1215 with pomalidomide and with whom even greater preclinical activity is seen; the all-oral 3-drug platform of AC1215, pomalidomide, and dexamethasone is, therefore, hoped to be a particularly important triplet going forward.

Heat-Shock Protein 90 Inhibitors

Heat-shock protein 90 (Hsp90) regulates cellular trafficking by facilitating the 3-dimensional folding of intracellular proteins implicated in cell proliferation and drug resistance.[47] In tumors, Hsp90s are an important target, as they act as a chaperone to mutated or overexpressed proteins that promote cell survival. In a phase I/II clinical trial, patients with RR MM were administered the hsp90 inhibitor tanespimycin

($100\text{–}340$ mg/m^2) and bortezomib ($0.7\text{–}1.3$ mg/m^2 IV) on days 1, 4, 8, and 11 in each 21-day cycle. Among the 67 evaluable patients, there were 2 (3%) complete responses and 8 (12%) PRs, for an ORR of 27%, including 8 (12%) MRs.[48] The most common AEs were diarrhea (60%), nausea (49%), fatigue (49%), thrombocytopenia (40%), transient elevations in AST (28%) and dizziness (28%). Most toxicities were grade 1 or grade 2. There was no reported grade 3/4 peripheral neuropathy.[48] Unfortunately, the tanespimycin program had to be closed prematurely because of insurmountable difficulties in producing adequate and high-quality amounts of the drug substance. Other studies of Hsp90 inhibition are ongoing, and early results show some promise (eg, AUY922).

Phosphoinosiide 3-kinase/Akt/Mammalian Target of Rapamycin Pathway Inhibitors

Akt modulates the phosphorylation of several downstream substrates involved in cellular growth and survival.[49] One of the most studied downstream protein kinases is the mammalian target of rapamycin, which has been implicated in the pathogenesis of several different cancers. In MM, the phosphoinosiide 3-kinase (PI3K)/Akt pathway is overactive, thus inhibiting apoptosis and allowing for clonal cell expansion. Hsu and colleagues[50] demonstrated, using immunohistochemistry, that Akt is frequently activated in MM cells and the frequency is directly proportional to the disease stage.[50] Interruption of the Akt pathway resulted in inhibition of MM cell growth in vitro.

Perifosine is a biologically available alkylphospholipid that inhibits the Akt pathway and, thus, promotes apoptosis in MM cells. In preclinical studies, baseline phosphorylation of Akt in MM cells was completely inhibited by perifosine in a time- and dose-dependent manner. Perifosine was also successful in inducing apoptosis even in MM cells adherent to BMSCs.[51] Perifosine was found to enhance the cytotoxic effects of novel agents, such as bortezomib.[51] Taken together, these data provided the rationale for clinical trials using Akt pathway inhibitors in the setting of patients with RR MM.

A phase I multicenter single-arm study was carried out looking at escalating doses of perifosine 50 to 100 mg in combination with lenalidomide plus dexamethasone 20 to 40 mg weekly. The most common AEs were grade 1 to 2 fatigue (48%) and diarrhea (45%), and grade 3 to 4 neutropenia (26%), hypophosphatemia (23%), thrombocytopenia (16%), and leucopenia (13%). MR or better was attained in 73% of evaluable patients, including 50% with a PR or better.

In a multicenter phase I/II study, perifosine was combined with bortezomib with or without dexamethasone in 84 patients with RR MM.[52] All patients were heavily pretreated, and many were resistant to bortezomib. The ORR (MR or better) was 41%, including an ORR of 32% in bortezomib-refractory patients. The median PFS was 6.4 months, with a median overall survival of 25 months. Treatment was well tolerated. Common treatment-related grade 1 and 2 AEs included nausea (63%), diarrhea (57%), fatigue (43%), musculoskeletal pain (42%), anorexia, and upper respiratory tract infections (33% each). All AEs were manageable with supportive care and dose reductions. Grade 3 or more toxicities included thrombocytopenia (23%), neutropenia (15%), anemia (14%), and pneumonia (12%).[52] Unfortunately, the pivotal prospective phase III study of perifosine, bortezomib, and dexamethasone versus placebo, bortezomib, and dexamethasone was closed prematurely as a result of resource constraints, slow accrual, and equivocal findings at interim analysis. Other studies with more potent Akt inhibitors are showing considerable promise (eg, GSK2110183). Most recently, Mimura and colleagues[53] also demonstrated anti-MM activities of a novel allosteric inhibitor TAS-117 alone and in combination with bortezomib.

BET Bromodomain Inhibitors

Myc plays a key role in the pathogenesis of many human cancers, including MM.[54] We have yet to discover therapeutic approaches to modulate the function of the c-Myc oncoprotein. Bromodomains are important recognition domains of coactivator proteins implicated in the initiation of transcription. Disruption of the bromodomains will interfere with signal transduction and, ultimately, will inhibit the transcription of the Myc oncoprotein. JQ1 is a selective small-molecule BET bromodomain inhibitor that downregulates Myc transcription and the expression of other Myc-dependent target genes.[55]

Antiproliferative activity of JQ1 was assessed using in vitro and xenograft models. MM cell proliferation was uniformly inhibited by JQ1. These samples included several cell lines resistant to Food and Drug Administration–approved agents. In primary cells isolated from a patient with RR MM, JQ1 treatment resulted in a time-dependent suppression of c-Myc expression.[55] It is hoped that clinical efficacy of the JQ1 inhibitor will be confirmed in human studies; clinical trials are now underway, with combination studies incorporating lenalidomide due to commence this year.

Deubiquitinating Enzyme Inhibitors

Ubiquitin regulates the degradation of proteins via proteasomes and lysosomes and modulates protein-protein interactions.[56,57] Deubiquitinating enzymes (DUBs) are a group of proteases that cleave the bond between ubiquitin and its substrate protein (see **Fig. 1**).[58] Inhibition of DUBs or proteasome results in the accumulation of ubiquitinated proteins.[59] The novel regulatory particle b-AP15 selectively blocks deubiquitinating activity without inhibiting proteasome activity. In preclinical studies, b-AP15 was shown to decrease viability in bortezomib-resistant MM cell lines and patient MM cells, even in the presence of BMSCs[60]; b-AP15 demonstrated good tolerability in human MM xenograft models. Combining b-AP15 with lenalidomide or dexamethasone induced synergistic anti-MM activity. DUB inhibitors will need to be further investigated as potential therapeutic agents to improve clinical outcomes in MM. To this end, clinical studies are planned and are expected to begin shortly.

Wnt, Hedgehog, Notch Inhibitors

Wnt

Wnt proteins are glycoproteins that serve as ligands to transmembrane receptors. Abnormal Wnt signaling has been described in MM.[61] Dickkopf 1 (DKK1) is a soluble antagonist of the Wnt pathway that is overexpressed by plasma cells in patients with osteolytic lesions. The overexpression of DKK1 blocks the differentiation of osteoblasts and, thus, inhibits the formation of bone.[62] BHQ880 is a fully human neutralizing antibody targeting DKK1. Preclinical studies have demonstrated that BHQ880 reduces IL-6 secretion and promotes osteoblastogenesis in vitro and in mouse models.[63] Preliminary data from a phase I study in patients with RR MM receiving both zoledronic acid and BHQ880 demonstrated an increase in bone density in some patients.[64] An open-label, multicenter, single-arm, phase II study designed to evaluate the safety and antimyeloma activity of BHQ880 in patients with high-risk smoldering MM (SMM) has recently been completed with excellent tolerability and some suggestion of activity seen.[65]

Notch

The Notch pathway regulates cell proliferation, cellular differentiation, and programmed cell death. It is implicated in the pathophysiology of multiple hematologic malignancies, including MM.[66] MRK003 is a γ-secretase inhibitor that has demonstrated in vitro anti-MM activity by blocking the Notch pathway.[67] There may be preclinical evidence that it also increases sensitivity to bortezomib,[68] and clinical evaluation is under consideration.

Hedgehog

The Hedgehog (Hh) pathway is necessary for cell growth and differentiation; its deregulation has been associated with several cancers, including MM.[69] NVP-LDE225 is a novel antagonist currently in development and has demonstrated an anti-MM activity in vitro by the downregulation of the Hh pathway.[70] Clinical studies in MM are also being considered and should soon be underway.

Kinesin Spindle Protein Inhibitors

Kinesin spindle protein (Ksp) inhibitor (ARRY-520) is a synthetic antimitotic agent that induces the death of actively dividing cells by targeting the Ksp, an essential component of mitosis. Ksp is a microtubule protein that is necessary in the formation of spindles.[71] ARRY-520 has shown promising activity not only as a single agent, but also in combination with bortezomib or lenalidomide in preclinical studies using MM cell lines and xenograft models.[72] These data also demonstrated the ability of ARRY-520 to downregulate mcl-1, a known driver in the development of dexamethasone resistance.[73] Based on phase I clinical studies in the RR setting,[74] a phase II study with ARRY-520 as a single agent and in combination with dexamethasone was carried out.[75] All patients had previously received an immunomodulator; 90% had received prior bortezomib, and 78% had prior autologous stem cell transplant. The most commonly reported treatment-emergent AEs were thrombocytopenia, anemia, neutropenia, and fatigue. The most frequent grade 3 or 4 AEs included neutropenia (62%) and thrombocytopenia (57%). Of the 32 patients in the single-agent arm, an MR or greater was observed in 6 patients (19%), 5 of which were PRs. Among patients who were bortezomib and lenalidomide refractory, a 15% ORR ($\geq$MR) was observed. Patients who received combination ARRY-520 and dexamethasone, the ORR was 28% (5 of 18), with 4 patients achieving a PR or greater.[75] There was no association between ARRY-520 and the development of peripheral neuropathy. Further evaluation of ARRY-520 in combination with other novel agents, such as bortezomib and carfilzomib, are underway.

Chromosome Region Maintenance 1

Chromosome region maintenance 1 (CMR1) is a nuclear export protein used to transfer proteins with leucine-rich nuclear sequences from the nucleus to the cytoplasm.[76] This shuttling system is very tightly regulated, given that its cargo includes tumor suppressor proteins, such as p53.[77,78]

The overexpression of CRM1 is responsible for the abnormal cellular localization of tumor suppressive proteins and has been implicated in the development of certain cancers.[79,80] Tai and colleagues[81] demonstrated that CRM1 is highly expressed in patients with MM, including those who are refractory to bortezomib. The overexpression of CRM1 was also correlated with lytic bone disease and a shorter survival. Irreversible selective inhibitors of nuclear export (SINE) targeting CRM1 (KPT-185, KPT-330) induced cell death in MM cells by the accumulation of CRM1 cargo tumor suppressor proteins, even in the presence of BMSCs or osteoclasts. In mice models with MM bone lesions, SINEs successfully inhibited bone lysis by impairing osteoclastogenesis and bone resorption by blocking the nuclear factor–κB pathway.[81] These results are convincing that CRM1 is an important therapeutic target and requires further investigation in human studies.

TARGETING THE BONE MARROW MICROENVIRONMENT

In MM, bone marrow microenvironmental factors play a crucial role in disease progression. Factors such as hypoxia, neoangiogenesis, and the critical interaction between plasma cells and bone marrow stroma are vitally important considerations when contemplating future drug targets in MM; these and other aspects of the tumor microenvironment, including the extramedullary milieu and cortical bone, constitute primary barriers to disease control.

Hypoxia

A hypoxic microenvironment has been associated with disease progression and drug resistance in MM.[82] TH-302 is a prodrug that is activated under tumor hypoxic conditions, a hallmark of MM where the bone marrow is often devoid of oxygen. TH-302 has demonstrated cytotoxicity against human cancer cell lines in vitro and was found to selectively target hypoxic MM cells in vivo, with promising early clinical activity seen in RR MM.[83]

Angiogenesis

Angiogenesis is governed by a balance between proangiogenic and antiangiogenic growth factors. Vascular endothelial growth factor (VEGF) is upregulated in MM. It is thought that active MM requires a vascular environment that contributes to clonal proliferation.[84] Studies looking at VEGF inhibitors have not been encouraging. Unfortunately, several phase II trials did not show any clinical responses in patients with RR MM.[85,86]

CXCR4

CXCR4 is a cell surface chemokine receptor expressed on the surface of normal and MM cells. The interaction between CXCR4 and its ligand stromal cell-derived factor 1 (SDF-1) plays a key role in adhesion and homing.[87] AMD3100 (plerixafor) is a CXCR4 inhibitor that blocks the interaction between MM cells and their bone marrow microenvironment.[88] Preliminary results from a phase I/II trial of plerixafor and bortezomib in RR MM demonstrated promising results.[89] Grade 3 toxicities included lymphopenia (40%), hypophosphatemia (20%), anemia (10%), hyponatremia (10%), and hypercalcemia (10%). Of the 10 evaluable patients, 1 (10%) achieved a VGPR, and 3 (30%) achieved PRs, with an ORR of 40% in this relapsed/refractory population.[89]

CELL CYCLE INHIBITORS
Aurora Kinase Inhibitors

The cell cycle is a very tightly organized process that involves the interaction of many regulatory proteins and enzymes. Aurora A kinases play a key role in the mitotic phase of the cell cycle by modulating chromosome configuration, spindle formation, and cytokinesis.[90–92] Inhibition of Aurora-A kinase gene expression in MM cells leads to apoptosis and cell death.[93,94] MLN8237 is the first orally available selective inhibitor of Aurora-A kinase. In preclinical studies, treatment of cultured MM cells with MLN8237 resulted in the inhibition of cell proliferation via apoptosis in addition to the upregulation of p53. When MLN8237 was combined with dexamethasone, doxorubicin, or bortezomib, anti-MM activity was amplified.[95] MLN8237 is currently under further investigation in phase I/II clinical trials in patients with RR MM, with encouraging tolerability and modest activity reported to date.

Cyclin-Dependent Kinase Inhibitors

Myeloma cells accumulate in the bone marrow because of impaired apoptosis.[96] Quiescent myeloma cells can become self-renewing by reentering the cell cycle, particularly during relapse. This deregulation of the cell cycle can be partially explained by the progression of MM cells through the G_1 phase by cyclin-dependent kinases (CDK).[97] Aberrant activation of Cdk4/Cdk6 is enhanced in advanced disease, regardless of previous treatment regimens or initial clinical presentation.[98] PD 0332991, an orally active inhibitor of recombinant Cdk4 and Cdk6, was shown to induce G_1 arrest in ex vivo myeloma cells and halted growth of tumor cells in human myeloma xenograft models.[99] Similarly, seliciclib (CYC202 or R-roscovitine) is a potent CDK inhibitor, which demonstrated compelling cytotoxicity against primary MM cells and cells resistant to conventional therapy. Seliciclib downregulated *Mcl-1* transcription and inhibited IL-6 transcription by tumor cells bound to BMSCs. The combination of seliciclib with bortezomib demonstrated synergism in vitro.[100] Early phase combination studies are now underway, and the results are anticipated with interest.

MONOCLONAL ANTIBODIES
Anti-CS1 (Elotuzumab)

CS1 is a cell surface glycoprotein and a member of the signaling lymphocyte-activating molecule-related receptor family (**Fig. 3**).[101] Using gene expression profiling, high CS1 expression was found in patients at all stages of MM, regardless of cytogenetics or previous lines of therapy.[102] There was little to no expression of CS1 in normal tissue,[102,103] which allows the opportunity for a potentially highly targeted therapy with a favorable therapeutic index.

Elotuzumab is a humanized monoclonal antibody (mAb) that targets CS1 and activates host natural killer (NK) cells to release perforin granules resulting in targeted myeloma cell death (see **Fig. 3**).[102,103] In preclinical studies, elotuzumab was successful in inducing antibody-dependent cell-mediated cytotoxicity (ADCC) in myeloma cells from patients known to be resistant to bortezomib[103,104] and also demonstrated inhibition of tumor growth in xenograft mouse models.[102,103] In other studies, the combination of elotuzumab with bortezomib or lenalidomide resulted in synergistically enhanced ADCC compared with any agent alone.[103,105]

Study 1703, a phase II trial, was conducted randomizing 73 patients with RR MM to either elotuzumab 10 mg/kg or 20 mg/kg IV once weekly in combination with lenalidomide at 25 mg (days 1–21) and low-dose oral dexamethasone.[106] At a median follow-up time of 20.8 months, the median PFS for elotuzumab 10 mg/kg arm was not reached, with a more recent estimate showing a median PFS of 33 months. Correlative studies confirmed equal saturation of the target at both doses on tumor obtained with serial bone marrow aspiration across treatment. Preliminary data established an ORR (PR or better) of 84% in all patients and 92% for patients treated with elotuzumab at a dose of 10 mg/kg IV. The median time to objective response was 1 month (range 0.7–19.2). Most common grade 3/4 treatment-emergent AEs were neutropenia (16%), thrombocytopenia (16%), and lymphopenia (16%). As commonly observed with other monoclonal antibodies, chills, pyrexia, flushing, and headache were the most common AEs. A premedication regimen with diphenhydramine, acetaminophen, and methylprednisolone reduced the incidence of infusion reactions subnstantially.[106] Based on these results, 10 mg/kg is now being taken forward in later phase studies.

Two phase III multicentered clinical trials have examined lenalidomide and low-dose oral dexamethasone with or without elotuzumab 10 mg/kg IV in patients with untreated MM (ELOQUENT 1) and in patients with RR MM (ELOQUENT 2). These trials

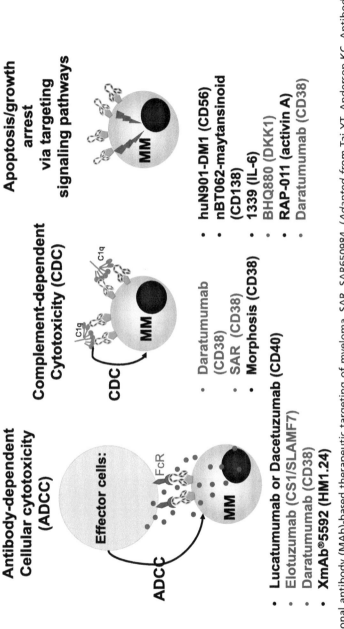

Fig. 3. Monoclonal antibody (MAb)-based therapeutic targeting of myeloma. SAR, SAR650984. (*Adapted from* Tai YT, Anderson KC. Antibody-based therapies in multiple myeloma. Bone Marrow Res 2011;2011:924058.)

assessed efficacy by measuring PFS, ORR, and overall survival. The studies are both completed and in the final stages of analysis, with results eagerly anticipated. Breakthrough status has been assigned to this agent because of these highly promising data, with regulatory approval hoped for within the next 12 months.

Anti-CD38

Daratumumab

CD38 is a 46-kDa single-chain, type II transmembrane glycoprotein with a short 20-aa N-terminal cytoplasmic tail and a 256-aa extracellular domain (see **Fig. 3**).[107] CD38 plays a role in receptor-mediated signaling events to regulate cell adhesion and also contributes to the intracellular mobilization of calcium.[108] CD38 is highly expressed on malignant plasma cells at all stages of MM.[109]

Daratumumab is a humanized monoclonal antibody targeting a unique epitope on the CD38 glycoprotein (see **Fig. 3**). It can effectively kill myeloma cells using ADCC, complement-dependent cytotoxicity (CDC), and apoptosis via cross-linking.[110] Preclinical studies demonstrated that daratumumab exhibited CDC and ADCC activity, even in the presence of BMSCs, which typically provide a protective microenvironment. The combination of lenalidomide and daratumumab demonstrated enhanced NK-mediated cytotoxicity in vitro using ADCC assays.[111]

In a phase I, first-in-human dose-escalation study, heavily pretreated patients with RR MM (median of 6 prior therapies; range 2–12) were treated with single-agent daratumumab over a period of 8 weeks. Ten cohorts were administered doses ranging from 0.005 mg/kg to 24.0 mg/kg. Of the 32 participants, 75% were refractory to both lenalidomide and bortezomib, 83% had previously undergone an autologous stem cell transplant, and 33% had undergone an allogeneic stem cell transplantation.[112–114] Preliminary efficacy data demonstrated a sizable reduction of bone marrow plasma cells by 80% to 100% in the cohorts receiving 4 mg/kg and onward. Overall, 42% of this heavily pretreated population of patients achieved at least a PR at doses 4 mg/kg or greater.[112]

Based on these very encouraging preliminary data, a phase I/II open-label multi-center study of daratumumab in combination with lenalidomide and oral dexamethasone is ongoing in the RR MM patient population. Daratumumab is being administered in dosages from 2 mg/kg to 16 mg/kg weekly for 8 weeks, twice a month for 16 weeks and once a month until disease progression, unmanageable toxicity or up to maximum 24 months. Preliminary data from 20 patients so far has shown a marked reduction in M protein, yielding a response rate of PR or better in 15 of the 20 patients (ORR 75%; CR = 3, VGPR = 6, PR = 6). Six AEs of grade 3 or more (5 events of neutropenia and 1 event of thrombocytopenia) were reported. Overall, daratumumab/lenalidomide/dexamethasone has also demonstrated a favorable safety profile with manageable toxicities, suggesting this combination has great promise for the future.[115] A broad range of studies in all phases are now underway as part of a comprehensive approval-finding strategy for daratumumab, and the agent was given breakthrough status in 2013.

SAR650984

SAR650984 (SAR) is a humanized IgG1 monoclonal antibody that also selectively targets the CD38 surface antigen on MM cells (see **Fig. 3**). SAR induces cell death by ADCC, CDC, and induction of apoptosis. SAR was investigated in a dose escalation phase I study in patients with selected CD38+ hematological malignancies, 27 of which had RR MM.[116] SAR was administered as a single-agent infusion every 2 weeks or weekly. After an initial accelerated dose-escalation schedule in phase I, all subsequent dosages (0.3 mg/kg, 1 mg/kg, 3 mg/kg, 5 mg/kg, 10 mg/kg, 20 mg/kg every 2 weeks and 10 mg/kg weekly) were administered following the classic 3 + 3 design based on DLT. DLTs were limited to grade 2 infusion reactions, which were mitigated with the introduction of a pretreatment regimen. The most common AEs were fatigue (46.9%), nausea (31.3%), pyrexia (28.1%), cough (25%), vomiting (21.9%), and hypercalcemia (18.8%), with headache, constipation, bone pain, chills, and diarrhea each occurring in 15.6% of patients. Responses included one PR at the 1 mg/kg (n = 3) and 5 mg/kg doses (n = 3). The 10 mg/kg dose demonstrated 3 PRs and 2 SDs among 6 patients with MM treated. The maximum tolerated dose was not reached with an every-other-week and an every-week schedule.[116] These data convincingly validate the targeting of CD38 in RR MM, and combination strategies are underway with particularly impressive response data already seen with lenalidomide and dexamethasone. Strategies combining SAR with pomalidomide and dexamethasone are now planned in advanced disease, targeting RR MM as an area of particular clinical need.

Anti–IL-6 (Siltuximab)

IL-6 is produced by stromal cells within the bone marrow and plays a crucial role in the proliferation and survival of MM cells.[117] IL-6 is implicated in chemotherapy resistance by its ability to protect against cell death.[118] Siltuximab is a chimeric monoclonal antibody targeting IL-6. Preclinical studies were encouraging with synergistic cytotoxic activity when siltuximab was combined with other agents, such as bortezomib,[118,119] and when considered as part of a rationale for targeting the tumor milieu.

A phase I dose-escalating study was conducted using single-agent siltuximab in relapsed/refractory patients. Although the drug was well tolerated, no responses were recorded.[120] A phase II trial evaluated siltuximab as a single agent and in combination with dexamethasone in RR MM.[121] As monotherapy, 62% of patients achieved SD at best; but when administered with dexamethasone, a PR rate of 19% and an MR rate 28% was seen, although the numbers were relatively small. Infections of any grade were seen in 57% of patients and grade 3 and 4 in 12% and 6% of patients, respectively.[121] A randomized phase II trial evaluated the addition of siltuximab to velcade, melphalan, prednisone (VMP) therapy in patients with untreated MM, but unfortunately no clinical benefit was seen.[122] Studies of siltuximab in other settings are being explored, including Castleman disease, with randomized studies showing a striking benefit in the latter, which suggests this agent may have a niche role when disease is highly IL-6 dependent.

NOVEL CYTOTOXICS
Melflufen

Melphalan-flufenamide (melflufen) is a prodrug that enhances the cytotoxic potential of melphalan by allowing a more rapid and superior incorporation of melphalan into the tumor cells resulting in intracellular hydrolysis and cell death.[123–125] Using in vitro and in vivo models, preclinical studies have demonstrated that melflufen has more potent antimyeloma activity than equimolar doses of melphalan and can induce apoptosis even in bortezomib and melphalan-resistant MM cells.[126] Melflufen exerts its anti-MM activity by the activation of caspases and through the induction of DNA damage. The combination of melflufen with other novel or conventional MM agents, such as bortezomib, lenalidomide, or dexamethasone, enhanced its cytotoxic effects.[126] These preclinical data provided the impetus for pursuing clinical trials evaluating the safety and efficacy of melflufen in the RR setting. An open-label phase I/IIa study of melflufen in combination with dexamethasone in patients with relapsed or RR MM is currently ongoing. Early data have shown promising activity in this heavily pretreated population, with myelosuppression as one of the more commonly reported AEs but otherwise favorable tolerability to date.

SUMMARY

New, next-generation targeted treatment strategies are urgently required to improve outcomes in patients with MM. Monoclonal antibodies, cell signaling inhibitors, and selective therapies targeting the bone marrow microenvironment have demonstrated encouraging results with generally manageable toxicity in therapeutic trials of patients with RR disease, each critically informed by preclinical studies. A combination approach of these newer agents with immunomodulators and/or PIs as part of a treatment platform seems to consistently improve the efficacy of anti-MM regimens, even in heavily pretreated patients. Future studies continue to be required to better understand the complex mechanisms of drug resistance in MM. Incorporating molecular correlates to further personalize treatment and to, thus, better integrate these agents into clinical practice is a clear priority. There is a broad and very promising armamentarium, which also includes immune-based therapies (discussed elsewhere), now available against this hitherto incurable disease; the hope of durable long-term remission in an increasing proportion of our patients is, therefore, becoming a reality.

REFERENCES

1. Kupperman E, Lee EC, Cao Y, et al. Evaluation of the proteasome inhibitor MLN9708 in preclinical models of human cancer. Cancer Res 2010;70(5):1970–80.
2. Chauhan D, Tian Z, Zhou B, et al. In vitro and in vivo selective antitumor activity of a novel orally bioavailable proteasome inhibitor MLN9708 against multiple myeloma cells. Clin Cancer Res 2011;17(16):5311–21.
3. Gupta N, Saleh M, Venkatakrishnan K. Flat-dosing versus BSA-based dosing for MLN9708, an investigational proteasome inhibitor: population pharmacokinetic (PK) analysis of pooled data from 4 phase-1 studies. ASH Annual Meeting Abstracts 2011;118(21):1433.
4. Kumar S, Bensinger W, Reeder CB, et al. Weekly dosing of the investigational oral proteasome inhibitor MLN9708 in patients (pts) with relapsed/refractory multiple myeloma (MM): a phase I study. J Clin Oncol 2012;30(Suppl) [abstract: 8034].
5. Lonial S, Baz RC, Wang M, et al. Phase I study of twice-weekly dosing of the investigational oral proteasome inhibitor MLN9708 in patients (pts) with relapsed and/or refractory multiple myeloma (MM). J Clin Oncol 2012;30(Suppl) [abstract: 8017].
6. Richardson PG, Hofmeister CC. Twice-weekly oral MLN9708 (Ixazomib Citrate), an investigational proteasome inhibitor, in combination with lenalidomide (Len) and dexamethasone (Dex) in patients (Pts) with newly diagnosed multiple myeloma (MM): final phase 1 results and phase 2 data. ASH Annual Meeting Abstracts 2013;122(21) [abstract: 535].
7. Kuhn DJ, Chen Q, Voorhees PM, et al. Potent activity of carfilzomib, a novel, irreversible inhibitor of the ubiquitin-proteasome pathway, against preclinical models of multiple myeloma. Blood 2007;110(9):3281–90.
8. Demo SD, Kirk CJ, Aujay MA, et al. Antitumor activity of PR-171, a novel irreversible inhibitor of the proteasome. Cancer Res 2007;67(13):6383–91.

9. Chauhan D, Singh AV, Aujay M, et al. A novel orally active proteasome inhibitor ONX 0912 triggers in vitro and in vivo cytotoxicity in multiple myeloma. Blood 2010;116(23):4906–15.

10. Zhou J, Geng G, Shi Q, et al. Design and synthesis of androgen receptor antagonists with bulky side chains for overcoming antiandrogen resistance. J Med Chem 2009;52(17):5546–50.

11. US National Institute of Health. ClinicalTrial.gov. 2012. Available at: http://clinicaltrials.gov/. Accessed July 31, 2012.

12. Papadopoulos KP, Mendelson DS, Tolcher AW, et al. A phase I, open-label, dose-escalation study of the novel oral proteasome inhibitor (PI) ONX 0912 in patients with advanced refractory or recurrent solid tumors. J Clin Oncol 2011;29(Suppl) [abstract: 3075].

13. Chauhan D, Tian Z, Nicholson B, et al. A small molecule inhibitor of ubiquitin-specific protease-7 induces apoptosis in multiple myeloma cells and overcomes bortezomib resistance. Canc Cell 2012;22(3):345–58.

14. Chauhan D, Singh A, Brahmandam M, et al. Combination of proteasome inhibitors bortezomib and NPI-0052 trigger in vivo synergistic cytotoxicity in multiple myeloma. Blood 2008;111(3):1654–64.

15. Chauhan D, Singh AV, Ciccarelli B, et al. Combination of novel proteasome inhibitor NPI-0052 and lenalidomide trigger in vitro and in vivo synergistic cytotoxicity in multiple myeloma. Blood 2010;115(4):834–45.

16. Richardson PG, Spencer A, Cannell P, et al. Phase 1 clinical evaluation of twice-weekly marizomib (NPI-0052), a novel proteasome inhibitor, in patients with relapsed/refractory multiple myeloma (MM). ASH Annual Meeting Abstracts 2011;118(21):302.

17. Jaenisch R, Bird A. Epigenetic regulation of gene expression: how the genome integrates intrinsic and environmental signals. Nat Genet 2003;33(Suppl): 245–54.

18. Sterner DE, Berger SL. Acetylation of histones and transcription-related factors. Microbiol Mol Biol Rev 2000;64(2):435–59.

19. de Ruijter AJ, van Gennip AH, Caron HN, et al. Histone deacetylases (HDACs): characterization of the classical HDAC family. Biochem J 2003;370(Pt 3):737–49.

20. Roth SY, Denu JM, Allis CD. Histone acetyltransferases. Annu Rev Biochem 2001;70:81–120.

21. Bolden JE, Peart MJ, Johnstone RW. Anticancer activities of histone deacetylase inhibitors. Nat Rev Drug Discov 2006;5(9):769–84.

22. Sasakawa Y, Naoe Y, Inoue T, et al. Effects of FK228, a novel histone deacetylase inhibitor, on tumor growth and expression of p21 and c-myc genes in vivo. Cancer Lett 2003;195(2):161–8.

23. Lin HY, Chen CS, Lin SP, et al. Targeting histone deacetylase in cancer therapy. Med Res Rev 2006;26(4):397–413.

24. Marks PA, Richon VM, Rifkind RA. Histone deacetylase inhibitors: inducers of differentiation or apoptosis of transformed cells. J Natl Cancer Inst 2000; 92(15):1210–6.

25. Fandy TE, Shankar S, Ross DD, et al. Interactive effects of HDAC inhibitors and TRAIL on apoptosis are associated with changes in mitochondrial functions and expressions of cell cycle regulatory genes in multiple myeloma. Neoplasia 2005; 7(7):646–57.

26. Qian DZ, Kato Y, Shabbeer S, et al. Targeting tumor angiogenesis with histone deacetylase inhibitors: the hydroxamic acid derivative LBH589. Clin Cancer Res 2006;12(2):634–42.

27. Shao W, Growney JD, Feng Y, et al. Potent anticancer activity of the pan-deacetylase inhibitor panobinostat (LBH589) as a single agent in in vitro and in vivo tumor models. 99th American Association of Cancer Research Annual Meeting [abstract: 6244]. 2008.

28. Atadja P. Development of the pan-DAC inhibitor panobinostat (LBH589): successes and challenges. Cancer Lett 2009;280(2):233–41.

29. Catley L, Weisberg E, Kiziltepe T, et al. Aggresome induction by proteasome inhibitor bortezomib and alpha-tubulin hyperacetylation by tubulin deacetylase (TDAC) inhibitor LBH589 are synergistic in myeloma cells. Blood 2006; 108(10):3441–9.

30. Ocio EM, Vilanova D, Atadja P, et al. In vitro and in vivo rationale for the triple combination of panobinostat (LBH589) and dexamethasone with either bortezomib or lenalidomide in multiple myeloma. Haematologica 2010;95(5): 794–803.

31. Wolf JL, Siegel D, Goldschmidt H, et al. Phase II trial of the pan-deacetylase inhibitor panobinostat as a single agent in advanced relapsed/refractory multiple myeloma. Leuk Lymphoma 2012;53(9):1820–3.

32. Hideshima T, Richardson PG, Anderson KC, et al. Intracellular protein degradation and its therapeutic implications. Clin Cancer Res 2005;11(24 Pt 1):8530–3.

33. San-Miguel JF, Richardson PG, Gunther A, et al. Phase Ib study of panobinostat and bortezomib in relapsed or relapsed and refractory multiple myeloma. J Clin Oncol 2013;31(29):3696–703.

34. Richardson PG, Schlossman RL, Alsina M, et al. PANORAMA 2: panobinostat in combination with bortezomib and dexamethasone in patients with relapsed and bortezomib-refractory myeloma. Blood 2013;122(14):2331–7.

35. Richardson PG, Hofmeister CC. Panorama 1: a randomized, double-blind, phase 3 study of panobinostat or placebo plus bortezomib and dexamethasone in relapsed or relapsed and refractory multiple myeloma. J Clin Oncol 2014; 30(Suppl) [abstract: 8017].

36. Xu WS, Parmigiani RB, Marks PA. Histone deacetylase inhibitors: molecular mechanisms of action. Oncogene 2007;26(37):5541–52.

37. Mitsiades CS, Mitsiades NS, McMullan CJ, et al. Transcriptional signature of histone deacetylase inhibition in multiple myeloma: biological and clinical implications. Proc Natl Acad Sci U S A 2004;101(2):540–5.

38. Mitsiades N, Mitsiades CS, Richardson PG, et al. Molecular sequelae of histone deacetylase inhibition in human malignant B cells. Blood 2003;101(10):4055–62.

39. Kaufman JL, Shah JJ, Laubach JP. Lenalidomide, bortezomib, and dexamethasone (RVD) in combination with vorinostat as front-line therapy for patients with multiple myeloma (MM): results of a phase 1 study. ASH Annual Meeting Abstracts 2012;120:336.

40. Siegel DS, Richardson P, Dimopoulos M, et al. Vorinostat in combination with lenalidomide and dexamethasone in patients with relapsed or refractory multiple myeloma. Blood Cancer J 2014;4:e202.

41. Dimopoulos M, Siegel DS, Lonial S, et al. Vorinostat or placebo in combination with bortezomib in patients with multiple myeloma (VANTAGE 088): a multi-centre, randomised, double-blind study. Lancet Oncol 2013;14(11):1129–40.

42. Hideshima T, Bradner JE, Wong J, et al. Small-molecule inhibition of proteasome and aggresome function induces synergistic antitumor activity in multiple myeloma. Proc Natl Acad Sci U S A 2005;102(24):8567–72.

43. McConkey D. Proteasome and HDAC: who's zooming who? Blood 2010;116(3): 308–9.

44. Santo L, Hideshima T, Kung AL, et al. Preclinical activity, pharmacodynamic, and pharmacokinetic properties of a selective HDAC6 inhibitor, ACY-1215, in combination with bortezomib in multiple myeloma. Blood 2012;119(11): 2579–89.

45. Raje NS, Vogl DT, Hari PN, et al. ACY-1215, a selective histone deacetylase (HDAC) 6 inhibitor: interim results of combination therapy with bortezomib in patients with multiple myeloma (MM). ASH Annual Meeting Abstracts 2013;122(21) [abstract: 3190].

46. Yee AJ, Vorhees P, Bensinger WI, et al. ACY-1215, a selective histone deacetylase (HDAC) 6 inhibitor, in combination with lenalidomide and dexamethasone (dex), is well tolerated without dose limiting toxicity (DLT) in patients (Pts) with multiple myeloma (MM) at doses demonstrating biologic activity: interim results of a phase 1b Trial. ASH Annual Meeting Abstracts 2013;122(21) [abstract: 3190].

47. Drysdale MJ, Brough PA, Massey A, et al. Targeting Hsp90 for the treatment of cancer. Curr Opin Drug Discov Dev 2006;9(4):483–95.

48. Richardson PG, Chanan-Khan AA, Lonial S, et al. Tanespimycin and bortezomib combination treatment in patients with relapsed or relapsed and refractory multiple myeloma: results of a phase 1/2 study. Br J Haematol 2011;153(6):729–40.

49. Liu P, Cheng H, Roberts TM, et al. Targeting the phosphoinositide 3-kinase pathway in cancer. Nat Rev Drug Discov 2009;8(8):627–44.

50. Hsu J, Shi Y, Krajewski S, et al. The AKT kinase is activated in multiple myeloma tumor cells. Blood 2001;98(9):2853–5.

51. Hideshima T, Catley L, Raje N, et al. Inhibition of Akt induces significant down-regulation of survivin and cytotoxicity in human multiple myeloma cells. Br J Haematol 2007;138(6):783–91.

52. Richardson PG, Wolf J, Jakubowiak A, et al. Perifosine plus bortezomib and dexamethasone in patients with relapsed/refractory multiple myeloma previously treated with bortezomib: results of a multicenter phase I/II trial. J Clin Oncol 2011;29(32):4243–9.

53. Mimura N, Hideshima T, Shimomura T, et al. Selective and potent Akt inhibition triggers anti-myeloma activities and enhances fatal endoplasmic reticulum stress induced by proteasome inhibition. Cancer Res 2014 [Epub ahead of print]. Accessed June 16, 2014.

54. Dang CV, Le A, Gao P. MYC-induced cancer cell energy metabolism and therapeutic opportunities. Clin Cancer Res 2009;15(21):6479–83.

55. Delmore JE, Issa GC, Lemieux ME, et al. BET bromodomain inhibition as a therapeutic strategy to target c-Myc. Cell 2011;146(6):904–17.

56. Glickman MH, Ciechanover A. The ubiquitin-proteasome proteolytic pathway: destruction for the sake of construction. Physiol Rev 2002;82(2):373–428.

57. Schnell JD, Hicke L. Non-traditional functions of ubiquitin and ubiquitin-binding proteins. J Biol Chem 2003;278(38):35857–60.

58. Reyes-Turcu FE, Ventii KH, Wilkinson KD. Regulation and cellular roles of ubiquitin-specific deubiquitinating enzymes. Annu Rev Biochem 2009;78: 363–97.

59. Menendez-Benito V, Verhoef LG, Masucci MG, et al. Endoplasmic reticulum stress compromises the ubiquitin-proteasome system. Hum Mol Genet 2005; 14(19):2787–99.

60. Tian Z, D'Arcy P, Wang X, et al. A novel small molecule inhibitor of deubiquitylating enzyme USP14 and UCHL5 induces apoptosis in multiple myeloma and overcomes bortezomib resistance. Blood 2014;123(5):706–16.

61. Takebe N, Harris PJ, Warren RQ, et al. Targeting cancer stem cells by inhibiting Wnt, Notch, and Hedgehog pathways. Nat Rev Clin Oncol 2011;8(2):97–106.

62. Tian E, Zhan F, Walker R, et al. The role of the Wnt-signaling antagonist DKK1 in the development of osteolytic lesions in multiple myeloma. N Engl J Med 2003; 349(26):2483–94.

63. Fulciniti M, Tassone P, Hideshima T, et al. Anti-DKK1 mAb (BHQ880) as a potential therapeutic agent for multiple myeloma. Blood 2009;114(2):371–9.

64. Padmanabhan S, Beck JT, Kelly KR, et al. A phase I/II study of BHQ880, a novel osteoblast activating, anti-dkk1 human monoclonal antibody, in relapsed and refractory multiple myeloma (MM) patients treated with zoledronic acid (Zol) and anti-myeloma therapy (MM Tx). Blood (ASH Annual Meeting Abstracts) 2009;114(21):750.

65. Munshi N, Abonour R, Beck JT, et al. Early evidence of anabolic bone activity of BHQ880, a fully human anti-DKK1 neutralizing antibody: results of a phase 2 study in previously untreated patients with smoldering multiple myeloma at risk for progression. Blood (ASH Annual Meeting Abstracts) 2012;120(21):331.

66. Mirandola L, Comi P, Cobos E, et al. Notch-ing from T-cell to B-cell lymphoid malignancies. Cancer Lett 2011;308(1):1–13.

67. Ramakrishnan V, Ansell S, Haug J, et al. MRK003, a gamma-secretase inhibitor exhibits promising in vitro pre-clinical activity in multiple myeloma and non-Hodgkin's lymphoma. Leukemia 2012;26(2):340–8.

68. Xu D, Hu J, De Bruyne E, et al. Dll1/notch activation contributes to bortezomib resistance by upregulating CYP1A1 in multiple myeloma. Biochem Biophys Res Commun 2012;428(4):518–24.

69. Davies FE, Dring AM, Li C, et al. Insights into the multistep transformation of MGUS to myeloma using microarray expression analysis. Blood 2003;102(13): 4504–11.

70. Blotta S, Jakubikova J, Calimeri T, et al. Canonical and noncanonical Hedgehog pathway in the pathogenesis of multiple myeloma. Blood 2012;120(25): 5002–13.

71. Kapoor TM, Mayer TU, Coughlin ML, et al. Probing spindle assembly mechanisms with monastrol, a small molecule inhibitor of the mitotic kinesin, Eg5. J Cell Biol 2000;150(5):975–88.

72. Woessner R, Tunquist BJ, Cox A, et al. Combination of the KSP inhibitor ARRY-520 with bortezomib or revlimid causes sustained tumor regressions and significantly increased time to regrowth in models of multiple myeloma. ASH Annual Meeting Abstracts 2011 2009;114:2858.

73. Tunquist BJ, Woessner RD, Walker DH. Mcl-1 stability determines mitotic cell fate of human multiple myeloma tumor cells treated with the kinesin spindle protein inhibitor ARRY-520. Mol Cancer Ther 2010;9(7):2046–56.

74. Shah JJ, Zonder J, Cohen A, et al. ARRY-520 shows durable responses in patients with relapsed/refractory multiple myeloma in a phase 1 dose-escalation study. ASH Annual Meeting Abstracts 2011 2011;118:1860.

75. Shah JJ, Zonder J, Cohen A, et al. The novel KSP inhibitor ARRY-520 is active both with and without low-dose dexamethasone in patients with multiple myeloma refractory to bortezomib and lenalidomide: results from a phase 2 study. ASH Annual Meeting Abstracts 2012;120(449).

76. Xu D, Grishin NV, Chook YM. NESdb: a database of NES-containing CRM1 cargoes. Mol Biol Cell 2012;23(18):3673–6.

77. Turner JG, Dawson J, Sullivan DM. Nuclear export of proteins and drug resistance in cancer. Biochem Pharmacol 2012;83(8):1021–32.

78. Brodie KM, Henderson BR. Characterization of BRCA1 protein targeting, dynamics, and function at the centrosome: a role for the nuclear export signal, CRM1, and Aurora A kinase. J Biol Chem 2012;287(10):7701–16.
79. Yao Y, Dong Y, Lin F, et al. The expression of CRM1 is associated with prognosis in human osteosarcoma. Oncol Rep 2009;21(1):229–35.
80. Huang WY, Yue L, Qiu WS, et al. Prognostic value of CRM1 in pancreas cancer. Clin Invest Med 2009;32(6):E315.
81. Tai YT, Landesman Y, Acharya C, et al. CRM1 inhibition induces tumor cell cytotoxicity and impairs osteoclastogenesis in multiple myeloma: molecular mechanisms and therapeutic implications. Leukemia 2014;28(1):155–65.
82. Azab AK, Hu J, Quang P, et al. Hypoxia promotes dissemination of multiple myeloma through acquisition of epithelial to mesenchymal transition-like features. Blood 2012;119(24):5782–94.
83. Hu J, Van Valckenborgh E, Xu D, et al. Synergistic induction of apoptosis in multiple myeloma cells by bortezomib and hypoxia-activated prodrug TH-302, in vivo and in vitro. Mol Cancer Ther 2013;12(9):1763–73.
84. de la Puente P, Muz B, Azab F, et al. Cell trafficking of endothelial progenitor cells in tumor progression. Clin Cancer Res 2013;19(13):3360–8.
85. Prince HM, Honemann D, Spencer A, et al. Vascular endothelial growth factor inhibition is not an effective therapeutic strategy for relapsed or refractory multiple myeloma: a phase 2 study of pazopanib (GW786034). Blood 2009;113(19):4819–20.
86. Kovacs MJ, Reece DE, Marcellus D, et al. A phase II study of ZD6474 Zactima, a selective inhibitor of VEGFR and EGFR tyrosine kinase in patients with relapsed multiple myeloma–NCIC CTG IND.145. Invest New Drugs 2006;24(6):529–35.
87. Alsayed Y, Ngo H, Runnels J, et al. Mechanisms of regulation of CXCR4/SDF-1 (CXCL12)-dependent migration and homing in multiple myeloma. Blood 2007;109(7):2708–17.
88. Azab AK, Runnels JM, Pitsillides C, et al. CXCR4 inhibitor AMD3100 disrupts the interaction of multiple myeloma cells with the bone marrow microenvironment and enhances their sensitivity to therapy. Blood 2009;113(18):4341–51.
89. Ghobrial I, Shain K, Hanlon C, et al. Phase I/II trial of plerixafor and bortezomib as a chemosensitization strategy in relapsed or relapsed/refractory multiple myeloma. ASH Annual Meeting Abstracts 2013;120:336.
90. Barr AR, Gergely F. Aurora-A: the maker and breaker of spindle poles. J Cell Sci 2007;120(Pt 17):2987–96.
91. Fu J, Bian M, Jiang Q, et al. Roles of Aurora kinases in mitosis and tumorigenesis. Mol Canc Res 2007;5(1):1–10.
92. Marumoto T, Honda S, Hara T, et al. Aurora-A kinase maintains the fidelity of early and late mitotic events in HeLa cells. J Biol Chem 2003;278(51):51786–95.
93. Evans R, Naber C, Steffler T, et al. Aurora A kinase RNAi and small molecule inhibition of Aurora kinases with VE-465 induce apoptotic death in multiple myeloma cells. Leuk Lymphoma 2008;49(3):559–69.
94. Dutta-Simmons J, Zhang Y, Gorgun G, et al. Aurora kinase A is a target of Wnt/beta-catenin involved in multiple myeloma disease progression. Blood 2009;114(13):2699–708.
95. Gorgun G, Calabrese E, Hideshima T, et al. A novel Aurora-A kinase inhibitor MLN8237 induces cytotoxicity and cell-cycle arrest in multiple myeloma. Blood 2010;115(25):5202–13.

96. Greipp PR, Witzig TE, Gonchoroff NJ, et al. Immunofluorescence labeling indices in myeloma and related monoclonal gammopathies. Mayo Clin Proc 1987;62(11):969–77.

97. Sherr CJ, Roberts JM. CDK inhibitors: positive and negative regulators of G1-phase progression. Genes Dev 1999;13(12):1501–12.

98. Ely S, Di Liberto M, Niesvizky R, et al. Mutually exclusive cyclin-dependent kinase 4/cyclin D1 and cyclin-dependent kinase 6/cyclin D2 pairing inactivates retinoblastoma protein and promotes cell cycle dysregulation in multiple myeloma. Cancer Res 2005;65(24):11345–53.

99. Baughn LB, Di Liberto M, Wu K, et al. A novel orally active small molecule potently induces G1 arrest in primary myeloma cells and prevents tumor growth by specific inhibition of cyclin-dependent kinase 4/6. Cancer Res 2006;66(15): 7661–7.

100. Raje N, Kumar S, Hideshima T, et al. Seliciclib (CYC202 or R-roscovitine), a small-molecule cyclin-dependent kinase inhibitor, mediates activity via down-regulation of Mcl-1 in multiple myeloma. Blood 2005;106(3):1042–7.

101. Kumaresan PR, Lai WC, Chuang SS, et al. CS1, a novel member of the CD2 family, is homophilic and regulates NK cell function. Mol Immunol 2002;39(1–2):1–8.

102. Hsi ED, Steinle R, Balasa B, et al. CS1, a potential new therapeutic antibody target for the treatment of multiple myeloma. Clin Cancer Res 2008;14(9): 2775–84.

103. Tai YT, Dillon M, Song W, et al. Anti-CS1 humanized monoclonal antibody Hu-Luc63 inhibits myeloma cell adhesion and induces antibody-dependent cellular cytotoxicity in the bone marrow milieu. Blood 2008;112(4):1329–37.

104. Rice AG, Balasa B, Yun R, et al. Natural killer cell activation, cytokine production, and cytotoxicity in human PBMC/myeloma cell co-cultures exposed to elotuzumab alone or in combination with lenalidomide. 17th Congress of the European Hematology Association. 2013.

105. van Rhee F, Szmania SM, Dillon M, et al. Combinatorial efficacy of anti-CS1 monoclonal antibody elotuzumab (HuLuc63) and bortezomib against multiple myeloma. Mol Cancer Ther 2009;8(9):2616–24.

106. Richardson P, Jagannath S, Moreau P, et al. A phase 2 study of elotuzumab (Elo) in combination with lenalidomide and low-dose dexamethasone (Ld) in patients (pts) with relapsed/refractory multiple myeloma (R/R MM): updated results. Blood (ASH Annual Meeting Abstracts) 2012;120(21):202.

107. Malavasi F, Funaro A, Roggero S, et al. Human CD38: a glycoprotein in search of a function. Immunol Today 1994;15(3):95–7.

108. Mehta K, Malavasi F. Human CD38 and related molecules. Switzerland: Karger; 2000.

109. Lin P, Owens R, Tricot G, et al. Flow cytometric immunophenotypic analysis of 306 cases of multiple myeloma. Am J Clin Pathol 2004;121(4):482–8.

110. de Weers M, Tai YT, van der Veer MS, et al. Daratumumab, a novel therapeutic human CD38 monoclonal antibody, induces killing of multiple myeloma and other hematological tumors. J Immunol 2011;186(3):1840–8.

111. van der Veer MS, de Weers M, van Kessel B, et al. Towards effective immunotherapy of myeloma: enhanced elimination of myeloma cells by combination of lenalidomide with the human CD38 monoclonal antibody daratumumab. Haematologica 2011;96(2):284–90.

112. Plesner T, Lokhorst H, Gimsing P, et al. Daratumumab, a CD38 monoclonal antibody in patients with multiple myeloma - data from a dose-escalation phase I/II study. Blood (ASH Annual Meeting Abstracts) 2012;120(21):73.

113. Plesner T, Lokhorst H, Gimsing P, et al. Daratumumab, a CD38 mab, for the treatment of relapsed/refractory multiple myeloma patients: preliminary efficacy data from a multicenter phase I/II study. ASCO Meeting Abstr 2012;30(Suppl 15):8019.

114. Lokhorst HM, Plesner T, Gimsing P, et al. Phase I/II dose-escalation study of daratumumab in patients with relapsed or refractory multiple myeloma. ASCO Meeting Abstr 2013;31(Suppl):8512.

115. Plesner T, Arkenau T, Lokhorst H, et al. Preliminary safety and efficacy data of daratumumab in combination with lenalidomide and dexamethasone in relapsed or refractory multiple myeloma. ASH Annual Meeting Abstracts 2013;122(21) [abstract: 1986].

116. Martin TG III, Strickland SA, Glenn M, et al. SAR650984, a CD38 monoclonal antibody in patients with selected CD38 + hematological malignancies- data from a dose-escalation phase i study. ASH Annual Meeting Abstracts 2013; 122(21) [abstract: 1986].

117. Klein B, Zhang XG, Jourdan M, et al. Paracrine rather than autocrine regulation of myeloma-cell growth and differentiation by interleukin-6. Blood 1989;73(2):517–26.

118. Voorhees PM, Chen Q, Kuhn DJ, et al. Inhibition of interleukin-6 signaling with CNTO 328 enhances the activity of bortezomib in preclinical models of multiple myeloma. Clin Cancer Res 2007;13(21):6469–78.

119. Voorhees PM, Chen Q, Small GW, et al. Targeted inhibition of interleukin-6 with CNTO 328 sensitizes pre-clinical models of multiple myeloma to dexamethasone-mediated cell death. Br J Haematol 2009;145(4):481–90.

120. van Zaanen HC, Lokhorst HM, Aarden LA, et al. Chimaeric anti-interleukin 6 monoclonal antibodies in the treatment of advanced multiple myeloma: a phase I dose-escalating study. Br J Haematol 1998;102(3):783–90.

121. Voorhees PM, Manges RF, Sonneveld P, et al. A phase 2 multicentre study of siltuximab, an anti-interleukin-6 monoclonal antibody, in patients with relapsed or refractory multiple myeloma. Br J Haematol 2013;161(3):357–66.

122. San Miguel J, Bladé J, Samoilova OS, et al. Randomized, open label, phase 2 study of siltuximab (an anti-IL6 mab) and bortezomib-melphalan-prednisone versus bortezomib-melphalan-prednisone in patients with previously untreated multiple myeloma. EHA Abstracts 2013;98(Suppl I):97.

123. Gullbo J, Wallinder C, Tullberg M, et al. Antitumor activity of the novel melphalan containing tripeptide J3 (L-prolyl-L-melphalanyl-p-L-fluorophenylalanine ethyl ester): comparison with its m-L-sarcolysin analogue P2. Mol Cancer Ther 2003;2(12):1331–9.

124. Gullbo J, Lindhagen E, Bashir-Hassan S, et al. Antitumor efficacy and acute toxicity of the novel dipeptide melphalanyl-p-L-fluorophenylalanine ethyl ester (J1) in vivo. Invest New Drugs 2004;22(4):411–20.

125. Wickstrom M, Johnsen JI, Ponthan F, et al. The novel melphalan prodrug J1 inhibits neuroblastoma growth in vitro and in vivo. Mol Cancer Ther 2007;6(9):2409–17.

126. Chauhan D, Ray A, Viktorsson K, et al. In vitro and in vivo antitumor activity of a novel alkylating agent, melphalan-flufenamide, against multiple myeloma cells. Clin Cancer Res 2013;19(11):3019–31.

127. Chauhan D, Catley L, Li G, et al. A novel orally active proteasome inhibitor induces apoptosis in multiple myeloma cells with mechanisms distinct from Bortezomib. Cancer Cell 2005;8(5):407–19.

128. Hideshima T, Richardson P, Chauhan D, et al. The proteasome inhibitor PS-341 inhibits growth, induces apoptosis, and overcomes drug resistance in human multiple myeloma cells. Cancer Res 2001;61(7):3071–6.

Immunotherapy Strategies in Multiple Myeloma

Jooeun Bae, PhD*, Nikhil C. Munshi, MD, Kenneth C. Anderson, MD

KEYWORDS

- Multiple myeloma • Passive-specific immunotherapy
- Active-specific immunotherapy

KEY POINTS

- After several years of disappointing results, immunotherapy is now emerging as a promising therapeutic approach for different types of cancer.
- Various immunotherapeutic strategies, including antibodies, vaccines, and checkpoint inhibitors, are currently in evaluation in multiple clinical trials.
- The studies on multiple myeloma (MM) microenvironment unveiled a complex network driven by MM plasma cells, which progressively lead to functional impairment of host immune system and immunotherapeutic approach.
- Novel immune targets, new combinational approaches, and biomarkers are additional subjects of ongoing studies.
- These areas are rapidly progressing and will probably change the landscape of therapy in MM in the near future.

Multiple myeloma (MM) is a B-cell malignancy characterized by the clonal proliferation of malignant plasma cells in the bone marrow and the development of osteolytic bone lesions. Over the last decade, MM has emerged as a paradigm within the cancers for the success of drug discovery and translational medicine. Despite recent advances in the treatment of MM using conventional and novel therapeutics in combination with transplantation, the disease still remains incurable and most patients eventually relapse.[1–4] Thus, novel therapeutic approaches, which have a mechanism of action distinct from cytotoxic chemotherapy, are required to eradicate the tumor cells. Immunotherapy is an encouraging option for the goal of inducing effective and long-lasting therapeutic outcome and has become an important approach in the development of treatment strategies for MM.[5–7] Immunotherapy can be divided into two distinct approaches, passive or active immunotherapies, which target tumor-associated antigens (TAAs) and have shown promising results in multiple preclinical and clinical studies.

Dana-Farber Cancer Institute, Harvard Medical School, 450 Brookline Avenue, Boston, MA 02215, USA
* Corresponding author.
E-mail address: Jooeun_Bae@dfci.harvard.edu

Hematol Oncol Clin N Am 28 (2014) 927–943
http://dx.doi.org/10.1016/j.hoc.2014.07.002
0889-8588/14/$ – see front matter © 2014 Elsevier Inc. All rights reserved.

PASSIVE-SPECIFIC IMMUNOTHERAPY

The monoclonal antibodies (mAbs) bind directly to TAA on the surface of myeloma cells, and induce apoptosis directly or trigger antigen-dependent cellular cytotoxicity or complement-dependent cytotoxicity against the tumor cells.[8–11] A variety of mAbs are undergoing preclinical and clinical investigation in MM. Elotuzumab is a specific mAb directed toward CS1, a glycoprotein that is specific to plasma cells and highly expressed on MM cells, although the antigen may also be expressed in natural killer and CD8+ T cells.[12] The results in monotherapy were modest[13]; however, the combination of elotuzumab with lenalidomide and dexamethasone has given excellent results with greater than 80% partial remission in relapsed patients and prolonged progression-free survival.[14,15] As the proposed mechanism of action, lenalidomide would prepare the natural killer and lymphoid cells by changing the conformation of their cytoskeleton to favor the immune recognition and elotuzumab would modify the plasma cells to be more prone to be targeted by the immune cells. A phase III trial in relapsed myeloma comparing lenalidomide plus dexamethasone with the combination of lenalidomide, dexamethasone, and elotuzumab has recently been completed.

Anti-CD38 mAb (daratumumab, SAR650954, MOR101) has shown consistent cytotoxic activity against MM cells both in vitro and in vivo. Daratumumab as a single agent demonstrated a marked reduction of myeloma cells and bone marrow plasma cells in subjects with relapsed or refractory MM.[16] Remarkably, 42% of the subjects treated achieved partial responses at therapeutic levels in the dose-escalation study with daratumumab monotherapy. This encouraging result has prompted the recent development of other anti-CD38 mAbs, such as SAR650984 and MOR101.[17]

CD40, CD56, and CD138 are other antigens of the plasma cells that have been targeted by mAbs. Lorvotuzumab and nBT062 directed against CD56 and CD138, respectively, have in common that they are each conjugated with a cytotoxic agent (DM1 and DM4, respectively) that is released inside the cells once bound to it. The results of the phase 1 trials in monotherapy showed some minimal responses and partial responses in subjects who were heavily pretreated.[18,19] mAbs against CD40, dacetuzumab, and lucatumumab have shown some modest responses as monotherapy.[20,21] Some of these antibodies are currently being combined with other agents, including with lenalidomide and dexamethasone, for a potential immune synergy.

Boost of immune responses has been demonstrated with a mAb specific to programmed cell death 1 (PD-1) on T cells. Blockade of the interaction between PD-1 and PD-1L and effectiveness of anti-PD-1 has also been shown in promoting T-cell activation in MM.[22,23] Other targets with potential clinical relevance are undergoing investigations such as anti–vascular endothelial growth factor (VEGF) Ab,[24] anti-IL6,[25,26] or anti-inhibitory killer immunoglobulin–like receptors.[27] A wide variety of monoclonal antibodies (**Table 1**) are currently under evaluation in clinical trials to treat patients with multiple myeloma.

ACTIVE-SPECIFIC IMMUNOTHERAPY

Active-specific immunotherapy has the distinct advantage of inducing highly effective T lymphocytes with antitumor activities and memory functions.[28,29] Results from recent research have indicated that myeloma cells are susceptible to T cell–mediated cytotoxicity. Long-lasting disease remission has been achieved in patients with MM after infusion of donor lymphocytes in the postallograft relapse setting in which patients are chemotherapy refractory.[30] With the encouraging results of allogeneic transplantation as well as graft-versus-myeloma responses following donor

Table 1
Development of antibodies in multiple myeloma

Target Antigen	Antibody Type	Clinical Development	Remarks
CD20	Chimeric with a human IgG1 Fc	II (ongoing)	NCT00258206 (with cyclophosphamide), NCT00505895
CD20	Radioactive iodine 131 attaching to anti-CD20;muIgG2a (131)	II (ongoing)	NCT00135200
CD20	Mouse IgG1	I (ongoing)	NCT00477815
CD38	Human IgG1	I/II (ongoing)	NCT00574288
CD40	Humanized IgG1	I b (ongoing)	NCT00664898
CD40	Human IgG1	I (ongoing)	NCT00231166
CD52	Humanized	II (ongoing)	NCT00625144
CD56	Humanized (maytansine DM1 conjugation)	I (ongoing)	NCT00346255
CD74 (variant MHC II)	Humanized IgG1 or humanized IgG1 doxorubicin conjugate	I/II (ongoing)	NCT00421525
CD138	Chimeric (B-B4-maytansinoid DM4)	I (ongoing)	NCT00723359
Activin receptor type IIA (ActRIIA)	Human IgG1	I/IIa (ongoing)	NCT00747123
Alpha-4 integrin	Humanized IgG4	I/II (ongoing)	NCT00675428
CS1	Humanized	I /II (ongoing)	NCT00742560, NCT00726869
DKK	Human IgG1	I/II (ongoing)	NCT00741377
EGFR	Chimerized	II (ongoing)	NCT00368121
IGF-1R	Humanized	I/II (ongoing)	Descamps et al,[102] 2009
IGF-1R	Human IgG2	I	Lacy et al,[103] 2008
IL-6	Chimerized IgG1	I/II (ongoing)	NCT00401843, NCT00911859, NCT00402181
IL-6R	Humanized	II	N/A
KIR	Human IgG4	I/IIa (ongoing)	NCT00552396 (ASCO 2009, Abstract #: 09-AB-3032)
MHC II (HLA-DR)	Human IgG4	I	Carlo-Stella et al,[104] 2007
RANKL	Human IgG2	II/III (ongoing)	NCT00259740
TRAIL-R1(DR4)	Human	II (ongoing)	NCT00315757
VEGF	Humanized	II (ongoing)	NCT00428545
Target Antigen	**Antibody Type**	**Stage**	**References**
β2-microglobulin	Mouse	Preclincial	Yu et al,[105] 2013, Cao et al,[106] 2011
BCMA	Auristatin- BCMA mAb	Preclincial	Tai et al,[107] 2014, Ryan et al,[108] 2007
			(continued on next page)

Table 1
(continued)

Target Antigen	Antibody Type	Stage	References
BLyS	Fusion protein of an antibody tethered to a toxin	Preclincial	Lyu et al,[109] 2007
HLA class I	Single-chain Fv diabody	Preclincial	Sekimoto et al,[110] 2007
HLA-DR	Bispecific antibody, Human IgG1	Preclincial	Rossi et al,[111] 2010, Carlo-Stella et al,[104] 2007
HM1.24	Humanized	Preclincial	Amano et al,[112] 2010, Ozaki et al,[113] 1999
CD38	Human IgG1	Preclincial	Deckert et al,[114] 2014
CD70	Humanized IgG1	Preclincial	McEarchern et al,[115] 2008
CD138	Radiolabeled mouse IgG1 mAb, Maytansinoid immunoconjugate mouse IgG1 mAb	Preclincial	Chérel et al,[116] 2013, Tassone et al,[117] 2004
FGFR3	Human IgG1 mAb	Preclincial	Kamath et al,[118] 2012, Trudel et al,[119] 2006
Kininogen	Mouse mAb	Preclincial	Sainz et al,[120] 2006
ICAM-1	Human IgG1, chimeric IgG1	Preclincial	Veitonmäki et al,[121] 2013, Smallshaw et al,[122] 2004, Coleman et al,[123] 2006
IL-1beta	Human Engineered™ IgG2	Preclincial	Lust et al, 2010, AACR abstract #2449
IL-6	Human IgG1	Preclincial	Fulciniti et al,[124] 2009
IL-6R	Human IgG1 fusion	Preclincial	Yoshio-Hoshino et al,[125] 2007
TACI	Fusion protein	Preclincial	Yaccoby et al,[126] 2008
TRAILR1, TRAILR2	Human	Preclincial	Menoret et al,[127] 2006

lymphocytes infusion, different types of active-specific immunotherapy approaches are being evaluated to treat patients with MM.[31] Most active-specific immunotherapy protocols in development for MM have used tumor-specific idiotypic protein or whole tumor cells and used dendritic cells (DCs) to generate patient-specific vaccines.

Idiotype (Id) proteins are tumor-specific antigens that can be used for an active immunization against idiotypic determinants on malignant B cells and have been shown to induce resistance to tumor in murine models.[32,33] Additional studies have shown that T cells in patients with myeloma responded to peptides corresponding to complementarity-determining regions of heavy and light chains of the autologous M-component.[34,35] In general, most clinical trials conducted using Id-pulsed DCs showed immune responses against the tumor target cells. Interestingly, the Id-induced T-cell stimulation was more confined to the CD4$^+$ T cell subset than the CD8$^+$ subset in most of the subjects examined, especially with T_H2-specific response in subjects with advanced MM (stage II–III).[36,37] However, the clinical responses were unsatisfactory, mainly due to the poor immunogenicity of the Id protein.[38,39] To overcome the limitation of weak immunogenicity of Id antigen and to elicit a robust T-cell response, several Id vaccination strategies have been adopted: immunization of the purified M component together with adjuvant cytokines such as granulocyte-macrophage colony-stimulating factor (GM-CSF),[40] keyhole-limpet-hemocyanin-coupled paraprotein immunization,[41] and Id-loaded DC administration.[42] In addition, different DC sources such as Langerhans cells could be explored because they have been shown to be comparable to monocytes-derived DC in generating effector T cells specific to tumor cells.[43] More recent results demonstrated improved clinical response by DC-based Id vaccination. A commercial product is currently being tested in phase III trial. Mylovenge (APC8020) is conducted by pulsing autologous DC with the subject's Id and showed that the long-term survival in the subjects with MM who received the vaccine and underwent autologous hematopoietic stem cell transplant.[44]

An alternative DC-based vaccination approach involves the fusion of autologous DC with patient-derived tumor cells to enhance the immunogenicity of tumor antigens.[45] DC fusion cells can stimulate both helper and cytotoxic T-cell responses through the presentation of internalized and newly synthesized antigens.[46] Lenalidomide has been shown to further improve the immunogenicity of DC-MM fusion vaccines by polarizing T-cell responses into Th1 and reducing regulatory T cells and the expression of immune suppressive molecules on T cells.[47] Recently, phase II studies were undertaken in which subjects with MM were vaccinated with an autologous DC-tumor cell fusion in combination with GM-CSF administration on the day of DC vaccination following autologous stem cell transplantation (ASCT) to target minimal residual disease.[48] In the study, the second cohort of 12 subjects received a pre-transplant vaccine followed by posttransplant vaccinations. The posttransplant period was associated with reduction in general measures of cellular immunity; however, an increase in myeloma-specific CD4$^+$ and CD8$^+$ T cells was observed after ASCT and the specific effector cells were significantly expanded following posttransplant vaccination. A high proportion (78%) of MM patients achieved either a complete response or very good partial response following vaccination, thereby demonstrating the potential for a positive clinical outcome using vaccine immunotherapy to treat multiple myeloma.

In addition, whole tumor cells or tumor lysates have been used to improve the efficacy of the DC-based vaccine in subjects with MM. There have been increasing reports of alternative approaches such as DC pulsed with tumor lysates, apoptotic tumor cells,[49–51] or DC transfected with myeloma-derived RNA.[52] Apoptotic bodies were shown to be more effective than cell lysate at inducing cytotoxic T lymphocytes (CTLs) against autologous myeloma cells.[53] In addition, tumor-derived heat shock proteins (HSPs), such as HSP70 and gp96, demonstrated their immunogenic characteristics and the myeloma-derived gp96-loaded DC were used to generate tumor-specific CTLs that were able to lyse tumor cells in patients with MM in an major histocompatibility complex (MHC) class I–restricted manner.[54,55]

However, these approaches with patient-specific protocols are labor-intensive and cost-ineffective, making their general applicability challenging. To overcome this limitation, development of an off-the-shelf–based immunotherapy is necessary for treating patients more efficiently. Among several options, peptide-based vaccines offer distinct advantages over individualized vaccines with regards to safety, broader applicability, low toxicity, easy of production, and monitoring for tumor-specific immune response in patients.[56] In addition, this approach can successfully induce antitumor immune responses with the potential of epitope spreading, whereby lysed target cancer cells release new antigenic epitopes, which are then taken up, processed, and presented by antigen-presenting cells to a new repertoire of CTL, and thereby further tumor lysis.[57,58] Although there is MHC restriction in this peptide-specific vaccine approach, application of cocktails of immunogenic peptides to different HLA molecules would broaden the induction of CTL specific to tumor cells of multiple MHC classifications. Based on the recent progress on the discovery of TAA, epitopes have been identified from multiple potential antigens and evaluated for the development of vaccines by eliciting the antigen-specific CD8[+] T cell responses against MM cells. Strategies for further improvement in the efficacy of therapy, including combined use of chemotherapy drugs and molecular target-based drugs, are being proposed. Peptide vaccination in an "adjuvant setting" should be considered a promising treatment to protect against progression or relapse of malignancies with minimal residual disease.

Following are several types of TAA applied and progress made for the development of peptide-based vaccines in MM.

- X-box binding protein 1 (XBP1), a critical transcription activator in the unfolded protein response, regulates a subset of endoplasmic reticulum–resident chaperone genes essential for protein folding and maturation.[59,60] Genome-wide profiling, along with association studies and immunohistochemistry, demonstrated that XBP1 expression was induced in a variety of cancers, including hematological malignancies such as MM and solid tumors.[61–64] It has been reported that XBP1 is activated in primary mammary tumors, that its expression correlates with enhanced tumor growth, moreover, transformed cells with XBP1 deficiency were sensitized to hypoxia and underwent apoptosis, implicating XBP1 as a survival factor.[65,66] Thus, disrupting or targeting the XBP1 pathway is a rational approach for selective cancer cell killing, providing the basis for therapeutic strategies against multiple solid tumors. In MM, it is highly expressed in primary cells and cell lines, selectively induced by exposure to IL-6, and has been implicated in the proliferation of malignant plasma cells.[65,66] Based on these observations, Bae and colleagues[67] proposed the XBP1 as a unique therapeutic target antigen and identified two heteroclitic peptides, YISPWILAV and YLFPQLISV, with improved HLA-A2-binding and stability from their respective native peptides, XBP1$_{184-192}$ (NISPWILAV) and XBP1 SP$_{367-375}$ (ELFPQLISV). The XBP1 peptides-specific CTL showed distinct phenotypes and functional activities and demonstrated MM-specific and HLA-A2-restricted proliferation, interferon (IFN)-γ secretion, and/or cytotoxic activity in response to MM cell lines and primary MM cells. These data demonstrate the distinct immunogenic characteristics of unique heteroclitic XBP1 peptides, which induce MM-specific CTL.
- The CD138, also known as syndecan-1, is a transmembrane heparan sulfate–bearing proteoglycan expressed by most MM cells. CD138 is critical for the growth of tumor cells by mediating cell-cell adhesion, binding MM cells to molecules such as collagen and fibronectin in the extracellular matrix, as well as binding to growth factors and cytokines.[68,69] In patients with MM, shed syndecan-1 accumulates in the bone marrow, and soluble syndecan-1 facilitates MM tumor progression, angiogenesis, and metastasis in vivo. It has a cytoplasmic domain that is linked to cytoskeletal elements to potentiate anchorage of the cells and stabilize cell morphology, whereas their extracellular domain has up to three heparan sulfate chains that bind to numerous soluble and insoluble molecules, thus CD138 has critical roles for the growth of tumor cells.[68,69] Therefore, targeting CD138 on malignant plasma cells to

prevent or reduce high levels of syndecan-1 in the serum, an indicator of poor prognosis in MM,[70,71] may have a direct clinical benefit. A novel immunogenic HLA-A2-specific peptide, $CD138_{260-268}$ (GLVGLIFAV), identified by Bae and colleagues,[72] induces antigen-specific CTL, and the CD138 peptide-specific CTL displayed a unique immunologic phenotype, as well as HLA-A2-restricted responses and functional activities against both primary MM cells and MM cell lines expressing CD138 antigen.

- CS1 is a cell surface glycoprotein of the CD2 family, which is highly and uniformly expressed by malignant plasma cells and has restricted expression in normal tissues.[73,74] CS1 localizes to the uropods of polarized MM cells, where it mediates adhesion of MM cells to bone marrow stroma and other human MM cells.[12] CS1 expression was observed on MM cells from all subjects, including MM with high-risk and low-risk molecular profiles, and those with and without cytogenetic abnormalities, suggesting that this antigen is not restricted to any particular MM subgroup.[75] Equally important for the development of immunotherapy, CS1 expression is maintained on subjects' MM cells even after relapse of disease. Based on these findings, Bae and colleagues[76] identified a novel immunogenic HLA-A2-specific epitope, $CS1_{239-247}$ peptide (SLFVLGLFL), which is derived from the CS1 antigen and has the ability to evoke MM-specific CTL. With the findings of universal expression of these functional antigens on MM cells, the development of an immunotherapeutic strategy targeting XBP1, CD138, and CS1 antigens was proposed as a novel treatment option for MM, and the multipeptide was evaluated for its immunogenicity as a cocktail to induce the peptides-specific CTL from smoldering MM (SMM) subjects' T cells. The multipeptide-specific CTL generated from SMM subjects' T cells demonstrated dramatic phenotypic changes and effective anti-MM responses, including the upregulation of critical markers including CD69 and CD137 (4-1BB), CTL proliferation, IFN-γ production, and degranulation (CD107a) in an HLA-A2-restricted and peptide-specific manner. The results also suggest that this multipeptide cocktail has the potential to induce effective and durable memory membraneproteoglycan-CTL in SMM subjects. Therefore, these findings provide the rationale for clinical evaluation of a therapeutic vaccine to prevent or delay progression of SMM to active disease.[77] Clinical applicability of the peptides derived from these antigens is undergoing evaluation.

- Dickkopf-1 (DKK1) is a secreted protein that specifically inhibits the Wnt/[beta]-catenin signaling by interacting with the coreceptor Lrp-6.[78,79] In addition to its direct inhibitory effect of DKK1 on osteoblasts, DKK1 disrupts the Wnt3a-regulated osteoprotegerin and receptor activator of nuclear factor–kappaB ligand (RANKL) expression in osteoblasts and thus it indirectly enhances osteoclast function in MM.[80–83] Recent studies demonstrated that DKK1 in subjects with myeloma was associated with the presence of lytic bone lesions and DKK1 plays an important role in myeloma bone disease.[80] Qian and colleagues[84] identified HLA-A2-specific peptides derived from DKK1 that was capable of inducing DKK1-specific T-cell lines and clones from HLA-A2[+] normal donors and MM patients. These CTL showed peptide-specific and MM-specific responses in vitro and showed the therapeutic efficacy in vivo against established tumor cells in an HLA-A2 transgenic murine model. They detected low frequencies of DKK1 peptide-specific CD8[+] T cells in subjects with myeloma by using tetramers, peptide-specific T-cell lines, and clones generated from HLA-A2[+] blood donors or patients with myeloma. These T cells efficiently lysed peptide-pulsed but not unpulsed T2 or autologous DC, DKK1[+]/HLA-A2[+]

myeloma cell lines U266 and IM-9 as well as HLA-A2$^+$ primary myeloma cells from patients. Thus, these data show that DKK1 is a novel target for the management of myeloma patients with lytic bone disease.

- Receptor for hyaluronic acid mediated motility (RHAMM) is another immunogenic antigen that plays a critical role in tumorigenesis. It is highly expressed in hematological malignancies including MM and induces humoral and cellular immune responses.[85–87] RHAMM-R3 peptide has been identified and investigated as a vaccine in subjects with MM (Schmitt and colleagues[88] and Greiner and colleagues[89]). In their phase I trial, the RHAMM-R3 peptide (ILSLELMKL) was administered four times (300 µg or 1 mg/vaccination) subcutaneously at a biweekly interval to HLA-A2$^+$ MM subjects who were in partial remission or near complete remission after high-dose chemotherapy with melphalan and autologous stem cell transplantation. Encouraging immune monitoring results were detected: (1) an increase (>50%) in IFN-γ^+ and granzyme$^+$ spots in ELISPOT analyses, (2) an increase (>50%) in HLA-A2/R3-tetramer$^+$/CD8$^+$ T lymphocytes and with an increase (>25%) in RHAMM-R3-tetramer$^+$/CD8$^+$ T lymphocytes, and (3) CD8$^+$ T cell responsiveness. The MM patients who had a positive immune response showed an increase of CD8$^+$ tetramer$^+$/CD45RA$^+$/CCR7$^-$/CD27$^-$/CD28$^-$ effector T cells and RHAMM-R3-specific CD8$^+$ T cells. In this study, 50% (2 out of 4) subjects with MM showed a reduction of free light chain serum levels. High-dose RHAMM-R3 peptide vaccination induced positive clinical effects.
- Cancer testis antigens (CTAs) have been extensively investigated in MM for their expression and application as target antigens. DNA microarray analysis of gene expression of greater than 95% pure myeloma cells from more than 300 subjects showed that the genes of MAGE-3 and NY-ESO-1 antigens were expressed in the tumor cells, particularly from subjects with relapsed disease or abnormal cytogenetics (in 7%–20% of MGUS and newly diagnosed MM and in 40%–50% of relapsed subjects or in subjects with cytogenetic abnormalities).[90,91] In addition, the protein expression of these antigens were also demonstrated in the tumor cells of subjects with positive gene expression. The mechanisms that underlie this expression are unclear but are at least partially related to demethylation of gene promoter sequences.[92] The HLA-A1-restricted or HLA-A2-restricted MAGE-3- or NY-ESO-1-specific peptide have been identified and the tumor-specific CTL generated by the peptide were demonstrated against myeloma cells.[93,94] In addition, other antigens, such as MUC-1,[95,96] sperm protein 17 (Sp17),[97,98] and HM1.24[99,100] may also be expressed on myeloma cells, and MHC-restricted antigen-specific CTL have been generated from subjects with myeloma that were able to lyse myeloma cells. Recently, a phase I–II clinical trial has been initiated to examine the safety and efficacy of Sp17-pulsed DC vaccination in subjects with myeloma.[98] Anderson and colleagues[101] identified peptides derived from MAGE-C1 (CT-7), which is the most commonly expressed CTA found in MM. The CT-7-specific CTL recognizing two peptides targeted both MM cells as well as CT-7 gene-transduced tumor cells. They demonstrated that these epitopes are promising targets for developing an immunotherapy against myeloma or other CT-7$^+$ malignancies. Clinical applicability of the peptides derived from the cancer testis antigens are undergoing evaluation.

The current clinical trials using active-specific immunotherapy are shown in **Table 2** to treat the patients with multiple myeloma.

Table 2
Active-specific immunotherapy in clinical trials for multiple myeloma

Type of Vaccine, Tumor-Associated Antigen	Patient Number, Combination	Results, Specific Response	Clinical Trial, Done	Reference
DC vaccine, Idiotype				
Id + DC	27, following ASCT	6/27 CR, 2/27 PR, 19/27 SD, increase OS	II	Lacy et al,[128] 2009
Id + DC, Id + KLH	26, following ASCT	4/26 w. specific T cell proliferation	II	Liso et al,[129] 2006
Id + DC, Id + GM-CSF	11	4/10 T cell, 3/10 humoral	I	Titzer et al,[130] 2000
Id + DC, Id + KLH	12, following ASCT	1/12 CD8 T cell response	I	Reichardt et al,[131] 2003
Id + DC	15, w. previous ASCT	8/15 T cell response	I	Abdalla et al,[132] 2007
DC vaccine, Fusion				
DC/myeloma fusion cells	12, following ASCT	T cells	II	Rosenblatt et al,[133] 2013
Peptide vaccine, Target				
WT1-specific	1, Montanide	CD8+ T cells	I	Tsuboi et al,[134] 2007
RHAMM-R3-specific	3, Montanide	CD8+ T cells	I	Greiner et al,[135] 2010
XBP1, CD138, CS1-specific	22 Smoldering myeloma patients, Montanide, Hiltonol®, with/without Lenalidomide	CD8+ T cells	I, In-progress	N/A

FUTURE DIRECTIONS

After several years of disappointing results, immunotherapy is now emerging as a promising therapeutic approach for different types of cancer. Various immunotherapeutic strategies including antibodies, vaccines, and checkpoint inhibitors are currently under evaluation in multiple clinical trials. The studies on MM microenvironment unveiled a complex network driven by MM plasma cells, which progressively lead to functional impairment of the host immune system and immunotherapeutic approach. Novel immune targets, coupled with new combination approaches to overcome immune suppression, and biomarkers for patient selection are subjects of ongoing studies. These areas are rapidly progressing and will most likely change the landscape of therapy in MM in the near future.

REFERENCES

1. Kumar SK, Dispenzieri A, Lacy MQ, et al. Continued improvement in survival in multiple myeloma: changes in early mortality and outcomes in older patients. Leukemia 2014;28:1122–8.

2. Laubach JP, Richardson PG, Anderson KC. The evolution and impact of therapy in multiple myeloma. Med Oncol 2010;27(Suppl 1):S1–6.
3. Yi Q. Novel immunotherapies. Cancer J 2009;15:502–10.
4. Barlogie B, Jagannath S, Desikan KR, et al. Total therapy with tandem transplants for newly diagnosed multiple myeloma. Blood 1999;93:55–65.
5. Rapoport AP, Aqui NA, Stadtmauer EA, et al. Combination immunotherapy after ASCT for multiple myeloma using MAGE-A3/Poly-ICLC immunizations followed by adoptive transfer of vaccine-primed and costimulated autologous T cells. Clin Cancer Res 2014;20:1355–65.
6. Garcia-Marquez MA, Shimabukuro-Vornhagen A, Theurich S, et al. Vaccination with dendritic cell-tumor fusion cells in multiple myeloma patients: a promising strategy? Immunotherapy 2013;5:1039–42.
7. Bae J, Smith R, Daley J, et al. Myeloma-specific multiple peptides able to generate cytotoxic T lymphocytes: a potential therapeutic application in multiple myeloma and other plasma cell disorders. Clin Cancer Res 2012;18:4850–60.
8. Ocio EM, Richardson PG, Rajkumar SV, et al. New drugs and novel mechanisms of action in multiple myeloma in 2013: a report from the International Myeloma Working Group (IMWG). Leukemia 2014;28:525–42.
9. van de Donk NW, Kamps S, Mutis T, et al. Monoclonal antibody-based therapy as a new treatment strategy in multiple myeloma. Leukemia 2012;26:199–213.
10. Richardson PG, Lonial S, Jakubowiak AJ, et al. Monoclonal antibodies in the treatment of multiple myeloma. Br J Haematol 2011;154:745–54.
11. Rossi M, Botta C, Correale P, et al. Immunologic microenvironment and personalized treatment in multiple myeloma. Expert Opin Biol Ther 2013;13(Suppl 1): S83–93.
12. Tai YT, Dillon M, Song W, et al. Anti-CS1 humanized monoclonal antibody Hu-Luc63 inhibits myeloma cell adhesion and induces antibody-dependent cellular cytotoxicity in the bone marrow milieu. Blood 2008;112:1329–37.
13. Zonder JA, Mohrbacher AF, Singhal S, et al. A phase 1, multicenter, open-label, dose escalation study of elotuzumab in patients with advanced multiple myeloma. Blood 2012;120:552–9.
14. Lonial S, Vij R, Harousseau JL, et al. Elotuzumab in combination with lenalidomide and low-dose dexamethasone in relapsed or refractory multiple myeloma. J Clin Oncol 2012;30:1953–9.
15. Richardson PG, Jagannath S, Moreau P, et al. A phase 2 study of elotuzumab (Elo) in combination with lenalidomide and low-dose dexamethasone (Ld) in patients (pts) with relapsed/refractory multiple myeloma (R/R MM): updated results. ASH Ann Meet Abstr 2012;120:202.
16. Plesner T, Lokhorst H, Gimsing P, et al. Daratumumab, a CD38 monoclonal antibody in patients with multiple myeloma—data from a dose-escalation phase I/II study. ASH Ann Meet Abstr 2012;120:73.
17. Lokhorst HM, Plesner T, Gimsing P, et al. Phase I/II dose-escalation study of daratumumab in patients with relapsed or refractory multiple myeloma. ASCO Meet Abstr 2013;31(15 Suppl):8512.
18. Heffner LT, Jagannath S, Zimmerman TM, et al. BT062, an antibody-drug conjugate directed against CD138, given weekly for 3 weeks in each 4 week cycle: safety and further evidence of clinical activity. ASH Ann Meet Abstr 2012; 120:4042.
19. Jagannath S, Chanan-Khan A, Heffner LT, et al. BT062, an antibody-drug conjugate directed against CD138, Shows clinical activity in patients with relapsed or relapsed/refractory multiple myeloma. ASH Ann Meet Abstr 2011;118:305.

20. Bensinger W, Maziarz RT, Jagannath S, et al. A phase 1 study of lucatumumab, a fully human anti-CD40 antagonist monoclonal antibody administered intravenously to patients with relapsed or refractory multiple myeloma. Br J Haematol 2012;159:58–66.

21. Hussein M, Berenson JR, Niesvizky R, et al. A phase I multidose study of dacetuzumab (SGN-40; humanized anti-CD40 monoclonal antibody) in patients with multiple myeloma. Haematologica 2010;95:845–8.

22. Rosenblatt J, Glotzbecker B, Mills H, et al. PD-1 blockade by CT-011, anti-PD-1 antibody, enhances ex vivo T-cell responses to autologous dendritic cell/myeloma fusion vaccine. J Immunother 2011;34:409–18.

23. Benson DM Jr, Bakan CE, Mishra A, et al. The PD-1/PD-L1 axis modulates the natural killer cell versus multiple myeloma effect: a therapeutic target for CT-011, a novel monoclonal anti-PD-1 antibody. Blood 2010;116:2286–94.

24. White D, Kassim A, Bhaskar B, et al. Results from AMBER, a randomized phase 2 study of bevacizumab and bortezomib versus bortezomib in relapsed or refractory multiple myeloma. Cancer 2013;119:339–47.

25. Voorhees PM, Manges RF, Sonneveld P, et al. A phase 2 multicenter study of siltuximab, an anti-IL-6 monoclonal antibody, in patients with relapsed or refractory multiple myeloma. ASH Ann Meet Abstr 2011;118:3971.

26. Rossi JF, Manges RF, Sutherland HJ, et al. Preliminary results of CNTO 328, an anti-interleukin-6 monoclonal antibody, in combination with bortezomib in the treatment of relapsed or refractory multiple myeloma. ASH Ann Meet Abstr 2008;112:867.

27. Benson DM Jr, Hofmeister CC, Padmanabhan S, et al. A phase I trial of the anti-KIR antibody IPH2101 in patients with relapsed/refractory multiple myeloma. Blood 2012;120:4324–33.

28. Slezak SL, Worschech A, Wang E, et al. Analysis of vaccine-induced T cells in humans with cancer. Adv Exp Med Biol 2010;684:178–88.

29. Westers TM, van den Ancker W, Bontkes HJ, et al. Chronic myeloid leukemia lysate-loaded dendritic cells induce T-cell responses towards leukemia progenitor cells. Immunotherapy 2011;3:569–76.

30. Tricot G, Jagannath S, Vesole DH, et al. Hematopoietic stem cell transplants for multiple myeloma. Leuk Lymphoma 1996;22:25–36.

31. Verdonck LF, Lokhorst HM, Dekker AW, et al. Graft-versus-myeloma effect in two cases. Lancet 1996;347:800–1.

32. King CA, Spellerberg MB, Zhu D, et al. DNA vaccines with single-chain Fv fused to fragment C of tetanus toxin induce protective immunity against lymphoma and myeloma [see comment]. Nat Med 1998;4:1281–6.

33. Campbell MJ, Esserman L, Byars NE, et al. Idiotype vaccination against murine B cell lymphoma. Humoral and cellular requirements for the full expression of antitumor immunity. J Immunol 1990;145:1029–36.

34. Szea DM, Brown RD, Yang S, et al. Prediction of high affinity class I-restricted multiple myeloma idiotype peptide epitopes. Leuk Lymphoma 2003;44:1557–68.

35. Hansson L, Rabbani H, Fagerberg J, et al. T-cell epitopes within the complementarity-determining and framework regions of the tumor-derived immunoglobulin heavy chain in multiple myeloma. Blood 2003;101:4930–6.

36. Romagnani S. Human TH1 and TH2 subsets: regulation of differentiation and role in protection and immunopathology. Int Arch Allergy Immunol 1992;98:279–85.

37. Yi Q, Osterborg A, Bergenbrant S, et al. Idiotype-reactive T-cell subsets and tumor load in monoclonal gammopathies. Blood 1995;86:3043–9.

38. Röllig C, Schmidt C, Bornhäuser M, et al. Induction of cellular immune responses in patients with stage-I multiple myeloma after vaccination with autologous idiotype-pulsed dendritic cells. J Immunother 2011;34(1):100–6.

39. Yi Q, Szmania S, Freeman J, et al. Optimizing dendritic cell-based immunotherapy in multiple myeloma: intranodal injections of idiotype-pulsed CD40 ligand-matured vaccines led to induction of type-1 and cytotoxic T-cell immune responses in patients. Br J Haematol 2010;150(5):554–64.

40. Rasmussen T, Hansson L, Osterborg A, et al. Idiotype vaccination in multiple myeloma induced a reduction of circulating clonal tumor B cells. Blood 2003; 101:4607–10.

41. Massaia M, Borrione P, Battaglio S, et al. Idiotype vaccination in human myeloma: generation of tumor-specific immune responses after high-dose chemotherapy. Blood 1999;94:673–83.

42. Titzer S, Christensen O, Manzke O, et al. Vaccination of multiple myeloma patients with idiotype-pulsed dendritic cells: immunological and clinical aspects. Br J Haematol 2000;108:805–16.

43. Romano E, Rossi M, Ratzinger G, et al. Peptide-loaded Langerhans cells, despite increased IL15 secretion and T-cell activation in vitro, elicit antitumor T-cell responses comparable to peptide-loaded monocyte-derived dendritic cells in vivo. Clin Cancer Res 2011;17:1984–97.

44. Lacy MQ, Mandrekar S, Dispenzieri A, et al. Idiotype pulsed antigen presenting cells following autologous transplantation for multiple myeloma may be associated with prolonged survival. Am J Hematol 2009;84(12):799–802.

45. Gong J, Koido S, Chen D, et al. Immunization against murine multiple myeloma with fusions of dendritic and plasmacytoma cells is potentiated by interleukin 12. Blood 2002;99:2512–7.

46. Vasir B, Borges V, Wu Z, et al. Fusion of dendritic cells with multiple myeloma cells results in maturation and enhanced antigen presentation. Br J Haematol 2005;129(5):687–700.

47. Luptakova K, Rosenblatt J, Glotzbecker B, et al. Lenalidomide enhances antimyeloma cellular immunity. Cancer Immunol Immunother 2013;62:39–49.

48. Rosenblatt J, Avivi I, Vasir B, et al. Vaccination with dendritic cell/tumor fusions following autologous stem cell transplant induces immunologic and clinical responses in multiple myeloma patients. Clin Cancer Res 2013;19:3640–8.

49. Yang DH, Kim MH, Hong CY, et al. Alpha-type 1-polarized dendritic cells loaded with apoptotic allogeneic myeloma cell line induce strong CTL responses against autologous myeloma cells. Ann Hematol 2010;89(8):795–801.

50. Lee JJ, Choi BH, Kang HK, et al. Induction of multiple myeloma-specific cytotoxic T lymphocyte stimulation by dendritic cell pulsing with purified and optimized myeloma cell lysates. Leuk Lymphoma 2007;48(10):2022–31.

51. Wen YJ, Min R, Tricot G, et al. Tumor lysate-specific cytotoxic T lymphocytes in multiple myeloma: promising effector cells for immunotherapy. Blood 2002; 99(9):3280–5.

52. Milazzo C, Reichardt VL, Müller MR, et al. Induction of myeloma-specific cytotoxic T cells using dendritic cells transfected with tumor-derived RNA. Blood 2003;101(3):977–82.

53. Hayashi T, Hideshima T, Akiyama M, et al. Ex vivo induction of multiple myeloma-specific cytotoxic T lymphocytes. Blood 2003;102(4):1435–42.

54. Qian J, Hong S, Wang S, et al. Myeloma cell line-derived, pooled heat shock proteins as a universal vaccine for immunotherapy of multiple myeloma. Blood 2009;114(18):3880–9.

55. Qian J, Wang S, Yang J, et al. Targeting heat shock proteins for immunotherapy in multiple myeloma: generation of myeloma-specific CTL using dendritic cells pulsed with tumor-derived gp96. Clin Cancer Res 2005;11(24):8808–15.

56. Dudek NL, Perlmutter P, Aguilar MI, et al. Epitope discovery and their use in peptide based vaccines. Curr Pharm Des 2010;16:3149–57.

57. Disis ML, Bernhard H, Jaffee EM. Use of tumour-responsive T cells as cancer treatment. Lancet 2009;373:673–83.

58. Parvanova I, Rettig L, Knuth A, et al. The form of NY-ESO-1 antigen has an impact on the clinical efficacy of anti-tumor vaccination. Vaccine 2011;29: 3832–6.

59. Jagannath S, Kyle RA, Palumbo A, et al. The current status and future of multiple myeloma in the clinic. Clin Lymphoma Myeloma Leuk 2010;10:28–43.

60. Bensinger WI. Role of autologous and allogeneic stem cell transplantation in myeloma. Leukemia 2009;23:442–8.

61. Zeiser R, Finke J. Allogeneic haematopoietic cell transplantation for multiple myeloma: reducing transplant-related mortality while harnessing the graft-versus-myeloma effect. Eur J Cancer 2006;42:1601–11.

62. Abdalla AO, Kokhaei P, Hansson L, et al. Idiotype vaccination in patients with myeloma reduced circulating myeloma cells (CMC). Ann Oncol 2008;19: 1172–9.

63. Lee K, Tirasophon W, Shen X, et al. IRE1-mediated unconventional mRNA splicing and S2P-mediated ATF6 cleavage merge to regulate XBP1 in signaling the unfolded protein response. Genes Dev 2002;16:452–66.

64. Mori K. Frame switch splicing and regulated intramembrane proteolysis: key words to understand the unfolded protein response. Traffic 2003;4:519–28.

65. Bagratuni T, Wu P, Gonzalez de Castro D, et al. XBP1s levels are implicated in the biology and outcome of myeloma mediating different clinical outcomes to thalidomide-based treatments. Blood 2010;116:250–3.

66. Patterson J, Palombella VJ, Fritz C, et al. IPI-504, a novel and soluble HSP-90 inhibitor, blocks the unfolded protein response in multiple myeloma cells. Cancer Chemother Pharmacol 2008;61:923–32.

67. Bae J, Carrasco R, Lee AH, et al. Identification of novel myeloma-specific XBP1 peptides able to generate cytotoxic T lymphocytes: a potential therapeutic application in multiple myeloma. Leukemia 2011;25(10):1610–9.

68. Bharti AC, Shishodia S, Reuben JM, et al. Nuclear factor-kappaB and STAT3 are constitutively active in CD138+ cells derived from multiple myeloma patients, and suppression of these transcription factors leads to apoptosis. Blood 2004;103:3175–84.

69. Wolowiec D, Dybko J, Wrobel T, et al. Circulating sCD138 and some angiogenesis-involved cytokines help to anticipate the disease progression of early-stage B-cell chronic lymphocytic leukemia. Mediators Inflamm 2006;2006:42394–9.

70. Sanderson RD, Yang Y. Syndecan-1: a dynamic regulator of the myeloma microenvironment. Clin Exp Metastasis 2008;25:149–59.

71. Yang Y, Yaccoby S, Liu W, et al. Soluble syndecan-1 promotes growth of myeloma tumors in vivo. Blood 2002;100:610–7.

72. Bae J, Tai YT, Anderson KC, et al. Novel epitope evoking CD138 antigen-specific cytotoxic T lymphocytes targeting multiple myeloma and other plasma cell disorders. Br J Haematol 2011;155(3):349–61.

73. van Rhee F, Szmania SM, Dillon M, et al. Combinatorial efficacy of anti-CS1 monoclonal antibody elotuzumab (HuLuc63) and bortezomib against multiple myeloma. Mol Cancer Ther 2009;8:2616–24.

74. Hsi ED, Steinle R, Balasa B, et al. CS1, a potential new therapeutic antibody target for the treatment of multiple myeloma. Clin Cancer Res 2008;14:2775–84.

75. Zhan F, Sawyer J, Tricot G. The role of cytogenetics in myeloma. Leukemia 2006; 20:1484–6.

76. Bae J, Song W, Smith R, et al. A novel immunogenic CS1-specific peptide inducing antigen-specific cytotoxic T lymphocytes targeting multiple myeloma. Br J Haematol 2012;157:687–701.

77. Bae J, Voskertchian A, Prabhala R, et al. A multiepitope of XBP1, CD138 and CS1 peptides induces myeloma-specific cytotoxic T lymphocytes in T cells of smoldering myeloma patients. Leukemia 2014. http://dx.doi.org/10.1038/leu. 2014.159.

78. Zorn AM. Wnt signalling: antagonistic Dickkopfs. Curr Biol 2001;11:R592–5.

79. Mao B, Wu W, Li Y, et al. LDL-receptor-related protein 6 is a receptor for Dickkopf proteins. Nature 2001;411:321–5.

80. Tian E, Zhan F, Walker R, et al. The role of the Wnt-signaling antagonist DKK1 in the development of osteolytic lesions in multiple myeloma. N Engl J Med 2003; 349:2483–94.

81. Krupnik VE, Sharp JD, Jiang C, et al. Functional and structural diversity of the human Dickkopf gene family. Gene 1999;238:301–13.

82. Kohn MJ, Kaneko KJ, DePamphilis ML. DkkL1 (Soggy), a Dickkopf family member, localizes to the acrosome during mammalian spermatogenesis. Mol Reprod Dev 2005;71:516–22.

83. Hall CL, Bafico A, Dai J, et al. Prostate cancer cells promote osteoblastic bone metastases through Wnts. Cancer Res 2005;65:7554–60.

84. Qian J, Xie J, Hong S, et al. Dickkopf-1 (DKK1) is a widely expressed and potent tumor-associated antigen in multiple myeloma. Blood 2007;110:1587–94.

85. Giannopoulos K, Własiuk P, Dmoszyńska A, et al. Peptide vaccination induces profound changes in the immune system in patients with B-cell chronic lymphocytic leukemia. Folia Histochem Cytobiol 2001;49:161–7.

86. Giannopoulos K, Mertens D, Bühler A, et al. The candidate immunotherapeutical target, the receptor for hyaluronic acid-mediated motility, is associated with proliferation and shows prognostic value in B-cell chronic lymphocytic leukemia. Leukemia 2009;23:519–27.

87. Greiner J, Schmitt M, Li L, et al. Expression of tumor-associated antigens in acute myeloid leukemia: Implications for specific immunotherapeutic approaches. Blood 2006;108:4109–17.

88. Schmitt M, Schmitt A, Rojewski MT, et al. RHAMM-R3 peptide vaccination in patients with acute myeloid leukemia, myelodysplastic syndrome, and multiple myeloma elicits immunologic and clinical responses. Blood 2008;111: 1357–65.

89. Greiner J, Schmitt A, Giannopoulos K, et al. High-dose RHAMM-R3 peptide vaccination for patients with acute myeloid leukemia, myelodysplastic syndrome and multiple myeloma. Haematologica 2010;95:1191–7.

90. Pellat-Deceunynck C, Mellerin MP, Labarriere N, et al. The cancer germ-line genes MAGE-1, MAGE-3 and PRAME are commonly expressed by human myeloma cells. Eur J Immunol 2000;30:803–9.

91. Gupta SK, Shaughnessy J, Droojenbroeck JV, et al. NY-ESO-1 RNA and protein expression in multiple myeloma is highest in aggressive myeloma and is correlated with chromosomal abnormalities. Blood 2002;100:401a.

92. Simpson AJ, Caballero OL, Jungbluth A, et al. Cancer/testis antigens, gametogenesis and cancer. Nat Rev Cancer 2005;5:615–25.

93. Szmania SM, Bennett G, Batchu RB, et al. Dendritic cells pulsed with NY-ESO-1 and MAGE-3 peptide stimulate myeloma cytotoxic T lymphocytes. Blood 2002; 100:399a.
94. van Rhee F, Szmania SM, Zhan F, et al. NY-ESO-1 is highly expressed in poor-prognosis multiple myeloma and induces spontaneous humoral and cellular immune responses. Blood 2005;105:3939–44.
95. Akagi J, Nakagawa K, Egami H, et al. Induction of HLA-unrestricted and HLA-class-II restricted cytotoxic T lymphocytes against MUC-1 from patients with colorectal carcinomas using recombinant MUC-1 vaccinia virus. Cancer Immunol Immunother 1998;47:21–31.
96. Moore A, Medarova Z, Potthast A, et al. In vivo targeting of underglycosylated MUC-1 tumor antigen using a multimodal imaging probe. Cancer Res 2004; 64:1821–7.
97. Lim SH, Wang Z, Chiriva-Internati M, et al. Sperm protein 17 is a novel cancer-testis antigen in multiple myeloma. Blood 2001;97:1508–10.
98. Lim SH, Chiriva-Internati M, Wang Z, et al. Sperm protein 17 (Sp17) as a tumor vaccine for multiple myeloma. Blood 2002;100:673a.
99. Treon SP, Raje N, Anderson KC. Immunotherapeutic strategies for the treatment of plasma cell malignancies. Semin Oncol 2000;27:598–613.
100. Ohtomo T, Sugamata Y, Ozaki Y, et al. Molecular cloning and characterization of a surface antigen preferentially overexpressed on multiple myeloma cells. Biochem Biophys Res Commun 1999;258:583–91.
101. Anderson LD Jr, Cook DR, Yamamoto TN, et al. Identification of MAGE-C1 (CT-7) epitopes for T-cell therapy of multiple myeloma. Cancer Immunol Immunother 2011;60:985–97.
102. Descamps G, Gomez-Bougie P, Venot C, et al. A humanised anti-IGF-1R monoclonal antibody (AVE1642) enhances Bortezomib-induced apoptosis in myeloma cells lacking CD45. Br J Cancer 2009;100(2):366–9.
103. Lacy MQ, Alsina M, Fonseca R, et al. Phase I, pharmacokinetic and pharmacodynamic study of the anti-insulinlike growth factor type 1 Receptor monoclonal antibody CP-751,871 in patients with multiple myeloma. J Clin Oncol 2008; 26(19):3196–203.
104. Carlo-Stella C, Guidetti A, Di Nicola M, et al. IFN-gamma enhances the antimyeloma activity of the fully human anti-human leukocyte antigen-DR monoclonal antibody 1D09C3. Cancer Res 2007;67(7):3269–75.
105. Yu C, Liu Q, Gao W, et al. Monoclonal antibodies directed against chicken β2-microglobulin developed with a synthesized peptide. Monoclon Antib Immunodiagn Immunother 2013;32(3):205–10.
106. Cao Y, Lan Y, Qian J, et al. Targeting cell surface b2-microglobulin by pentameric IgM antibodies. Br J Haematol 2011;154(1):111–21.
107. Tai YT, Mayes PA, Acharya C, et al. Novel anti-B-cell maturation antigen antibody-drug conjugate (GSK2857916) selectively induces killing of multiple myeloma. Blood 2014;123(20):3128–38.
108. Ryan MC, Hering M, Peckham D, et al. Antibody targeting of B-cell maturation antigen on malignant plasma cells. Mol Cancer Ther 2007;6(11):3009–18.
109. Lyu MA, Cheung LH, Hittelman WN, et al. The rGel/BLyS fusion toxin specifically targets malignant B cells expressing the BLyS receptors BAFF-R, TACI, and BCMA. Mol Cancer Ther 2007;6(2):460–70.
110. Sekimoto E, Ozaki S, Ohshima T, et al. A single-chain Fv diabody against human leukocyte antigen-A molecules specifically induces myeloma cell death in the bone marrow environment. Cancer Res 2007;67(3):1184–92.

111. Rossi EA, Rossi DL, Stein R, et al. A bispecific antibody-IFNalpha2b immunocy-tokine targeting CD20 and HLA-DR is highly toxic to human lymphoma and multiple myeloma cells. Cancer Res 2010;70(19):7600–9.

112. Amano J, Masuyama N, Hirota Y, et al. Antigen-dependent internalization is related to rapid elimination from plasma of humanized anti-HM1.24 monoclonal antibody. Drug Metab Dispos 2010;38(12):2339–46.

113. Ozaki S, Kosaka M, Wakahara Y, et al. Humanized anti-HM1.24 antibody mediates myeloma cell cytotoxicity that is enhanced by cytokine stimulation of effector cells. Blood 1999;93(11):3922–30.

114. Deckert J, Wetzel MC, Bartle LM, et al. SAR650984, a novel humanized CD38-targeting antibody, demonstrates potent anti-tumor activity in models ofmultiple myeloma and other CD38+ hematologic malignancies. Clin Cancer Res 2014. pii:clincanres.0695.2014.

115. McEarchern JA, Smith LM, McDonagh CF, et al. Preclinical characterization of SGN-70, a humanized antibody directed against CD70. Clin Cancer Res 2008;14(23):7763–72.

116. Chérel M, Gouard S, Gaschet J, et al. 213Bi radioimmunotherapy with an anti-mCD138 monoclonal antibody in a murine model of multiple myeloma. J Nucl Med 2013;54(9):1597–604.

117. Tassone P, Goldmacher VS, Neri P, et al. Cytotoxic activity of the maytansinoid immunoconjugate B-B4-DM1 against CD138+ multiple myeloma cells. Blood 2004;104(12):3688–96.

118. Kamath AV, Lu D, Gupta P, et al. Preclinical pharmacokinetics of MFGR1877A, a human monoclonal antibody to FGFR3, and prediction of its efficacious clinical dose for the treatment of t(4;14)-positive multiple myeloma. Cancer Chemother Pharmacol 2012;69(4):1071–8.

119. Trudel S, Stewart AK, Rom E, et al. The inhibitory anti-FGFR3 antibody, PRO-001, is cytotoxic to t(4;14) multiple myeloma cells. Blood 2006;107(10):4039–46.

120. Sainz IM, Isordia-Salas I, Espinola RG, et al. Multiple myeloma in a murine syngeneic model:modulation of growth and angiogenesis by a monoclonal antibody to kininogen. Cancer Immunol Immunother 2006;55(7):797–807.

121. Veitonmäki N, Hansson M, Zhan F, et al. A human ICAM-1 antibody isolated by a function-first approach has potent macrophage-dependent antimyeloma activity in vivo. Cancer Cell 2013;23(4):502–15.

122. Smallshaw JE, Coleman E, Spiridon C, et al. The generation and anti-myeloma activity of a chimeric anti-CD54 antibody, cUV3. J Immunother 2004;27(6):419–24.

123. Coleman EJ, Brooks KJ, Smallshaw JE, et al. The Fc portion of UV3, an anti-CD54 monoclonal antibody, is critical for its antitumor activity in SCID mice with human multiple myeloma or lymphoma cell lines. J Immunother 2006;29(5):489–98.

124. Fulciniti M, Hideshima T, Vermot-Desroches C, et al. A high-affinity fully human anti-IL-6 mAb, 1339, for the treatment of multiple myeloma. Clin Cancer Res 2009;15(23):7144–52.

125. Yoshio-Hoshino N, Adachi Y, Aoki C, et al. Establishment of a new interleukin-6 (IL-6) receptor inhibitor applicable to the gene therapy for IL-6-dependent tumor. Cancer Res 2007;67(3):871–5.

126. Yaccoby S, Pennisi A, Li X, et al. Atacicept (TACI-Ig) inhibits growth of TACI(high) primary myeloma cells in SCID-hu mice and in coculture with osteoclasts. Leukemia 2008;22(2):406–13.

127. Menoret E, Gomez-Bougie P, Geffroy-Luseau A, et al. Mcl-1L cleavage is involved in TRAIL-R1- and TRAIL-R2-mediated apoptosis induced by HGS-ETR1 and HGS-ETR2 human mAbs in myeloma cells. Blood 2006;108(4): 1346–52.
128. Lacy MQ, Mandrekar S, Dispenzieri A, et al. Idiotype-pulsed antigen-presenting cells following autologous transplantation for multiple myeloma may be associated with prolonged survival. Am J Hematol 2009;84(12):799–802.
129. Liso A, Stockerl-Goldstein KE, Auffermann-Gretzinger S, et al. Idiotype vaccination using dendritic cells after autologous peripheral blood progenitor cell transplantation for multiple myeloma. Biol Blood Marrow Transplant 2000;6(6):621–7.
130. Titzer S, Christensen O, Manzke O, et al. Vaccination of multiple myeloma patients with idiotype-pulsed dendritic cells: immunological and clinical aspects. Br J Haematol 2000;108(4):805–16.
131. Reichardt VL, Milazzo C, Brugger W, et al. Idiotype vaccination of multiple myeloma patients using monocyte-derived dendritic cells. Haematologica 2003;88(10):1139–49.
132. Abdalla AO, Hansson L, Eriksson I, et al. Long-term effects of idiotype vaccination on the specific T-cell response in peripheral blood and bone marrow of multiple myeloma patients. Eur J Haematol 2007;79(5):371–81.
133. Rosenblatt J, Avivi I, Vasir B, et al. Vaccination with dendritic cell/tumor fusions following autologous stem cell transplant induces immunologic and clinical responses in multiple myeloma patients. Clin Cancer Res 2013;19(13):3640–8.
134. Tsuboi A, Oka Y, Nakajima H, et al. Wilms tumor gene WT1 peptide-based immunotherapy induced a minimal response in a patient with advanced therapy-resistant multiple myeloma. Int J Hematol 2007;86(5):414–7.
135. Greiner J, Schmitt A, Giannopoulos K, et al. High-dose RHAMM-R3 peptide vaccination for patients with acute myeloid leukemia, myelodysplastic syndrome and multiple myeloma. Haematologica 2010;95(7):1191–7.

Waldenström Macroglobulinemia

 CrossMark

Steven P. Treon, MD, MA, PhD[a],*, Zachary R. Hunter, PhD[a], Jorge J. Castillo, MD[a], Giampaolo Merlini, MD[b]

KEYWORDS

- Waldenström macroglobulinemia • Lymphoproliferative disorder • MYD88 L265P
- CXCR4 WHIM mutations • Morbidity • Treatment options

KEY POINTS

- Waldenström macroglobulinemia (WM) is an IgM-secreting B-cell lymphoproliferative disorder, with strong familial predisposition.
- Clinical manifestations of disease are related to both tumor cell infiltration and paraprotein production.
- Current treatment options include monoclonal antibodies, alkylating agents, nucleoside analogs, proteasome inhibitors, immunomodulatory drugs, and signal inhibitors.
- Both short- and long-term toxicities should be weighed in treatment decisions with use of these agents.
- Elucidation of the signaling pathways involved in WM are helping to advance targeted therapeutics for WM and include efforts directed at MYD88 and CXCR4 signaling.

INTRODUCTION

WM is a distinct clinicopathologic entity resulting from the accumulation, predominantly in the bone marrow, of clonally related lymphocytes, lymphoplasmacytic cells, and plasma cells that secrete a monoclonal IgM protein.[1] This condition is considered to correspond to the lymphoplasmacytic lymphoma (LPL) as defined by the World Health Organization classification system.[2] Most cases of LPL are WM, with less than 5% of cases made up of IgA, IgG, and nonsecreting LPL.

EPIDEMIOLOGY

WM is an uncommon disease, with a reported age-adjusted incidence rate of 3.4 per million among men and 1.7 per million among women in the United States, and a

[a] Bing Center for Waldenström's Macroglobulinemia, Dana-Farber Cancer Institute, Harvard Medical School, 450 Brookline Avenue, Boston, MA 02215, USA; [b] Department of Molecular Medicine, Amyloidosis Research and Treatment Center, University Hospital Policlinico San Matteo, Viale C. Golgi, 19, Pavia 27100, Italy
* Corresponding author.
E-mail address: steven_treon@dfci.harvard.edu

Hematol Oncol Clin N Am 28 (2014) 945–970
http://dx.doi.org/10.1016/j.hoc.2014.06.003
0889-8588/14/$ – see front matter © 2014 Elsevier Inc. All rights reserved.
hemonc.theclinics.com

geometric increase with age.[3] The incidence rate for WM is higher among whites, with African descendants representing only 5% of all patients. The incidence of WM may be higher for individuals of Ashkenazi Jewish descent.[4] Genetic factors seem important to the pathogenesis of WM. A common predisposition for WM with other malignancies has been raised,[4,5] with numerous reports of familiar clustering of individuals with WM alone and with other B-cell lymphoproliferative diseases.[6–10] In a large single-center experience, 26% of 924 consecutive patients with WM had a first- or second-degree relative with either WM or another B-cell disorder.[5]

BIOLOGY
Cytogenetics

Chromosome 6q deletions encompassing 6q21-25 have been observed in up to half of WM patients and at a comparable frequency among patients with and without a familial history.[7,11–13] The presence of 6q deletions has been suggested to discern patients with WM from those with IgM monoclonal gammopathy of unknown significance (MGUS) and to have potential prognostic significance, including impact on progression-free survival (PFS) after treatment response, although other investigators have reported no prognostic significance to the presence of 6q deletions in WM.[11,13,14] Other abnormalities by cytogenetic or fluorescence in situ hybridization analyses include deletions in 13q14, TP53, and ATM, and trisomy 4, 12, and 18.[14,15] IgH rearrangements are uncommon in WM and may be helpful in discerning cases of WM from IgM myeloma, wherein IgH switch region rearrangements are a prominent feature.[16]

Mutation in MYD88

A highly recurrent somatic mutation (MYD88 L265P) was first identified in WM patients by paired tumor/normal whole-genome sequencing and subsequently confirmed by multiple groups using Sanger sequencing and allele-specific (AS)–polymerase chain reaction (PCR) assays.[17] MYD88 L265P is expressed in 90% to 100% of WM cases when more sensitive AS-PCR has been used using both CD19 sorted and unsorted bone marrow cells.[18–22] By comparison, MYD88 L265P was absent in myeloma samples, including IgM myeloma, and was expressed in a small subset (6.5%) of marginal zone lymphoma patients, who surprisingly had many WM-related features.[18] By PCR assays, 50% to 80% of IgM MGUS patients also express MYD88 L265P, and expression of this mutation was associated with increased risk of malignant progression.[18,19,23] The presence of MYD88 L265P in IgM MGUS patient suggests that this somatic mutation is likely an early oncogenic driver and other mutations or copy number alterations that affect critical regulatory genes are likely to play a role in disease progression to WM.[24]

The role of MYD88 L265P in supporting growth and survival signaling in WM cells has been addressed in several studies (**Fig. 1**). Knockdown of MYD88 decreased survival of MYD88 L265P expressing WM cells, whereas survival was more enhanced by knock-in of MYD88 L265P versus wild-type MYD88.[25] The discovery of a mutation in MYD88 is of significance given its role as an adaptor molecule in Toll-like receptor (TLR) and interleukin 1 receptor (IL-1R) signaling.[26] All TLRs except TLR3 use MYD88 to facilitate their signaling. After TLR or IL-1R stimulation, MYD88 is recruited to the activated receptor complex as a homodimer, which then complexes with IRAK4 and activates IRAK1 and IRAK2.[27–29] Tumor necrosis factor receptor–associated factor 6 is then activated by IRAK1, leading to nuclear factor κB (NF-κB) activation via IκBα phosphorylation.[30] Use of inhibitors of MYD88 pathway led to decreased

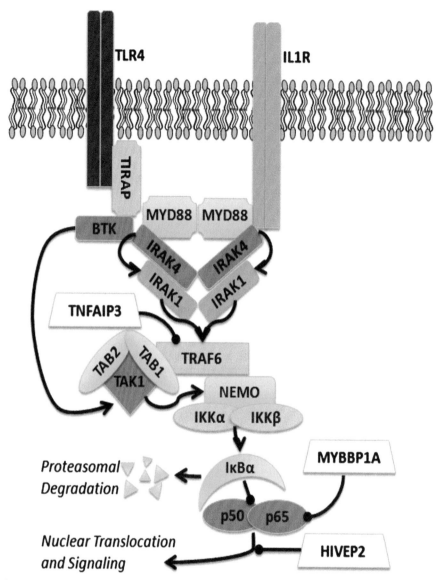

Fig. 1. The MYD88 L265P somatic mutation is present in greater than 90% of WM patients and triggers NF-κB signaling through BTK and IRAK 1/4. Monoallelic losses in TNFAIP3, MYBBP1A, and HIVEP2 may further enhance NF-κB signaling in certain WM patients.

IRAK1 and IκBα phosphorylation as well as survival of MYD88 L265P expressing WM cells. These observations are of particular relevance to WM because NF-κB signaling is important for WM growth and survival.[31] Recently, Yang and colleagues[25] showed that Bruton tyrosine kinase (BTK) was also activated by MYD88 L265P. Activated BTK coimmunoprecipated with MYD88 that could be abrogated by use of the BTK kinase inhibitor and overexpression of MYD88 L265P but not MYD88 wild-type triggered BTK activation. Moreover, knockdown of MYD88 by lentiviral tranfection or use of a MYD88 homodimer inhibitor in MYD88 L265P mutated WM cells abrogated BTK activation.

CXCR4 WHIM Mutations

Recently Hunter and colleagues[24] identified the first ever reported somatic mutations in human cancer involving CXCR4. These mutations were present in 30% of WM patients, and involve the C-terminus that contain serine phosphorylation sites which regulate signaling of CXCR4 by its only known ligand, stromal derived factor-1a (SDF-1a) (CXCL12). The location of somatic mutations in the C-terminal domain of WM patients are similar to those observed in the germline of patients with warts, hypogammaglobulinemia, infections, and myelokathexis (WHIM) syndrome, a congenital immunodeficiency disorder characterized by chronic noncyclic neutropenia.[32,33] Germline mutations in the C-terminus of CXCR4 in WHIM patients block receptor internalization after SDF-1a stimulation in myeloid cells that results in persistent CXCR4 activation and bone marrow (BM) myeloid cell trafficking.[34]

In WM patients, 2 classes of CXCR4 mutations occur in the C-terminus. These include nonsense ($CXCR4^{WHIM/NS}$) mutations that truncate the distal 15 to 20 amino acid region, and frameshift ($CXCR4^{WHIM/FS}$) mutations that compromise a region of up to 40 amino acids in the C- terminal domain.[24,35] Nonsense and frameshift mutations are almost equally divided among WM patients with CXCR4 somatic mutations, and more than 30 different types of CXCR4 WHIM mutations have been identified in WM patients. Preclinical studies with the most common $CXCR4^{WHIM/NS}$ mutation in WM (S338X) have shown enhanced and sustained AKT, ERK, and BTK signaling after SDF-1a relative to $CXCR4^{WT}$ as well increased cell migration, adhesion, growth, and survival of WM cells.[36,37]

Other recurrent somatic mutations described in WM include ARID1A, TRAF3, CD79B, TP53, and MYBBP1A as well as monoallelic deletions of PRDM2, BTG1, TNFAIP3, and HIVEP2.[24,38,39] Many of these mutations and/or losses have an impact on NF-κB regulation and may further enhance NF-κB signaling in response to MYD88 L265P (see **Fig. 1**).

CLINICAL FEATURES

The morbidity of WM is mediated by bone marrow and organ tumor infiltration as well as the IgM paraprotein by producing symptoms through increased serum viscosity, autoantibody effects, and tissue deposition.[40]

MORBIDITY MEDIATED BY THE EFFECTS OF IGM
Hyperviscosity Syndrome

Serum hyperviscosity is effected by increased serum IgM levels leading to hyperviscosity-related complications.[41] The mechanisms behind the marked increase in the resistance to blood flow and the resulting impaired transit through the microcirculatory system are complex.[41–43] The main determinants are (1) a high concentration of monoclonal IgMs, which may form aggregates and may bind water through their carbohydrate component, and (2) their interaction with blood cells. Monoclonal IgMs increase red cell aggregation (rouleaux formation) and red cell internal viscosity while also reducing deformability. The possible presence of cryoglobulins can contribute to increasing blood viscosity as well as to the tendency to induce erythrocyte aggregation. Serum viscosity is proportional to IgM concentration up to 30 g/L, then increases sharply at higher levels. Clinical manifestations are related to circulatory disturbances that are best appreciated by ophthalmoscopy, which result in distended and tortuous retinal veins, hemorrhages, and papilledema (**Fig. 2**).[44] Symptoms usually occur when the monoclonal IgM concentration exceeds 50 g/L or when

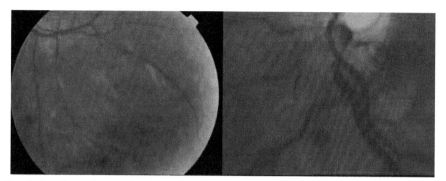

Fig. 2. Funduscopic examination of a patient with WM demonstrating hyperviscosity-related changes, including peripheral hemorrhages (*left*) and dilated retinal vessels (*right*).

serum viscosity is greater than 4.0 cP, but there is a great individual variability, with some patients showing no evidence of hyperviscosity even at 10 cp.[41] The most common symptoms are oronasal bleeding, visual disturbances due to retinal bleeding, and dizziness that may rarely lead to coma. Heart failure can be aggravated, particularly in the elderly, owing to increased blood viscosity, expanded plasma volume, and anemia. Inappropriate transfusion can exacerbate hyperviscosity and may precipitate cardiac failure.

Cryoglobulinemia

In up to 20% of WM patients, the monoclonal IgM can behave as a cryoglobulin (type I), but it is symptomatic in 5% or less of the cases.[45] Cryoprecipitation is mainly dependent on the concentration of monoclonal IgM; for this reason, plasmapheresis or plasma exchange is commonly effective in this condition. Symptoms result from impaired blood flow in small vessels and include Raynaud phenomenon; acrocyanosis; necrosis of the regions most exposed to cold, such as the tip of the nose, ears, fingers, and toes (**Fig. 3**); malleolar ulcers; purpura; and cold urticaria. Renal manifestations may occur but are infrequent.

IgM-Related Neuropathy

The presence of peripheral neuropathy has been estimated to range from 5% to 38% in WM patients.[46–50] The nerve damage is mediated by diverse pathogenetic mechanisms: IgM antibody activity toward nerve constituents causing demyelinating polyneuropathies; endoneurial granulofibrillar deposits of IgM without antibody activity, associated with axonal polyneuropathy; occasionally by tubular deposits in the endoneurium associated with IgM cryoglobulin; and, rarely, by amyloid deposits or by neoplastic cell infiltration of nerve structures.[51] Half of patients with IgM neuropathy have a distinctive clinical syndrome that is associated with antibodies against a minor 100-kDa glycoprotein component of nerve, myelin-associated glycoprotein (MAG). Anti-MAG antibodies are generally monoclonal IgMκ, and usually also exhibit reactivity with other glycoproteins or glycolipids that share antigenic determinants with MAG.[52–54] The anti-MAG–related neuropathy is typically distal and symmetric, affecting both motor and sensory functions; it is slowly progressive with a long period of stability.[47,55,56] Most patients present with sensory complaints (paresthesias, aching discomfort, dysesthesias, or lancinating pains); imbalance and gait ataxia, owing to lack proprioception; and leg muscle atrophy in advanced stage.

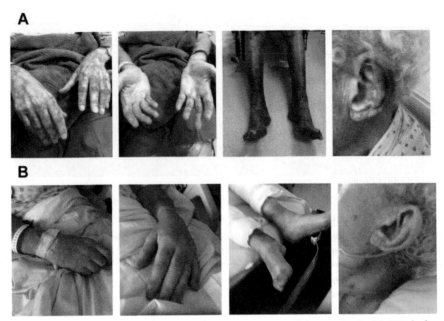

Fig. 3. Cryoglobulinemia manifesting with severe acrocyanosis in a patient with WM before (*A*) and after (*B*) warming and plasmapheresis.

Cold Agglutinin Hemolytic Anemia

Monoclonal IgM may present with cold agglutinin activity (ie, it can recognize specific red cell antigens at temperatures below physiologic, producing chronic hemolytic anemia). This disorder occurs in less than 10% of WM patients[57] and is associated with cold agglutinin titers greater than 1:1000 in most cases. The monoclonal component is usually an IgMκ and reacts most commonly with I/i antigens, with complement fixation and activation.[58,59] Mild chronic hemolytic anemia can be exacerbated after cold exposure but rarely does hemoglobin drop below 70 g/L. The hemolysis is usually extravascular (removal of C3b opsonized cells by the reticuloendotelial system, primarily in the liver) and rarely intravascular from complement destruction of red blood cell (RBC) membrane. The agglutination of RBCs in the cooler peripheral circulation also causes Raynaud syndrome, acrocyanosis, and livedo reticularis. Macroglobulins with the properties of both cryoglobulins and cold agglutinins with anti-Pr specificity have been reported. These properties may have as a common basis the immune binding of the sialic acid–containing carbohydrate present on RBC glycophorins and on Ig molecules. Several other macroglobulins with various antibody activities toward autologous antigens (phospholipids, tissue and plasma proteins and so forth) and foreign ligands have also been reported.

Amyloidosis and Other Deposition Disease

In addition to the precipitation of monoclonal IgM in tissues, as observed after cold exposure in cryoglobulinemia, the monoclonal protein or its fragments (light chains) can deposit in several organs determining their dysfunction. For instance, the monoclonal IgM can produce kidney injury characterized by a mesangiocapillary glomerulonephritis. IgM-associated AL amyloidosis is an uncommon complication of WM and presents distinctive clinical characteristics. Patients are older than non-IgM patients, have a higher frequency of lymph node involvement, and have significantly lower median proteinuria and less frequent and severe heart involvement.[60]

LABORATORY INVESTIGATIONS AND FINDINGS
Hematological Abnormalities

Anemia is the most common finding in patients with symptomatic WM and is caused by a combination of factors: myelosuppression due to bone marrow infiltration, hemolysis due to warm and cold antibodies, splenic entrapment, and hepcidin production. Leukocyte and platelet counts are usually within the reference range at presentation, although patients may occasionally present with severe thrombocytopenia. Monoclonal B-lymphocytes are uncommonly recognized by peripheral blood flow cytometry, although circulating clonal cells can be detected by AS-PCR testing for the MYD88 L265P mutation.

Biochemical Investigations

High-resolution electrophoresis combined with immunofixation of serum and urine is recommended for identification and characterization of the IgM monoclonal protein. The light chain of the monoclonal IgM is κ in 75% to 80% of patients. A few WM patients have more than one M component. The concentration of the serum monoclonal protein is variable but in most cases lies within the range of 15 to 45 g/L. Densitometry should be adopted to determine IgM levels for serial evaluations because nephelometry is unreliable and shows large intralaboratory as well as interlaboratory variation. The presence of cold agglutinins or cryoglobulins may affect determination of IgM levels and, therefore, testing for cold agglutinins and cryoglobulins should be performed at diagnosis. If present, subsequent serum samples should be analyzed under warm conditions for determination of serum monoclonal IgM level. Although Bence Jones proteinuria is frequently present, it exceeds 1 g/24 h in only 3% of cases. Although IgM levels are elevated in WM patients, IgA and IgG levels are most often depressed and do not demonstrate recovery even after successful treatment, suggesting that patients with WM harbor a defect that prevents normal plasma cell development and/or Ig heavy chain rearrangements.[61]

Serum Viscosity

Because of its large size (approximately 1,000,000 Da), most IgM molecules are retained within the intravascular compartment and can exert an undue effect on serum viscosity. Therefore, serum viscosity should be measured if the patient has signs or symptoms of hyperviscosity syndrome. Fundoscopy remains an excellent indicator of clinically relevant hyperviscosity. Among the first clinical signs of hyperviscosity, the appearance of peripheral and midperipheral dot and blot hemorrhages in the retina, which are best appreciated with indirect ophthalmoscopy and scleral depression.[44] In more severe cases of hyperviscosity, dot, blot, and flame-shaped hemorrhages can appear in the macular area along with markedly dilated and tortuous veins with focal constrictions resulting in venous sausaging, as well as papilledema.

Bone Marrow Findings

The bone marrow is always involved in WM. Central to the diagnosis of WM is the demonstration, by trephine biopsy, of bone marrow infiltration by a lymphoplasmacytic cell population constituted by small lymphocytes with evidence of plasmacytoid/plasma cell differentiation (**Fig. 4**). The pattern of bone marrow infiltration may be diffuse, interstitial, or nodular, usually showing an intertrabecular pattern of infiltration. A solely paratrabecular pattern of infiltration is unusual and should raise the possibility

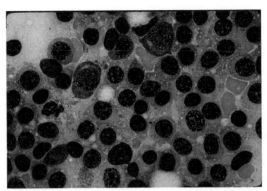

Fig. 4. Aspirate (Wright stain, 100× original magnification) from a patient with WM demonstrating excess mature lymphocytes, lymphoplasmacytic cells, and plasma cells. (*Courtesy of Marvin Stone, MD, Baylor Cancer Center, Dallas, TX, USA.*)

of follicular lymphoma. The bone marrow infiltration should routinely be confirmed by immunophenotypic studies (flow cytometry and/or immunohistochemistry) showing the following profile: sIgM⁺CD19⁺CD20⁺CD22⁺CD79⁺.[62–64] Up to 20% of cases may express CD5, CD10, or CD23.[65] In these cases, care should be taken to satisfactorily exclude chronic lymphocytic leukemia and mantle cell lymphoma. Intranuclear periodic acid–Schiff–positive inclusions (Dutcher-Fahey bodies) consisting of IgM deposits in the perinuclear space and sometimes, in intranuclear vacuoles, may be seen occasionally in lymphoid cells in WM. An increased number of mast cells, usually in association with the lymphoid aggregates, are commonly found in WM, and their presence may help in differentiating WM from other B-cell lymphomas.[1,2] AS-PCR testing for MYD88 L265P is particularly helpful in discerning WM from other overlapping IgM-secreting B-cell malignancies, including marginal zone lymphomas, IgM myeloma, and chronic lymphocytic leukemia, which rarely express this somatic mutation.[17,18]

PROGNOSIS AND RISK STRATIFICATION

WM typically presents as an indolent disease though considerable variability in prognosis can be seen. Castillo and colleagues[66] recently examined trends in relative survival (RS) and overall survival (OS) in patients with WM from the Surveillance, Epidemiology, and End Results database. A total of 6231 patients diagnosed with WM between 1980 and 2010 were included in their analysis. The median OS times were 5.6 and 7.3 years for the 1980 to 2000 and the 2001 to 2010 cohorts, respectively. The 5-year RS rates for the 1980 to 2000 and 2001 to 2010 cohorts were 67% and 78%, and the 5-year OS rates were 56% and 65%, respectively. In the multivariate analysis, survival benefits were identified for the 2001 to 2010 cohort in almost every stratum analyzed, with exception of patients less than 40 years and greater than or equal to 80 years. These results are consistent with a 1555-patient Swedish population-based study that also showed that outcome of patients with WM has improved over the period 1980 to 2005.[67]

Age has been consistently an important prognostic factor (>60–70 years),[68–71] although unrelated morbidities often have an impact. Anemia, which can be multifactorial, is an adverse prognostic factor in WM, with hemoglobin levels of less than 9 to 12 g/dL associated with decreased survival in several series.[68,69,71,72] Cytopenias have also been regularly identified as a significant predictor of survival. The number of cytopenias in a given patient may predict survival.[69] Serum albumin levels have correlated with survival in WM patients in certain but not all studies using multivariate analyses.[65,69] High-serum β_2-microglobulin (>3–3.5 g/dL) levels,[71–73] high-serum IgM M-protein (>7 g/dL),[71] low-serum IgM M-protein (<4 g/dL),[73] the presence of cryoglobulins,[73] and the presence of a familial disease background[74] have also been reported to confer adverse outcomes. The presence of 6q deletion as an adverse marker remains controversial.[11,13] In one study, the presence of MYD88 wild-type correlated with poor survival, whereas the presence of nonsense CXCR4 WHIM mutations was associated with more aggressive presentation but did not have an impact on survival relative to those patients with wild-type CXCR4.[35]

There have been several attempts to organize prognostic factors into prognostic systems for the risk stratification of patients with WM and as a tool for the comparison between studies. A multicenter collaborative project analyzed a large number of previously untreated, symptomatic patients and 5 adverse covariates (age >65 years, hemoglobin $\leq$11.5 g/dL, platelet count $\leq$100 $\times$ 109/L, β_2-microglobulin >3 mg/L, and serum monoclonal protein concentration >70 g/L) was used to define 3 risk groups (low-, intermediate-, and high-risk, respectively).[71] This International Prognostic Scoring System for WM (ISSWM) has been externally validated in independent cohorts. Although results per ISSWM risk category are increasingly reported in phase II studies and are used for the stratification of patients in randomized clinical trials, its use in making treatment decisions remains to be delineated.

TREATMENT OF WALDENSTRÖM MACROGLOBULINEMIA
Treatment Indications

Consensus guidelines on indications for treatment intitiation were formulated as part of the Second International Workshop on Waldenström's Macroglobulinemia.[70] Initiation of therapy should not be based only on the IgM levels because they may not correlate with either disease burden nor symptomatic status.[75,76] Initiation of therapy is appropriate for patients with constitutional symptoms, such as recurrent fever, night sweats, fatigue due to anemia, or weight loss. The presence of progressive, symptomatic lymphadenopathy or splenomegaly provides additional reasons to begin therapy. The presence of anemia with a hemoglobin value of less than or equal to 10 g/dL or a platelet count less than or equal to 100 $\times$ 10^9/L on this basis of disease is also a reasonable indication for treatment initiation. Certain complications of WM, such as hyperviscosity syndrome, symptomatic sensorimotor peripheral neuropathy, systemic amyloidosis, renal insufficiency, and symptomatic cryoglobulinemia, are also indications for therapy.

Treatment Options

A precise therapeutic algorithm for therapy for WM remains to be defined given the paucity of randomized clinical trials. Active agents include monoclonal antibodies (rituximab and ofatumumab), alkylators (chlorambucil, cyclophosphamide, and bendamustine), nucleoside analogs (cladribine and fludarabine), proteasome inhibitors (bortezomib and carfilzomib), immunomodulatory drugs (thalidomide, lenalidomide, and pomalidomide), and signal inhibitors (everolimus and ibrutinib).[77] Combination regimens particularly with rituximab commonly have been used to treat WM. Individual patient considerations, including the presence of cytopenias, need for more rapid disease control, age, and candidacy for autologous transplant therapy, should be taken into account in making the choice of a first-line agent. For patients who are candidates for autologous transplant therapy, exposure to continuous chlorambucil or nucleoside analog therapy should be limited given potential for stem cell damage. The use of nucleoside analogs may also increase risk for histologic transformation to diffuse large B-cell lymphoma as well as myelodysplasia and acute myelogenous leukemia.[77]

Monoclonal antibodies

Rituximab is a chimeric monoclonal antibody that targets CD20, a widely expressed antigen on lymphoplasmacytic cells in WM. The use of rituximab at standard dosimetry (ie, 4 weekly infusions at 375 mg/m^2) induces partial or better responses in approximately 27% to 35% of previously treated and untreated patients.[78,79] Patients who achieved even minor responses (MRs), however, benefited from rituximab as evidenced by improved hemoglobin and platelet counts and reduction of lymphadenopathy and/or splenomegaly.[78] The median time to treatment failure in these studies was found to range from 8 to 27+ months. Studies evaluating an extended rituximab schedule consisting of 4 weekly courses at 375 mg/m^2/wk, repeated 3 months later by another 4-week course, have demonstrated higher major response rates of 44% to 48%, with time to progression estimates exceeding 29 months.[80,81]

In many WM patients, a transient increase of serum IgM (IgM flare) may be noted immediately after initiation of rituximab treatment.[82–84] The IgM flare in response to rituximab does not herald treatment failure, and although most patients return to their baseline serum IgM level by 12 weeks, some patients may flare for months despite having tumor responses in their bone marrow. Patients with baseline serum IgM levels of greater than 40 g/dL or serum viscosity of greater than 3.5 cp may be particularly at risk for a hyperviscosity-related event and in such patients plasmapheresis should be considered or rituximab omitted for the first few cycles of therapy until IgM levels decline to safer levels.[74] Because of the decreased likelihood of response in patients with higher IgM levels as well as the possibility that serum IgM and viscosity levels may abruptly rise, rituximab monotherapy should not be used as sole therapy for the treatment of patients at risk for hyperviscosity symptoms. Intolerance to rituximab is common in WM patients, with an estimated frequency of 10%. Ofatumumab is a fully humanized CD20-directed monoclonal antibody that targets the small loop of CD20, an epitope that is different from rituximab. An overall response rate (ORR) of 59% was observed in a series of 37 symptomatic WM patients after ofatumumab administration, which included untreated and previously treated patients.[85] Responses were higher among rituximab-naïve patients. An IgM flare with symptomatic hyperviscosity was also observed in 2 (5%) patients in this series who required plasmapheresis. Ofatumumab has also been successfully administered to WM patients who demonstrated intolerance to rituximab.[85,86]

Alkylating agents

Oral alkylating drugs, alone and in combination therapy with steroids, have been extensively evaluated in the upfront treatment of WM. The greatest experience with oral alkylator therapy has been with chlorambucil, which has been administered on both a continuous (ie, daily dose) as well as an intermittent schedule. Patients receiving chlorambucil on a continuous schedule typically receive 0.1 mg/kg per day, whereas on the intermittent schedule patients typically receive 0.3 mg/kg for 7 days, every 6 weeks. In a prospective randomized study, Kyle and colleagues[87] reported no significant difference in the ORR between these schedules, although the median response duration was greater for patients receiving intermittent versus continuously dosed chlorambucil (46 vs 26 months). Despite the favorable median response duration in this study for use of the intermittent schedule, no difference in the median OS was observed. Moreover, an increased incidence for development of myelodysplasia and acute myelogenous leukemia with the intermittent (3 of 22 patients) versus the continuous (0 of 24 patients) chlorambucil schedule prompted the investigators of this study to express preference for use of continuous chlorambucil dosing. In a study of 414 patients, including 339 with WM, 37 with non–mucosa-associated lymphoid tissue marginal zone lymphoma, and 38 with LPL, patients were randomized to receive chlorambucil or fludarabine.[88] On the basis of intent-to-treat analysis, the ORR was 47.8% in the fludarabine arm versus 38.6% in the chlorambucil arm. With a median follow-up of 36 months, median PFS was significantly higher in those patients who received fludarabine (36.3 months) compared with chlorambucil arm (27.1 months). Moreover, in patients with WM, median OS was not reached in the fludarabine arm versus 69.8 months in the chlorambucil arm. Grade 3 to 4 neutropenia was significantly higher among patients treated with fludarabine (36%) compared with patients treated with chlorambucil (18%). However, secondary malignancies were significantly more frequent with chlorambucil versus fludarabine, with a 6-year cumulative incidence rate of 21% and 4%, respectively. Additional factors to be taken into account in considering chlorambucil therapy for patients with WM include necessity for more rapid disease control given the slow nature of response to this agent as well as consideration for preserving stem cells in patients who are candidates for autologous transplant therapy. Chlorambucil should, therefore, be reserved for nontransplant candidates with more indolent disease.

The combination of cyclophosphamide, doxorubicin, vincristine, prednisone (CHOP) with rituximab (CHOP-R) was investigated in a randomized frontline study by the German Low Grade Lymphoma Study Group involving 69 patients, most of whom had WM.[89] The addition of rituximab to CHOP resulted in a higher ORR (94% vs 67%) and median time to progression (63 vs 22 months) in comparison to patients treated with CHOP alone. Dimopoulos and colleagues[90] investigated the combination of rituximab, dexamethasone, and oral cyclophosphamide as primary therapy in 72 patients with WM. At least a major response was observed in 74% of patients in this study, and the 2-year PFS was 67%. Therapy was well tolerated, although 1 patient died of interstitial pneumonia. In the salvage setting, the use of CHOP-R has been investigated in relapsed/refractory WM patients.[91] Among 13 evaluable patients, 10 patients achieved a major response (77%), including 3 CR and 7 PR, and 2 patients achieved an MR. In a retrospective study, Ioakimidis and colleagues[92] examined the outcomes of symptomatic WM patients who received CHOP-R, Cyclophosphamide, Vincristine, Prednisone, Rituximab (CVP-R), or Cyclophosphamide, Prednisone, Rituximab (CP-R). Baseline characteristics for all 3 cohorts were similar for age, prior therapies, bone marrow involvement, hematocrit, platelet count, and serum β_2-microglobulin, although serum IgM levels were higher in patients treated with CHOP-R. The ORRs to therapy were comparable for all 3 treatments: CHOP-R (96%), CVP-R (88%), and CP-R (95%), although more CRs were observed among patients treated with either CVP-R or CHOP-R. Comparison of adverse events for these regimens showed a higher incidence for neutropenic fever as well as treatment-related neuropathy in patients receiving CHOP-R and CVP-R versus CPR. These studies suggest that in WM, the use of doxorubicin and vincristine may be omitted to minimize treatment-related complications. Therefore, more intense cyclophosphamide-based regimens, such as CHOP-R or CVP-R, should be avoided.

Bendamustine is a recently approved agent for the treatment of relapsed/refractory indolent non-Hodgkin lymphoma. Bendamustine has structural similarities to both alkylating agents and purine analogs.[93] The use of bendamustine in combination with rituximab was explored by Rummel and colleagues[94] in the frontline therapy for WM. As part of a randomized study, patients received 6 cycles of bendamustine plus rituximab (Benda-R) or CHOP-R. A total of 546 patients were enrolled in this study for indolent non-Hodgkin lymphoma patients and included 40 patients with WM. Patients in the Benda-R arm received bendamustine at 90 mg/m^2 on days 1 and 2 and rituximab at 375 mg/m^2 on day 1 with the frequency of 4 weeks for each cycle. The ORR was 96% for Benda-R and 94% for CHOP-R treated patients. With a median observation period of 26 months, 20/23 (87%) Benda-R versus 9/17 (53%) CHOP-R–treated WM patients remain free of progression. Benda-R was associated with a lower incidence of grade 3 or 4 neutropenia, infectious complications, and alopecia. In the salvage setting, the outcome of 30 WM patients with relapsed/refractory disease who received bendamustine alone or with a CD20-directed antibody showed an ORR of 83.3% and a median PFS of 13.2 months.[86] Overall, therapy was well tolerated in this study although prolonged myelosuppression occurred in patients who received prior nucleoside analog therapy. Cytoreduction, including extramedullary disease, is particulary good with bendamustine-based therapy and can be considered in patients presenting with bulky adenopathy or splenomegaly or who have other symptomatic extramedullary disease.

Nucleoside analogs

Both cladribine and fludarabine have been evaluated in untreated as well as previously treated WM patients. Cladribine administered as a single agent by continuous intravenous (IV) infusion, by 2-hour daily infusion or by subcutaneous bolus injections for 5 to 7 days has resulted in major responses in 40% to 90% of patients who received primary therapy, whereas in the salvage setting responses have ranged from 38% to 54%.[95–98] The ORR with daily infusional fludarabine therapy administered mainly on 5-day schedules in previously untreated and treated WM patients has ranged from 38% to 100% and 30% to 40%, respectively, on par with the response data for single-agent cladribine.[99,100] In general, response rates and durations of responses have been greater for patients receiving nucleoside analogs as first-line agents, although in one large study that included both untreated and previously treated patients, no substantial difference in the overall response to fludarabine was observed.[72] Myelosuppression commonly occurred after prolonged exposure to either of the nucleoside analogs, as did lymphopenia with sustained depletion of both CD4$^+$ and CD8$^+$ T lymphocytes observed in WM patients 1 year after initiation of therapy. Treatment-related mortality due to myelosuppression and/or opportunistic infections attributable to immunosuppression occurred in up to 5% of all treated patients in some series with either nucleoside analog.

Combination therapy with nucleoside analogs has been investigated as both first-line and salvage therapy in WM. Weber and colleagues[101] administered rituximab along with cladribine and cyclophosphamide to 17 previously untreated patients with WM. At least a partial response was documented in 94% of WM patients, including a complete response (CR) in 18%. With a median follow-up of 21 months, no patient has relapsed. Laszlo and colleagues[102] evaluated the combination of subcutaneous cladribine with rituximab in 29 WM patients with either untreated or previously treated disease. Intended therapy consisted of rituximab on day 1 followed by subcutaneous cladribine, 0.1 mg/kg, for 5 consecutive days, administered monthly for 4 cycles. With a median follow-up of 43 months, the ORR observed was 89.6%, with 7 CRs, 16 partial responses, and 3 MRs. Response activity was similar between untreated and previously treated patients. No major infections were observed despite the lack of antimicrobial prophylaxis. In a study by the Waldenström's Macroglobulinemia Clinical Trials Group (WMCTG), a combination of rituximab and fludarabine was administered to 43 WM patients, 32 (75%) of whom were previously untreated.[103] The ORR was 95.3%, and 83% of patients achieved a major response. The median time to progression was 51.2 months in this series and was longer for those patients who were previously untreated and for those achieving at least a very good partial response (VGPR). Hematological toxicity was common, in particular neutropenia and thrombocytopenia. Two deaths occurred in this study due to non–*Pneumocystis carinii* pneumonia. Secondary malignanices, including transformation to aggressive lymphoma and development of myelodysplasia or acute myeloid leukemia, were observed in 6 patients in this series. The addition of rituximab to fludarabine and cyclophosphamide has also been explored in the salvage setting by Tam and colleagues[104] wherein 4 of 5 patients demonstrated a response. Hensel and colleagues[105] administered rituximab along with pentostatin and cyclophosphamide to 13 patients with untreated and previously treated WM or LPL. A major response was observed in 77% or patients. The addition of alkylating agents to nucleoside analogs has also been explored in WM. Dimopoulos and colleagues[106] examined fludarabine in combination with IV cyclophosphamide and observed partial responses in 6 of 11 (55%) patients with primary refractory disease or who relapsed on treatment. The combination of fludarabine plus cyclosphosphamide was also evaluated in a recent study by Tamburini and colleagues[107] involving 49 patients, 35 of whom were previously treated. Seventy-eight percent of the patients in this study achieved a response and median time to treatment failure was 27 months. Hematological toxicity was commonly observed and 3 patients died of treatment-related toxicities. Findings in this study included the development of acute leukemia in 2 patients, histologic transformation to diffuse large cell lymphoma in 1 patient, 2 cases of solid malignancies (prostate and melanoma), and failure to mobilize stem cells in 4 of 6 patients. Tedeschi and colleagues[108] recently completed a multicenter study with fludarabine, cyclophosphamide, and rituximab in symptomatic WM patients with untreated or relapsed/refractory disease to 1 line of chemotherapy. Treatment consisted of rituximab at 375 mg/m^2 on day 1, fludarabine at 25 mg/m^2, and cyclophosphamide at 250 mg/m^2 by IV administration on days 2 to 4 every 4 weeks. Forty-three patients were accrued to this study. The ORR was 89%, with 83% of patients attaining a major remission and 14% a CR. Prolonged neutropenia was observed in up to one-third of patients. With a median follow-up of 15 months, the median PFS for this study has not been reached.

The safety of nucleoside analogs has been the subject of investigation in several recent studies. Thomas and colleagues[109] recently reported their experiences in harvesting stem cells in 21 patients with symptomatic WM in whom autologous peripheral blood stem cell collection was attempted. Autologous stem cell collection succeeded on the first attempt in 14 of 15 patients who received non-nucleoside analog-based therapy versus 2 of 6 patients who received a nucleoside analog. The long-term safety of nucleoside analogs in WM was recently examined by Leleu and colleagues[110] in a large series of WM patients. A 7-fold increase in transformation to an aggressive lymphoma and a 3-fold increase in the development of acute myelogenous leukemia/myelodysplasia were observed among patients who received a nucleoside analog versus other therapies for their WM. A recent metanalysis by Leleu and colleagues[111] of several trials using nucleoside analogs in WM patients, which included patients who had previously received an alkylator agent, showed a crude incidence of 6.6% to 10% for development of disease transformation and 1.4% to 8.9% for development of myelodysplasia or acute myelogenous leukemia. None of the studied risk factors (ie, gender, age, family history of WM or B-cell malignancies, typical markers of tumor burden and prognosis, type of nucleoside analog therapy [cladribine vs fludarabine], time from diagnosis to nucleoside analog use, nucleoside analog treatment as primary or salvage therapy, and treatment with an oral alkylator [ie, chlorambucil]) predicted for the occurrence of transformation or development of myelodysplasia/acute myelogenous leukemia for WM patients treated with a nucleoside analog. Nucleoside analogs should, therefore, be avoided in younger patients given the constellation of short- as well as long-term toxicity risks.

Proteasome inhibitors

Bortezomib has been extensively investigated in WM. In a multicenter study of the WMCTG, 27 patients received up to 8 cycles of bortezomib at 1.3 mg/m^2 on days 1, 4, 8, and 11.[112] All but 1 patient had relapsed/or refractory disease. After therapy, median serum IgM levels declined from 4660 mg/dL to 2092 mg/dL (P<.0001). The ORR was 85%, with 10 and 13 patients achieving a MR and major response, respectively. Responses were prompt and occurred at median of 1.4 months. The median time to progression for all responding patients in this study was 7.9 months, and the most common grade III/IV toxicities occurring in greater than or equal to 5% of patients were sensory neuropathies (22.2%), leukopenia (18.5%), neutropenia (14.8%), dizziness (11.1%), and thrombocytopenia (7.4%). Importantly, sensory neuropathies resolved or improved in nearly all patients after cessation of therapy. As part of a National Cancer Institute of Canada study, Chen and colleagues[113] treated 27 patients with both untreated (44%) and previously treated (56%) disease. Patients in this study received bortezomib using the standard schedule until they demonstrated progressive disease or 2 cycles beyond a CR or stable disease. The ORR in this study was 78%, with major responses observed in 44% of patients. Sensory neuropathy occurred in 20 patients, 5 with grade greater than 3, and occurred after 2 to 4 cycles of therapy. Among the 20 patients developing a neuropathy, 14 patients resolved and 1 patient demonstrated a 1-grade improvement at 2 to 13 months. In addition to these experiences with bortezomib monotherapy in WM, Dimopoulos and colleagues[114] observed major responses in 6 of 10 (60%) previously treated WM patients. The combination of bortezomib, dexamethasone, and rituximab (BDR) has been investigated as primary therapy in WM patients by the WMCTG. An ORR of 96%, major response rate of 83%, and complete attainment in 22% was observed with BDR.[115] The updated median PFS in this study was greater than 56.1 months. The incidence of grade 3 neuropathy was 30% in this study, which used a twice-a-week schedule for bortezomib administration at 1.3 mg/m^2. Peripheral neuropathy from bortezomib was reversible in most patients in this study after discontinuation of therapy, and patients benefitted from pregabalin. An increased incidence of herpes zoster was also observed with BDR, prompting the use of prophylactic antiviral therapy. An alternative schedule for bortezomib administration (ie, weekly at 1.6 mg/m^2) in combination with rituximab and/or dexamethasone has been investigated in several studies with ORRs of 80% to 90%.[116,117] A lower incidence of peripheral neuropathy was observed in studies with weekly dosed bortzomib.[116] In a hybrid study by the European Myeloma Network, patients received twice-weekly bortezomib for the first cycle, then weekly bortezomib for cycles 2 to 5 with dexamethasone and rituximab. An ORR of 85%, with VGPR or better in 10% of patients, was observed.[118] The median PFS was 43 months, and patients with VGPR/CR had longer PFS. Grade greater than or equal to 2 treatment–related peripheral neuropathy occurred in 24% of patients and led to bortezomib discontinuation in 8% of patients.

Because bortezomib frequently produces severe treatment-related peripheral neuropathy in WM, the WMCTG investigated the use of carfilzomib, a neuropathy-sparing proteasome-inhibitor, in combination with rituximab and dexamethasone (CaRD) in symptomatic WM patients naïve to bortezomib and rituximab.[119] Protocol therapy consisted of IV carfilzomib 20 mg/m^2 (cycle 1); 36 mg/m^2 (cycles 2–6) with IV dexamethasone 20 mg on days 1, 2, 8, 9; and rituximab 375 mg/m^2 on days 2 and 9 every

21 days. Maintenance therapy followed 8 weeks later with IV carfilzomib 36 mg/m^2 and IV dexamethasone 20 mg on days 1 and 2 and rituximab 375 mg/m^2 on day 2 every 8 weeks for 8 cycles. Post-therapy, median serum IgM levels declined from 3375 to 749 mg/dL (P<.0001); bone marrow disease declined from 60% to 5% (P<.0001); hematocrit rose from 32.3% to 41.3% (P<.0001). ORR was 87.1% (1 CR, 10 VGPRs, 10 PRs, and 6 MRs) and was not impacted by MYD88^{L265P} or CXCR4^{WHIM} mutation status. With a median follow-up of 15.4 months, 20 patients remain progression-free, including 8 on maintenance-therapy. Grade greater than or equal to 2 toxicities included asymptomatic hyperlipasemia (41.9%), reversible neutropenia (12.9%), and cardiomyopathy in 1 patient (3.2%) with multiple risk factors. Declines in serum IgA and IgG were common and were associated with recurring infections necessitating IVIG therapy in several patients.

Immunomodulatory agents

Thalidomide as monotherapy and in combination with dexamethasone and/or clarithromycin has been examined in WM. Dimopoulos and colleagues[120] demonstrated a major response in 5 of 20 (25%) previously untreated and treated patients who received single-agent thalidomide. Dose escalation from the thalidomide start dose of 200 mg daily was hindered by development of side effects, including the development of peripheral neuropathy in 5 patients, obligating discontinuation or dose reduction. Low doses of thalidomide (50 mg orally daily) in combination with dexamethasone (40 mg orally once a week) and clarithromycin (250 mg orally twice a day) have also been examined, with 10 of 12 (83%) previously treated patients demonstrating at least a major response.[121] In a follow-up study by Dimopoulos and colleagues,[122] however, using a higher thalidomide dose (200 mg orally daily) along with dexamethasone (40 g orally once a week) and clarithromycin (500 mg orally twice a day), only 2 of 10 (20%) previously treated patients responded. The combination of immunomodulator agents (thalidomide, lenalidomide, and pomalidomide) with rituximab was investigated by the WMCTG. Thalidomide was administered at 200 mg daily for 2 weeks, followed by 400 mg daily and thereafter for 1 year. Patients received 4 weekly infusions of rituximab at 375 mg/m^2 beginning 1 week after initiation of thalidomide, followed by 4 additional weekly infusions of rituximab at 375 mg/m^2 beginning at week 13. The ORR and major response rate were 72% and 64%, respectively, and the median time to progression was 38 months in this series.[123] Dose reduction and/or discontinuation of thalidomide was common and mainly attributed to treatment-related neuropathy. The investigators concluded in this study that lower doses of thalidomide (ie, 50–100 mg/d) should be considered in this patient population. The combination of lenalidomide with rituximab was investigated by the WMCTG using lenalidomide at 25 mg daily on a syncopated schedule wherein therapy was administered for 3 weeks, followed by a 1-week pause for an intended duration of 48 weeks.[124] Patients received 1 week of therapy with lenalidomide, after which rituximab (375 mg/m^2) was administered weekly on weeks 2 through 5, then 13 through 16. The ORR and a major response rates in this study were 50% and 25%, respectively, and a median time to progression for responders was 18.9 months. In 2 patients with bulky disease, significant reduction in extramedullary disease was observed. An acute decrease in hematocrit was observed, however, during first 2 weeks of lenalidomide therapy in 13 of 16 (81%) patients, with a median absolute decrease in hematocrit of 4.8%, resulting in anemia-related complications and hospitalizations in 4 patients. Despite dose reduction, most patients in this study continued to demonstrate aggravated anemia with lenalidomide. There was no evidence of hemolysis or more general myelosuppression with lenalidomide in this study. Pomalidomide was recently investigated in a dose-escalating phase 1 study with rituximab.[125] Patients showed intolerance at doses above 1 mg daily, and rituximab flaring led to symptomatic hyperiscosity and emergent plasmapheresis in 3 of 7 patients. The ORR in this study was 43% with median response duration of 15 months.

Everolimus

Everolimus is an oral inhibitor of the Akt-mTOR pathway. Inhibition of this pathway leads to apoptosis of primary WM cells and WM cell lines.[126] Sixty patients with a median of 3 prior therapies were treated with everolimus in a joint Dana-Farber/Mayo Clinic study.[127] The ORR was 73%, with 50% of patients attaining a major response. The median PFS in this study was 21 months. Grade 3 or higher related toxicities were observed in 67% of patients, with cytopenias constituting the most common toxicity. Pulmonary toxicity occurred in 5% of patients, and dose reductions due to toxicity occurred in 52% of patients. A clinical trial examining the activity of everolimus in 33 previously untreated patients with WM was recently reported by the WMCTG that included serial bone marrow biopsies in response assessment.[128] The ORR in this study was 72%, including partial or better responses in 60% of patients. Discordance between serum IgM levels, on which consensus criteria for response are based, and BM disease response were common and complicated response assessment. At 6-month assessments, in 10 of 22 (45.5%) patients for whom both serum IgM and BM assessments were performed, discordance between serum IgM and BM disease involvement were observed. Among these patients, 2 had no change and 8 had increased bone marrow disease involvement despite decreases in serum IgM levels. Grade greater than or equal to 2 hematologic and nonhematologic toxicities related to everolimus were predominately hematological, including anemia (39.4%), thrombocytopenia (12%), and neutropenia (18.2%). Nonhematological toxicities included oral ulcerations (27.3%), which improved with oral dexamethasone swish and spit solution, and pneumonitis (15%), the latter leading to treatment discontinuation in 5 patients.

Ibrutinib

BTK is a target of MYD88 L265P mutation, which leads to its activation.[25] Furthermore, ibrutinib inhibits BTK and in vitro induces apoptosis of WM cells bearing MYD88 L265P. Given these preclinical findings, symptomatic WM patients who received at least 1 prior treatment were enrolled on a prospective clinical trial examining the safety and efficacy of daily dosed ibrutinib.[129] Intended therapy consisted of 420 mg of oral ibrutinib daily for 2 years or until progression or unacceptable toxicity. Sixty-three patients, including 17 with refractory disease, were enrolled. With a short median follow-up of 6 cycles, the best ORR was 81% (4 VGPR, 32 PR, and 15 MR), with a major response rate (PR or better) of 57.1% and a median time to response of 4 weeks. Grade greater than 2 treatment-related toxicities include thrombocytopenia (14.3%) and neutropenia (19.1%), which occurred mainly in heavily pretreated patients. Responses were impacted by mutations in CXCR4 in those patients who underwent tumor genotypic. The major response rate was 77% for patients with wild-type CXCR4 versus 30% in those with WHIM-like CXCR4 mutations. Decreases in serum IgM as well as improvements in hemoglobin were also greater in patients with wild-type CXCR4. Patients with wild-type CXCR4 also had increased peripheral lymphocytosis after ibrutinib treatment versus those with WHIM-like CXCR4 mutations.

MAINTENANCE THERAPY

A role for maintenance rituximab in WM patients after response to a rituximab-containing regimen was reviewed in a retrospective study examining the outcome of

248 WM rituximab-naïve patients who were either observed or received maintenance rituximab.[130] In this study, categorical responses improved in 16 of 162 (10%) of observed patients and in 36 of 86 (41.8%) of patients who received maintenance rituximab after induction therapy. Both PFS (56.3 vs 28.6 months) and OS (>120 vs 116 months) were longer in patients who received maintenance rituximab. Improved PFS was evident despite previous treatment status, induction with rituximab alone, or in combination therapy. Best serum IgM response was lower and hematocrit higher in those patients receiving maintenance rituximab. Among patients receiving maintenance rituximab, an increased number of infectious events, predominantly sinusitis and bronchitis, were observed, although mainly grade 1 or 2. A prospective study examining the role of maintenance rituximab was initiated by the German STiL group[131]; 162 patients received up to 6 cycles of Benda-R, and responders randomized to either observation or maintenance rituximab every 2 months for 2 years. Enrollment for this study is complete, and response outcome for maintenance is awaited.

HIGH-DOSE THERAPY AND STEM CELL TRANSPLANTATION

The use of stem cell transplantion (SCT) therapy has also been explored in patients with WM. Many small series of patient have been previously reported for both autologous and allogeneic experiences, with variable outcomes. Kyriakou and colleagues[132] reported the largest SCT experience using European Bone Marrow Transplant (EBMT) registry data for WM patients receiving an autologous or allogeneic SCT. Among 158 WM patients receiving an autologous SCT, which included primarily relapsed or refractory patients, the 5-year PFS and OS rates were 39.7% and 68.5%, respectively. Nonrelapse mortality at 1 year was 3.8%. Chemorefractory disease and the number of prior lines of therapy at time of the autologous SCT were the most important prognostic factors for PFS and OS. The achievement of a negative immunofixation after autologous SCT had a positive impact on PFS. When used as consolidation at first response, autologous transplantation provided a PFS of 44% at 5 years. In the allogeneic SCT experience from the EBMT, the long-term outcome of 86 WM patients was reported.[133] A total of 86 patients received allograft by either myeloablative (n = 37) or reduced-intensity (n = 49) conditioning. The median age of patients in this series was 49 years, and 47 patients had 3 or more previous lines of therapy. Eight patients failed prior autologous SCT. Fifty-nine patients (68.6%) had chemotherapy-sensitive disease at the time of allogeneic SCT. Nonrelapse mortality at 3 years was 33% for patients receiving a myeloablative transplant and 23% for those who received reduced-intensity conditioning. The ORR was 75.6%. The relapse rates at 3 years were 11% for myeloablative and 25% for reduced-intensity conditioning recipients. Five-year PFS and OS rates for WM patients who received a myeloablative allogenic SCT were 56% and 62%, respectively, and for patients who received reduced intensity conditioning were 49% and 64%, respectively. The occurrence of chronic graft-versus-host disease was associated with improved PFS and suggested the existence of a clinically relevant graft-versus-WM effect in this study.

RESPONSE CRITERIA IN WALDENSTRÖM MACROGLOBULINEMIA

The consensus response criteria for WM were recently revised and are presented in **Table 1**. Response assessment is often complicated due to the use of IgM as a surrogate marker of disease, which often fluctuates independent of tumor cell killing, particularly with biologically targeted agents, such as rituximab, bortezomib, everolimus, and ibrutinib.[82–84,112,128,129,134] Rituximab induces a spike or flare in serum IgM levels, which can occur when used as monotherapy and in combination with other

---

Table 1
Summary of updated response criteria adopted at the Sixth International Workshop on Waldenström's Macroglobulinemia

Complete response (CR)	IgM in normal range and disappearance of monoclonal protein by immunofixation; no histological evidence of bone marrow involvement, and resolution of any adenopathy/organomegaly (if present at baseline), along with no signs or symptoms attributable to WM. Reconfirmation of the CR status is required by repeat immunofixation studies.
Very good partial response (VGPR)	A ≥90% reduction of serum IgM and decrease in adenopathy/organomegaly (if present at baseline) on physical examination or on CT scan. No new symptoms or signs of active disease.
Partial response (PR)	A ≥50% reduction of serum IgM and decrease in adenopathy/organomegaly (if present at baseline) on physical examination or on CT scan. No new symptoms or signs of active disease.
Minor response (MR)	A ≥25% but <50% reduction of serum IgM. No new symptoms or signs of active disease.
Stable disease (SD)	A <25% reduction and <25% increase of serum IgM without progression of adenopathy/organomegaly, cytopenias or clinically significant symptoms due to disease and/or signs of WM.
Progressive disease (PD)	A ≥25% increase in serum IgM by protein confirmed by a second measurement or progression of clinically significant findings due to disease (ie, anemia, thrombocytopenia, leukopenia, bulky adenopathy/organomegaly) or symptoms (unexplained recurrent fever ≥38.4°C, drenching night sweats, ≥10% body weight loss, or hyperviscosity, neuropathy, symptomatic cryoglobulinemia or amyloidosis) attributable to WM.

From Owen RG, Kyle RA, Stone MJ, et al. Response assessment in Waldenstrom macroglobulinaemia: update from the VIth International Workshop. Br J Haematol 2013;160(2):171–6.

---

agents, including cyclophosphamide, nucleoside analogs, thalidomide, and lenalidomide and last for several weeks to months,[82–84,92,123,124,134] whereas bortezomib, everolimus, and ibrutinib can suppress IgM levels independent of tumor cell killing in certain patients.[112,128,129,135] Moreover, Varghese and colleagues[136] showed that in patients treated with selective B-cell depleting agents, such as rituximab and alemtuzumab, residual IgM producing plasma cells are spared and continue to persist, thus potentially skewing the relative response and assessment to treatment. Therefore, in circumstances where the serum IgM levels seem out of context with the clinical progress of the patient, a bone marrow biopsy should be considered to clarify the patient's underlying disease burden. Soluble CD27 may serve as an alternative surrogate marker in WM and remains a faithful marker of disease in patients experiencing a rituximab-related IgM flare as well as plasmapheresis.[137] More recently, quantitative AS-PCR assessment of MYD88 L265P for both peripheral blood and bone marrow samples has been used to assess disease burden in WM patients who carry this somatic mutation with encouraging results.[18,20,138] Further studies are needed to validate the use of soluble CD27 and quantitative AS-PCR testing for MYD88 L265P for response assessment.

SUMMARY

WM is an IgM-secreting B-cell lymphoproliferative disorder, with strong familial predisposition. MYD88 L265P and CXCR4 WHIM mutations are common in patients with WM and support the growth and survival of WM cells. Clinical manifestations of disease are related to both tumor cell infiltration and paraprotein production. Current treatment options include monoclonal antibodies, alkylating agents, nucleoside analogs, proteasome inhibitors, immunomodulatory drugs, and signal inhibitors. Both short- and long-term toxicities should be weighed in treatment decisions with use of these agents. Elucidation of the signaling pathways involved in WM is helping to advance targeted therapeutics for WM and includes efforts directed at MYD88 and CXCR4 signaling.

REFERENCES

1. Owen RG, Treon SP, Al-Katib A, et al. Clinicopathological definition of Waldenström's macroglobulinemia: consensus panel recommendations from the Second International Workshop on Waldenström's macroglobulinemia. Semin Oncol 2003;30:110–5.
2. Campo E, Swerdlow SH, Harris NL, et al. The 2008 WHO classification of lymphoid neoplasms and beyond: evolving concepts and practical applications. Blood 2011;117(19):5019–32.
3. Groves FD, Travis LB, Devesa SS, et al. Waldenström's macroglobulinemia: incidence patterns in the United States, 1988–1994. Cancer 1998;82: 1078–81.
4. Hanzis C, Ojha RP, Hunter Z, et al. Associated malignancies in patients with Waldenström's macroglobulinemia and their kin. Clin Lymphoma Myeloma Leuk 2011;11:88–92.
5. Varettoni M, Tedesci A, Arcaini L, et al. Risk of second cancers in Waldenstrom macroglobulinemia. Ann Oncol 2011;23(2):411–5.
6. Renier G, Ifrah N, Chevailler A, et al. Four brothers with Waldenstrom's macroglobulinemia. Cancer 1989;64:1554–9.
7. Treon SP, Hunter ZR, Aggarwal A, et al. Characterization of familial Waldenstrom's macroglobulinemia. Ann Oncol 2006;17:488–94.
8. Kristinsson SY, Bjorkholm M, Goldin LR, et al. Risk of lymphoproliferative disorders among first-degree relatives of lymphoplasmacytic lymphoma/Waldenstrom's macroglobulinemia patients: a population-based study in Sweden. Blood 2008;112:3052–6.
9. McMaster ML, Csako G, Giambarresi TR, et al. Long-term evaluation of three multiple-case Waldenstrom's macroglobulinemia families. Clin Cancer Res 2007;13:5063–9.
10. Ogmundsdottir HM, Sveinsdottir S, Sigfusson A, et al. Enhanced B cell survival in familial macroglobulinaemia is associated with increased expression of Bcl-2. Clin Exp Immunol 1999;117:252–60.
11. Schop RF, Kuehl WM, Van Wier SA, et al. Waldenström macroglobulinemia neoplastic cells lack immunoglobulin heavy chain locus translocations but have frequent 6q deletions. Blood 2002;100:2996–3001.
12. Ocio EM, Schop RF, Gonzalez B, et al. 6q deletion in Waldenstrom's macroglobulinemia is associated with features of adverse prognosis. Br J Haematol 2007; 136:80–6.
13. Chang H, Qi C, Trieu Y, et al. Prognostic relevance of 6q deletion in Waldenstrom's macroglobulinemia. Clin Lymph Myeloma 2009;9:36–8.
14. Nguyen-Khac F, Lejeune J, Chapiro E, et al. Cytogenetic abnormalities in a cohort of 171 patients with Waldenström macroglobulinemia before treatment: clinical and biological correlations. Blood 2010;116 [abstract: 801].

15. Rivera AI, Li MM, Beltran G, et al. Trisomy 4 as the sole cytogenetic abnormality in a Waldenstrom macroglobulinemia. Cancer Genet Cytogenet 2002;133: 172–3.

16. Avet-Loiseau H, Garand R, Lode L, et al. 14q32 translocations discriminate IgM multiple myeloma from Waldenstrom's macroglobulinemia. Semin Oncol 2003; 30:153–5.

17. Treon SP, Xu L, Zhou Y, et al. Whole genome sequencing reveals a widely expressed mutation (MYD88 L265P) with oncogenic activity in Waldenstrom's macroglobulinemia. Blood 2011;118 [abstract: 300].

18. Xu L, Hunter Z, Yang G, et al. MYD88 L265P in Waldenstrom macroglobulinemia, immunoglobulin M monoclonal gammopathy, and other B-cell lymphoproliferative disorders using conventional and quantitative allele-specific polymerase chain reaction. Blood 2013;121(11):2051–8.

19. Varettoni M, Arcaini L, Zibellini S, et al. Prevalence and clinical significance of the MYD88 L265P somatic mutation in Waldenstrom macroglobulinemia, and related lymphoid neoplasms. Blood 2013;121:2522–8.

20. Jiménez C, Sebastián E, Del Carmen Chillón M, et al. MYD88 L265P is a marker highly characteristic of, but not restricted to, Waldenström's macroglobulinemia. Leukemia 2013;27(8):1722–8.

21. Poulain S, Roumier C, Decambron A, et al. MYD88 L265P mutation in Waldenstrom's macroglobulinemia. Blood 2013;121(22):4504–11.

22. Ansell SM, Hodge LS, Secreto FJ, et al. Activation of TAK1 by MYD88 L265P drives malignant B-cell growth in Non-Hodgkin lymphoma. Blood Cancer J 2014;4:e183.

23. Landgren O, Staudt L. MYD88 L265P somatic mutation in IgM MGUS. N Engl J Med 2012;367:2255–6.

24. Hunter ZR, Xu L, Yang G, et al. The genomic landscape of Waldenstöm's macroglobulinemia is characterized by highly recurring MYD88 and WHIM-like CXCR4 mutations, and small somatic deletions associated with B-cell lymphomagenesis. Blood 2014;123(11):1637–46.

25. Yang G, Zhou Y, Liu X, et al. A mutation in MYD88 (L265P) supports the survival of lymphoplasmacytic cells by activation of Bruton tyrosine kinase in Waldenstrom macroglobulinemia. Blood 2013;122(7):1222–32.

26. Watters T, Kenny EF, O'Neill LA. Structure, function and regulation of the Toll/IL-1 receptor adaptor proteins. Immunol Cell Biol 2007;85:411–9.

27. Cohen L, Henzel WJ, Baeuerie PA. IKAP is a scaffold protein of the IkappaB kinase complex. Nature 1998;395:292–6.

28. Loiarro M, Gallo G, Fanto N, et al. Identification of critical residues of the MYD88 death domain involved in the recruitment of downstream kinases. J Biol Chem 2009;284:28093–281023.

29. Lin SC, Lo YC, Wu H. Helical assembly in the MYD88-IRAK4-IRAK2 complex in TLR/IL-1R signaling. Nature 2010;465:885–91.

30. Kawagoe T, Sato S, Matsushita K, et al. Sequential control of Toll-like receptor dependent responses by IRAK1 and IRAK2. Nat Immunol 2008;9:684–91.

31. Leleu X, Eeckhoute J, Jia X, et al. Targeting NF-kappaB in Waldenstrom macroglobulinemia. Blood 2008;111:5068–77.

32. Busillo JM, Benovic JL. Regulation of CXCR4 signalling. Biochim Biophys Acta 2007;1768(4):952–63.

33. Busillo JM, Amando S, Sengupta R, et al. Site-specific phosphorylation of CXCR4 is dynamically regulated by multiple kinases and results in differential modulation of CXCR4 signalling. J Biol Chem 2010;285(10):7805–17.

34. Dotta L, Tassone L, Badolato R. Clinical and genetic features of Warts, Hypogammaglobulinemia, Infections and Myelokathexis (WHIM) syndrome. Curr Mol Med 2011;11(4):317–25.

35. Treon SP, Cao Y, Xu L, et al. Somatic mutations in MYD88 and CXCR4 are determinants of clinical presentation and overall survival in Waldenstrom macroglobulinemia. Blood 2014;123(18):2791–6.

36. Cao Y, Hunter ZR, Liu X, et al. The WHIM-like CXCR4^{S338x} somatic mutation activates AKT and ERK, and promotes resistance to ibrutinib and other agents used in the treatment of Waldenstrom's macroglobulinemia. Leukemia 2014. [Epub ahead of print].

37. Roccaro A, Sacco A, Jiminez C, et al. C1013G/CXCR4 acts as a driver mutation of tumor progression and modulator of drug resistance in lymphoplasmacytic lymphoma. Blood 2014;123(26):4120–31.

38. Braggio E, Keats JJ, Leleu X, et al. Identification of copy number abnormalities and inactivating mutations in two negative regulators of nuclear factor-kappaB signaling pathways in Waldenstrom's macroglobulinemia. Cancer Res 2009; 69(8):3579–88.

39. Poulain S, Roumier C, Galiègue-Zouitina S, et al. Genome Wide SNP Array identified multiple mechanisms of genetic changes in Waldenstrom macroglobulinemia. Am J Hematol 2013;88(11):948–54.

40. Dimopoulos MA, Kyle RA, Anagnostopoulos A, et al. Diagnosis and management of Waldenstrom's macroglobulinemia. J Clin Oncol 2005;23(7):1564–77.

41. Mackenzie MR, Babcock J. Studies of the hyperviscosity syndrome. II. Macroglobulinemia. J Lab Clin Med 1975;85:227–34.

42. Gertz MA, Kyle RA. Hyperviscosity syndrome. J Intensive Care Med 1995;10: 128–41.

43. Kwaan HC, Bongu A. The Hyperviscosity syndromes. Semin Thromb Hemost 1999;25:199–208.

44. Menke MN, Feke GT, McMeel JW, et al. Hyperviscosity-related retinopathy in Waldenstrom's macroglobulinemia. Arch Opthalmol 2006;124:1601–6.

45. Merlini G, Baldini L, Broglia C, et al. Prognostic factors in symptomatic Waldenström's macroglobulinemia. Semin Oncol 2003;30:211–5.

46. Dellagi K, Dupouey P, Brouet JC, et al. Waldenström's macroglobulinemia and peripheral neuropathy: a clinical and immunologic study of 25 patients. Blood 1983;62:280–5.

47. Nobile-Orazio E, Marmiroli P, Baldini L, et al. Peripheral neuropathy in macroglobulinemia: incidence and antigen-specificity of M proteins. Neurology 1987;37:1506–14.

48. Nemni R, Gerosa E, Piccolo G, et al. Neuropathies associated with monoclonal gammapathies. Haematologica 1994;79:557–66.

49. Ropper AH, Gorson KC. Neuropathies associated with paraproteinemia. N Engl J Med 1998;338:1601–7.

50. Treon SP, Hanzis CA, Ioakimidis LI, et al. Clinical characteristics and treatment outcome of disease-related peripheral neuropathy in Waldenstrom's macroglobulinemia. Proc Am Soc Clin Oncol 2010;28 [abstract: 8114].

51. Vital A. Paraproteinemic neuropathies. Brain Pathol 2001;11:399–407.

52. Latov N, Braun PE, Gross RB, et al. Plasma cell dyscrasia and peripheral neuropathy: identification of the myelin antigens that react with human paraproteins. Proc Natl Acad Sci U S A 1981;78:7139–42.

53. Chassande B, Leger JM, Younes-Chennoufi AB, et al. Peripheral neuropathy associated with IgM monoclonal gammopathy: correlations between M-protein

antibody activity and clinical/electrophysiological features in 40 cases. Muscle Nerve 1998;21:55–62.

54. Weiss MD, Dalakas MC, Lauter CJ, et al. Variability in the binding of anti-MAG and anti-SGPG antibodies to target antigens in demyelinating neuropathy and IgM paraproteinemia. J Neuroimmunol 1999;95:174–84.

55. Latov N, Hays AP, Sherman WH. Peripheral neuropathy and anti-MAG antibodies. Crit Rev Neurobiol 1988;3:301–32.

56. Dalakas MC, Quarles RH. Autoimmune ataxic neuropathies (sensory gangliono-pathies): are glycolipids the responsible autoantigens? Ann Neurol 1996;39: 419–22.

57. Crisp D, Pruzanski W. B–cell neoplasms with homogeneous cold-reacting antibodies (cold agglutinins). Am J Med 1982;72:915–22.

58. Pruzanski W, Shumak KH. Biologic activity of cold-reacting autoantibodies (first of two parts). N Engl J Med 1977;297:538–42.

59. Pruzanski W, Shumak KH. Biologic activity of cold-reacting autoantibodies (second of two parts). N Engl J Med 1977;297:583–9.

60. Palladini G, Russo P, Bosoni T, et al. AL amyloidosis associated with IgM monoclonal protein: a distinct clinical entity. Clin Lymphoma Myeloma 2009;9(1):80–3.

61. Hunter ZR, Manning RJ, Hanzis C, et al. IgA and IgG hypogammaglobulinemia in Waldenstrom's Macroglobulinemia. Haematologica 2010;95:470–5.

62. Owen RG, Barrans SL, Richards SJ, et al. Waldenström macroglobulinemia. Development of diagnostic criteria and identification of prognostic factors. Am J Clin Pathol 2001;116:420–8.

63. Feiner HD, Rizk CC, Finfer MD, et al. IgM monoclonal gammopathy/Waldenström's macroglobulinemia: a morphological and immunophenotypic study of the bone marrow. Mod Pathol 1990;3:348–56.

64. San Miguel JF, Vidriales MB, Ocio E, et al. Immunophenotypic analysis of Waldenstrom's macroglobulinemia. Semin Oncol 2003;30:187–95.

65. Hunter ZR, Branagan AR, Manning R, et al. CD5, CD10, CD23 expression in Waldenstrom's macroglobulinemia. Clin Lymph 2005;5:246–9.

66. Castillo JJ, Olzewski AJ, Cronin AM, et al. Survival trends in patients with Waldenstrom's macroglobulinemia: an analysis of the Surveillance, Epidemiology, and End Results database. Blood 2014;123(25):3999–4000.

67. Kristinsson SY, Eloranta S, Dickman PW, et al. Patterns of survival in lymphoplasmacytic lymphoma/Waldenström macroglobulinemia: a population-based study of 1,555 patients diagnosed in Sweden from 1980 to 2005. Am J Hematol 2013; 88:60–5.

68. Gobbi PG, Bettini R, Montecucco C, et al. Study of prognosis in Waldenström's macroglobulinemia: a proposal for a simple binary classification with clinical and investigational utility. Blood 1994;83:2939–45.

69. Morel P, Monconduit M, Jacomy D, et al. Prognostic factors in Waldenström macroglobulinemia: a report on 232 patients with the description of a new scoring system and its validation on 253 other patients. Blood 2000;96:852–8.

70. Kyle RA, Treon SP, Alexanian R, et al. Prognostic markers and criteria to initiate therapy in Waldenström's macroglobulinemia: consensus panel recommendations from the Second International Workshop on Waldenström's macroglobulinemia. Semin Oncol 2003;30:116–20.

71. Morel P, Duhamel A, Gobbi P, et al. International prognostic scoring system for Waldenstrom macroglobulinemia. Blood 2009;113:4163–70.

72. Dhodapkar MV, Jacobson JL, Gertz MA, et al. Prognostic factors and response to fludarabine therapy in patients with Waldenström macroglobulinemia: results

of United States intergroup trial (Southwest Oncology Group S9003). Blood 2001;98:41–8.

73. Dimopoulos M, Gika D, Zervas K, et al. The international staging system for multiple myeloma is applicable in symptomatic Waldenstrom's macroglobulinemia. Leuk Lymphoma 2004;45:1809–13.

74. Treon SP. Treatment with a Bortezomib-containing regimen is associated with better therapeutic outcomes in patients with Waldenstrom's macroglobulinemia who have familial disease predisposition. Blood 2011;118 [abstract: 1643].

75. Treon SP. How i treat Waldenstrom's macroglobulinemia. Blood 2009;114:419–31.

76. Dimopoulos MA, Gertz MA, Kastritis E, et al. Update on treatment recommendations from the Fourth International Workshop on Waldenstrom's macroglobulinemia. J Clin Oncol 2009;27:120–6.

77. Anderson KC, Alsina M, Bensinger W, et al. Waldenström's macroglobulinemia/lymphoplasmacytic lymphoma, version 2.2013. J Natl Compr Canc Netw 2012; 10(10):1211–9.

78. Treon SP, Agus DB, Link B, et al. CD20-Directed antibody-mediated immunotherapy induces responses and facilitates hematologic recovery in patients with Waldenstrom's macroglobulinemia. J Immunother 2001;24:272–9.

79. Gertz MA, Rue M, Blood E, et al. Multicenter phase 2 trial of rituximab for Waldenstrom macroglobulinemia (WM): an Eastern Cooperative Oncology Group Study (E3A98). Leuk Lymphoma 2004;45:2047–55.

80. Dimopoulos MA, Zervas C, Zomas A, et al. Treatment of Waldenstrom's macroglobulinemia with rituximab. J Clin Oncol 2002;20:2327–33.

81. Treon SP, Emmanouilides C, Kimby E, et al. Extended rituximab therapy in Waldenström's macroglobulinemia. Ann Oncol 2005;16:132–8.

82. Donnelly GB, Bober-Sorcinelli K, Jacobson R, et al. Abrupt IgM rise following treatment with rituximab in patients with Waldenstrom's macroglobulinemia. Blood 2001;98:240b.

83. Treon SP, Branagan AR, Anderson KC. Paradoxical increases in serum IgM levels and serum viscosity following rituximab therapy in patients with Waldenstrom's macroglobulinemia. Ann Oncol 2004;15:1481–3.

84. Ghobrial IM, Fonseca R, Greipp PR, et al. The initial "flare" of IgM level after rituximab therapy in patients diagnosed with Waldenstrom macroglobulinemia: an Eastern Cooperative Oncology Group Study. Cancer 2004;101:2593–8.

85. Furman RR, Eradat H, Switzky JC, et al. A phase II trial of ofatumumab in subjects with Waldenstrom's macroglobulinemia. Blood 2011;118 [abstract: 3701].

86. Treon SP, Hanzis C, Tripsas C, et al. Bendamustine therapy in patients with relapsed or refractory Waldenström's macroglobulinemia. Clin Lymphoma Myeloma Leuk 2011;11:133–5.

87. Kyle RA, Greipp PR, Gertz MA, et al. Waldenström's macroglobulinaemia: a prospective study comparing daily with intermittent oral chlorambucil. Br J Haematol 2000;108:737–42.

88. Leblond V, Johnson S, Chevret S, et al. Results of a randomized trial of chlorambucil versus fludarabine for patients with untreated Waldenström macroglobulinemia, marginal zone lymphoma, or lymphoplasmacytic lymphoma. J Clin Oncol 2013;31(3):301–7.

89. Buske C, Hoster E, Dreyling MH, et al. The addition of rituximab to front-line therapy with CHOP (R-CHOP) results in a higher response rate and longer time to treatment failure in patients with lymphoplasmacytic lymphoma: results of a randomized trial of the German Low-Grade Lymphoma Study Group (GLSG). Leukemia 2009;23:153–61.

90. Dimopoulos MA, Anagnostopoulos A, Kyrtsonis MC, et al. Primary treatment of Waldenstrom's macroglobulinemia with dexamethasone, rituximab and cyclophosphamide. J Clin Oncol 2007;25:3344–9.

91. Treon SP, Hunter Z, Branagan A. CHOP plus rituximab therapy in Waldenström's macroglobulinemia. Clin Lymphoma 2005;5:273–7.

92. Ioakimidis L, Patterson CJ, Hunter ZR, et al. Comparative outcomes following CP-R, CVP-R and CHOP-R in Waldenstrom's macroglobulinemia. Clin Lymphoma Myeloma 2009;9:62–6.

93. Cheson BD, Rummel MJ. Bendamustine: rebirth of an old drug. J Clin Oncol 2009;27:1492–501.

94. Rummel M, Niederle N, Maschmeyer G, et al. Bendamustine plus rituximab versus CHOP plus rituximab as first-line treatment for patients with indolent and mantle-cell lymphomas: an open-label, multicentre, randomised, phase 3 non-inferiority trial. Lancet 2013;381(9873):1203–10.

95. Dimopoulos MA, Kantarjian H, Weber D, et al. Primary therapy of Waldenström's macroglobulinemia with 2-chlorodeoxyadenosine. J Clin Oncol 1994;12:2694–8.

96. Liu ES, Burian C, Miller WE, et al. Bolus administration of cladribine in the treatment of Waldenström macroglobulinaemia. Br J Haematol 1998;103:690–5.

97. Hellmann A, Lewandowski K, Zaucha JM, et al. Effect of a 2-hour infusion of 2-chlorodeoxyadenosine in the treatment of refractory or previously untreated Waldenström's macroglobulinemia. Eur J Haematol 1999;63:35–41.

98. Betticher DC, Hsu Schmitz SF, Ratschiller D, et al. Cladribine (2-CDA) given as subcutaneous bolus injections is active in pretreated Waldenström's macroglobulinaemia. Swiss Group for Clinical Cancer Research (SAKK). Br J Haematol 1997;99:358–63.

99. Dimopoulos MA, O'Brien S, Kantarjian H, et al. Fludarabine therapy in Waldenström's macroglobulinemia. Am J Med 1993;95:49–52.

100. Foran JM, Rohatiner AZ, Coiffier B, et al. Multicenter phase II study of fludarabine phosphate for patients with newly diagnosed lymphoplasmacytoid lymphoma, Waldenström's macroglobulinemia, and mantle-cell lymphoma. J Clin Oncol 1999;17:546–53.

101. Weber DM, Dimopoulos MA, Delasalle K, et al. 2-chlorodeoxyadenosine alone and in combination for previously untreated Waldenstrom's macroglobulinemia. Semin Oncol 2003;30:243–7.

102. Laszlo D, Andreola G, Rigacci L, et al. Rituximab and subcutaneous 2-chloro-2'-deoxyadenosine combination treatment for patients with Waldenstrom macroglobulinemia: clinical and biologic results of a phase II multicenter study. J Clin Oncol 2010;28:2233–8.

103. Treon SP, Branagan AR, Ioakimidis L, et al. Long term outcomes to fludarabine and rituximab in Waldenström's macroglobulinemia. Blood 2009;113:3673–8.

104. Tam CS, Wolf MM, Westerman D, et al. Fludarabine combination therapy is highly effective in first-line and salvage treatment of patients with Waldenstrom's macroglobulinemia. Clin Lymphoma Myeloma 2005;6:136–9.

105. Hensel M, Villalobos M, Kornacker M, et al. Pentostatin/cyclophosphamide with or without rituximab: an effective regimen for patients with Waldenstrom's macroglobulinemia/lymphoplasmacytic lymphoma. Clin Lymphoma Myeloma 2005;6:131–5.

106. Dimopoulos MA, Hamilos G, Efstathiou E, et al. Treatment of Waldenstrom's macroglobulinemia with the combination of fludarabine and cyclophosphamide. Leuk Lymphoma 2003;44:993–6.

107. Tamburini J, Levy V, Chateilex C, et al. Fludarabine plus cyclophosphamide in Waldenstrom's macroglobulinemia: results in 49 patients. Leukemia 2005;19:1831–4.

108. Tedeschi A, Benevolo G, Varettoni M, et al. Fludarabine plus cyclophosphamide and rituximab in Waldenstrom macroglobulinemia: an effective but myelosuppressive regimen to be offered to patients with advanced disease. Cancer 2012;118:434–43.
109. Treon SP, Patterson CJ, Kimby E, et al. Advances in the biology and treatment of Waldenström's macroglobulinemia: a report from the 5th International Workshop on Waldenström's Macroglobulinemia. Stockholm, Sweden: Clin Lymphoma Myeloma 2009;9(1):10–5.
110. Leleu XP, Manning R, Soumerai JD, et al. Increased incidence of transformation and myelodysplasia/acute leukemia in patients with Waldenström macroglobulinemia treated with nucleoside analogs. J Clin Oncol 2009;27:250–5.
111. Leleu X, Tamburini J, Roccaro A, et al. Balancing risk versus benefit in the treatment of Waldenstrom's macroglobulinemia patients with nucleoside analogue based therapy. Clin Lymph Myeloma 2009;9:71–3.
112. Treon SP, Hunter ZR, Matous J, et al. Multicenter clinical trial of bortezomib in relapsed/refractory Waldenstrom's macroglobulinemia: results of WMCTG trial 03-248. Clin Cancer Res 2007;13:3320–5.
113. Chen CI, Kouroukis CT, White D, et al. Bortezomib is active in patients with untreated or relapsed Waldenstrom's macroglobulinemia: a phase II study of the National Cancer Institute of Canada Clinical Trials Group. J Clin Oncol 2007;25:1570–5.
114. Dimopoulos MA, Anagnostopoulos A, Kyrtsonis MC, et al. Treatment of relapsed or refractory Waldenstrom's macroglobulinemia with bortezomib. Haematologica 2005;90:1655–7.
115. Treon SP, Ioakimidis L, Soumerai JD, et al. Primary therapy of Waldenstrom's macroglobulinemia with Bortezomib, Dexamethasone and Rituximab: results of WMCTG clinical trial 05-180. J Clin Oncol 2009;27:3830–5.
116. Ghobrial IM, Xie W, Padmanabhan S, et al. Phase II trial of weekly bortezomib in combination with rituximab in untreated patients with Waldenström macroglobulinemia. Am J Hematol 2010;85:670–4.
117. Agathocleous A, Rohatiner A, Rule S, et al. Weekly versus twice weekly bortezomib given in conjunction with rituximab, in patients with recurrent follicular lymphoma, mantle cell lymphoma and Waldenström macroglobulinaemia. Br J Haematol 2010;151:346–53.
118. Dimopoulos MA, García-Sanz R, Gavriatopoulou M, et al. Primary therapy of Waldenstrom macroglobulinemia (WM) with weekly bortezomib, low-dose dexamethasone, and rituximab (BDR): long-term results of a phase 2 study of the European Myeloma Network (EMN). Blood 2013;122(19):3276–82.
119. Treon SP, Tripsas CK, Meid K, et al. Carfilzomib, rituximab and dexamethasone (CaRD) is active and offers a neuropathy-sparing approach for proteasome-inhibitor based therapy in Waldenstrom's macroglobulinemia. Blood 2014; 124(4):503–10. [Epub ahead of print].
120. Dimopoulos MA, Zomas A, Viniou NA, et al. Treatment of Waldenström's macroglobulinemia with thalidomide. J Clin Oncol 2001;19:3596–601.
121. Coleman C, Leonard J, Lyons L, et al. Treatment of Waldenström's macroglobulinemia with clarithromycin, low-dose thalidomide and dexamethasone. Semin Oncol 2003;30:270–4.
122. Dimopoulos MA, Zomas K, Tsatalas K, et al. Treatment of Waldenström's macroglobulinemia with single agent thalidomide or with combination of clarithromycin, thalidomide and dexamethasone. Semin Oncol 2003;30:265–9.
123. Treon SP, Soumerai JD, Branagan AR, et al. Thalidomide and rituximab in Waldenstrom's macroglobulinemia. Blood 2008;112:4452–7.

124. Treon SP, Soumerai JD, Branagan AR, et al. Lenalidomide and rituximab in Waldenström's macroglobulinemia. Clin Cancer Res 2008;15:355–60.

125. Treon SP, Tripsas CK, Warren D, et al. Phase I study of pomalidomide, dexamethasone and rituximab in patients with relapsed or refractory Waldenstrom's macroglobulinemia. Hematol Oncol 2013;31:267.

126. Leleu X, Jia X, Runnels J, et al. The Akt pathway regulates survival and homing in Waldenstrom macroglobulinemia. Blood 2007;110:4417–26.

127. Ghobrial IM, Witzig TE, Gertz M, et al. Long-term results of the phase II trial of the oral mTOR inhibitor everolimus (RAD001) in relapsed or refractory Waldenstrom macroglobulinemia. Am J Hematol 2014;89(3):237–42.

128. Treon SP, Tripsas CK, Meid K, et al. Prospective, multicenter study of the mtor inhibitor everolimus (RAD001) as primary therapy in Waldenstrom's macroglobulinemia. Blood 2013;122:1822.

129. Treon SP, Tripsas C, Yang G, et al. A Prospective Multicenter Study Of The Bruton's Tyrosine Kinase Inhibitor Ibrutinib In Patients With Relapsed Or Refractory Waldenstrom's Macroglobulinemia. Proc. of the American Society of Hematology. Blood 2013;122(21):251.

130. Treon SP, Hanzis C, Manning RJ, et al. Maintenance rituximab is associated with improved clinical outcome in rituximab naïve patients with Waldenstrom's macroglobulinemia who respond to a rituximab containing regimen. Br J Haematol 2011;154:357–62.

131. Rummel MJ, Lerchenmüller C, Greil R, et al. Bendamustin-rituximab induction followed by observation or rituximab maintenance for newly diagnosed patients with Waldenström's macroglobulinemia: results from a prospective, randomized, multicenter study (StiL NHL 7–2008). Blood 2012;120:2739.

132. Kyriakou C, Canals C, Sibon D, et al. High-dose therapy and autologous stem-cell transplantation in Waldenstrom macroglobulinemia: the Lymphoma Working Party of the European Group for Blood and Marrow Transplantation. J Clin Oncol 2010;28:2227–32.

133. Kyriakou C, Canals C, Cornelissen JJ, et al. Allogeneic stem-cell transplantation in patients with Waldenström macroglobulinemia: report from the Lymphoma Working Party of the European Group for Blood and Marrow Transplantation. J Clin Oncol 2010;28:4926–34.

134. Nichols GL, Savage DG. Timing of rituximab/fludarabine in Waldenstrom's macroglobulinemia may avert hyperviscosity. Blood 2004;104:237b.

135. Strauss SJ, Maharaj L, Hoare S, et al. Bortezomib therapy in patients with relapsed or refractory lymphoma: potential correlation of in vitro sensitivity and tumor necrosis factor alpha response with clinical activity. J Clin Oncol 2006;24:2105–12.

136. Varghese AM, Rawstron AC, Ashcroft AJ, et al. Assessment of bone marrow response in Waldenström's macroglobulinemia. Clin Lymph Myeloma 2009;9:53–5.

137. Ciccarelli BT, Yang G, Hatjiharissi E, et al. Soluble CD27 is a faithful marker of disease burden and is unaffected by the rituximab induced IgM flare, as well as plasmapheresis in patients with Waldenstrom's macroglobulinemia. Clin Lymphoma Myeloma 2009;9:56–8.

138. Xu L, Hunter Z, Yang G, et al. Detection of MYD88 L265P in peripheral blood from patients with Waldenström's macroglobulinemia and IgM monoclonal gammopathy of undetermined significance. Leukemia 2014. [Epub ahead of print].

Index

Note: Page numbers of article titles are in **boldface** type.

Hematol Oncol Clin N Am 28 (2014) 971–981
http://dx.doi.org/10.1016/S0889-8588(14)00096-3
0889-8588/14/$ – see front matter © 2014 Elsevier Inc. All rights reserved.

United States Postal Service

Statement of Ownership, Management, and Circulation
(All Periodicals Publications Except Requestor Publications)

1. Publication Title

Hematology/Oncology Clinics of North America

2. Publication Number 0 0 2 - 4 7 3

3. Filing Date 9/14/14

4. Issue Frequency Feb, Apr, Jun, Aug, Oct, Dec

5. Number of Issues Published Annually 6

6. Annual Subscription Price $385.00

7. Complete Mailing Address of Known Office of Publication (*Not printer*) (*Street, city, county, state, and ZIP+4®*)

Elsevier Inc.
360 Park Avenue South
New York, NY 10010-1710

Contact Person Stephen R. Bushing

Telephone (Include area code) 215-239-3688

8. Complete Mailing Address of Headquarters or General Business Office of Publisher (*Not printer*)

Elsevier Inc., 360 Park Avenue South, New York, NY 10010-1710

9. Full Names and Complete Mailing Addresses of Publisher, Editor, and Managing Editor (*Do not leave blank*)

Publisher (*Name and complete mailing address*)

Linda Belfus, Elsevier Inc., 1600 John F. Kennedy Blvd., Suite 1800, Philadelphia, PA 19103-2899

Editor (*Name and complete mailing address*)

Jessica McCool, Elsevier Inc., 1600 John F. Kennedy Blvd., Suite 1800, Philadelphia, PA 19103-2899

Managing Editor (*Name and complete mailing address*)

Adrianne Brigido, Elsevier Inc., 1600 John F. Kennedy Blvd., Suite 1800, Philadelphia, PA 19103-2899

10. Owner (*Do not leave blank. If the publication is owned by a corporation, give the name and address of the corporation immediately followed by the names and addresses of all stockholders owning or holding 1 percent or more of the total amount of stock. If not owned by a corporation, give the names and addresses of the individual owners. If owned by a partnership or other unincorporated firm, give its name and address as well as those of each individual owner. If the publication is published by a nonprofit organization, give its name and address.*)

Full Name	Complete Mailing Address
Wholly owned subsidiary of	1600 John F. Kennedy Blvd, Ste. 1800
Reed/Elsevier, US holdings	Philadelphia, PA 19103-2899

11. Known Bondholders, Mortgagees, and Other Security Holders Owning or Holding 1 Percent or More of Total Amount of Bonds, Mortgages, or Other Securities. If none, check box ☐ None

Full Name	Complete Mailing Address
N/A	

12. Tax Status (*For completion by nonprofit organizations authorized to mail at nonprofit rates*) (*Check one*)
The purpose, function, and nonprofit status of this organization and the exempt status for federal income tax purposes:
☐ Has Not Changed During Preceding 12 Months
☐ Has Changed During Preceding 12 Months (*Publisher must submit explanation of change with this statement*)

PS Form 3526, August 2012 (Page 1 of 3 (Instructions Page 3)) PSN 7530-01-000-9931 PRIVACY NOTICE: See our Privacy policy in www.usps.com

---

13. Publication Title Hematology/Oncology Clinics of North America

14. Issue Date for Circulation Data Below June 2014

15. Extent and Nature of Circulation

			Average No. Copies Each Issue During Preceding 12 Months	No. Copies of Single Issue Published Nearest to Filing Date
a.	Total Number of Copies (*Net press run*)		674	717
b. Paid Circulation (By Mail and Outside the Mail)	(1)	Mailed Outside-County Paid Subscriptions Stated on PS Form 3541. (*Include paid distribution above nominal rate, advertiser's proof copies, and exchange copies*)	261	226
	(2)	Mailed In-County Paid Subscriptions Stated on PS Form 3541 (*Include paid distribution above nominal rate, advertiser's proof copies, and exchange copies*)		
	(3)	Paid Distribution Outside the Mails Including Sales Through Dealers and Carriers, Street Vendors, Counter Sales, and Other Paid Distribution Outside USPS®	145	131
	(4)	Paid Distribution by Other Classes Mailed Through the USPS (e.g. First-Class Mail®)		
c.	Total Paid Distribution (*Sum of 15b (1), (2), (3), and (4)*)		406	357
d. Free or Nominal Rate Distribution (By Mail and Outside the Mail)	(1)	Free or Nominal Rate Outside-County Copies Included on PS Form 3541	133	175
	(2)	Free or Nominal Rate In-County Copies Included on PS Form 3541		
	(3)	Free or Nominal Rate Copies Mailed at Other Classes Through the USPS (e.g. First-Class Mail)		
	(4)	Free or Nominal Rate Distribution Outside the Mail (Carriers or other means)		
e.	Total Free or Nominal Rate Distribution (*Sum of 15d (1), (2), (3) and (4)*)		133	175
f.	Total Distribution (*Sum of 15c and 15e*)		539	532
g.	Copies not Distributed (*See instructions to publishers #4 (page #3)*)		135	185
h.	Total (*Sum of 15f and g*)		674	717
i.	Percent Paid (*15c divided by 15f times 100*)		75.32%	67.11%

16 Total circulation includes electronic copies. Report circulation on PS Form 3526-X worksheet.

17. Publication of Statement of Ownership
If the publication is a general publication, publication of this statement is required. Will be printed in the October 2014 issue of this publication.

18. Signature and Title of Editor, Publisher, Business Manager, or Owner

Stephen R. Bushing – Inventory Distribution Coordinator

Date September 14, 2014

I certify that all information furnished on this form is true and complete. I understand that anyone who furnishes false or misleading information on this form or who omits material or information requested on the form may be subject to criminal sanctions (including fines and imprisonment) and/or civil sanctions (including civil penalties).

PS Form 3526, August 2012 (Page 2 of 3)

Moving?

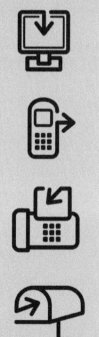

Printed and bound by CPI Group (UK) Ltd, Croydon, CR0 4YY

03/10/2024

01040494-0001